JOURNAL OF REPRODUCTION AND FERTILITY

SUPPLEMENT No. 37

MATERNAL RECOGNITION OF PREGNANCY AND MAINTENANCE OF THE CORPUS LUTEUM

Proceedings of a Workshop held in
Jerusalem, Israel
March 1988

EDITED BY
M. Shemesh and Barbara J. Weir

Journal of Reproduction & Fertility

1989

First published 1989

ISSN 0449-3087
ISBN 0 906545 15 3

Published by **The Journals of Reproduction and Fertility Ltd.**

Agents for distribution: **The Biochemical Society Book Depot, P.O. Box 32, Commerce Way, Whitehall Industrial Estate, Colchester, CO2 8HP, Essex, U.K.**

Printed in Great Britain by
Henry Ling Ltd., at
The Dorset Press, Dorchester, Dorset

CONTENTS

J. Reprod. Fert., Suppl. **37** (1989), v

Printed in Great Britain
© 1989 Journals of Reproduction & Fertility Ltd

Preface

Early embryonic mortality is a major cause of reproductive loss in man as well as in classes of farm animals. These large embryonic death losses occur at or near the time of the maternal recognition or pregnancy in cattle and other domestic animal species. Trophoblastic cells which migrate to the endometrial endothelium or their products are a potential vehicle for early communication between the mother and the embryo. An essential requirement for the establishment and maintenance of pregnancy is that the normal ovarian cycle be changed and the functional activity of the corpus luteum prolonged. Maintenance and function of the corpus luteum are the results of the trophic action of pituitary LH and, in some species, prolactin. During gestation, there is an additional feto-placental control. The survival and demise of the corpus luteum depends on a delicate balance between trophic factors and luteolytic agents: the process of luteolysis is not controlled exclusively by luteolytic factors.

To date, we still do not understand the mechanism by which the developing conceptus signals its presence to the mother. There is evidence of at least 3 possible modes of action of the conceptus to avoid the early death of the corpus luteum. (1) Both progesterone and oestrogen produced by the blastocysts may act directly or indirectly respectively to suppress the uterine release of PGF-2α. (2) Blastocysts may secrete an anti-prostaglandin synthetase or a substance which blocks the release of uterine arachidonic acid. (3) Chorionic gonadotrophin-like activity produced by the blastocyst could act locally to stimulate progesterone secretion directly or indirectly through increasing blastocyst steroidogenesis.

In the cow, sheep and pig, the signal for pregnancy recognition is transmitted to the mother even before the embryonic tissue becomes intimately attached to the uterine epithelia and is therefore clearly distinct from implantation. Such findings have led to the concept that the blastocyst might participate in the events leading to its own implantation by signalling its presence to the uterus. In the cow, the early effect of the conceptus on plasma progesterone concentration is evident as early as the 10th day of gestation. In species such as the pig, the blastocyst, while it remains free in the uterine lumen, may produce some substance that is capable of diffusing into the uterine fluids and across the lumen, exerting a local effect on the uterine tissue.

The main object of this workshop was to discuss the question: how does an animal know that it is pregnant? Emphasis is given to the ways by which the life-span and function of the corpus luteum is prolonged by the presence of an embryo. This 'maternal recognition of pregnancy' not only describes the rescue of the corpus luteum but also the maternal adjustments to the allogeneic embryo that allow its retention in the uterus rather than its rejection as foreign tissue.

A full list of Sponsors is given overleaf but we should particularly like to thank the Binational (US–Israel) Agricultural Research and Development Fund (BARD) for sponsoring the Workshop.

M. Shemesh

Sponsors

MAJOR SPONSOR
BARD—Binational (US–Israel) Agricultural Research and Development Fund

ACADEMIC AND ORGANIZATIONAL SPONSORS
Israel Academy of Sciences and Humanities
Israel National Council for Research and Development
Israel Milk Marketing Board
Kimron Veterinary Institute
Koret School of Veterinary Medicine

ACADEMIC AUSPICES
Israel Endocrine Society
Israel Society for the Immunology of Reproduction
Israel Society for the Study of Fertility

CORPORATE SPONSORS
Clonatec, France
Vitamed Ltd, Israel
Smithkline Beckman Animal Health Products, USA
Koffolk Ltd, Israel

LUTEOTROPHIC COMPOUNDS

Chairmen

G. King
A. Eshkol

J. Reprod. Fert., Suppl. **37** (1989), 1–10

Printed in Great Britain
© 1989 Journals of Reproduction & Fertility Ltd

Regulation of the human chorionic gonadotrophin β subunit genes

I. Boime*†, T. Otani*, F. Otani* and D. Chaplin‡§

Departments of *Pharmacology, †Obstetrics and Gynecology and ‡Medicine, and §Howard Hughes Medical Institute, Washington University School of Medicine, 660 South Euclid Avenue, St Louis, Missouri 63110, U.S.A.

Keywords: hCGβ promoter; trophoblast; differentiation; regulation

Introduction

One of the unique features of the human placenta is its continued differentiation during gestation. We have previously shown, by in-situ hybridization, that human chorionic gonadotrophin (hCG) α- and β-subunit mRNAs are expressed in the syncytiotrophoblast regions and some cytotrophoblasts of the placenta whereas human placental lactogen mRNA was expressed primarily in the syncytial region. The hCG-α mRNA is 6-fold greater in first trimester placenta compared to term, and hCG-β mRNA falls to undetectable levels at term (Boothby *et al.*, 1983). Human placental lactogen, on the other hand, attains maximal levels at term although the amount of mRNA per gram of tissue is not greatly altered (Hoshina *et al.*, 1982). Based on these data we proposed that the hCG and human placental lactogen genes are activated at different stages of placental differentiation (Hoshina *et al.*, 1982, 1983, 1985). We also suggested that hCG-α and -β subunit expression is dependent on the presence of proliferating cytotrophoblasts whereas placental lactogen expression is sustained constitutively in differentiated syncytium.

Our findings in normal placenta were supported by probing trophoblastic neoplasms with the placental lactogen and hCG-α and -β subunit cDNA. Choriocarcinoma consists of clusters of cytotrophoblast-like cells and large multinucleated cells. Signals corresponding to hCG-α and -β mRNAs were seen predominantly in the latter. By contrast, no significant placental lactogen signal was observed. Hydatidiform mole tissue, which maintains villous morphology, gave positive signals for all 3 mRNAs (Hoshina *et al.*, 1983). These findings are consistent with the following model: hCG and placental lactogen genes remain unexpressed in proliferating cytotrophoblasts. The next stage, commitment of cytotrophoblasts to syncytiotrophoblast, is associated with activation of the hCG-α and then -β subunit genes. Such intermediates, especially those bearing the hCGβ subunit, are transient; they differentiate further, at which point hCG-α and -β mRNAs decline while maximal expression of human placental lactogen is coincident with syncytial formation.

Using a cell culture system of human trophoblasts (McQueen *et al.*, 1987) we examined the differentiation of cytotrophoblasts *in vitro* to test some predictions of the above model. The essential feature associates activation of hCG and placental lactogen genes with different stages of differentiation. We would propose that there are at least 3 steps in the pathway (McQueen & Boime, 1986); (1) commitment of progenitor cytotrophoblasts to syncytium; these cells initiate subunit synthesis; (2) fusion of cytotrophoblasts occurs and this activates expression of the β-gene; (3) further differentiation of these fused cells leads to cessation of β subunit synthesis; coincident with or subsequent to this step synthesis of placental lactogen ensues.

Alternatively, regulation of hCG-β gene expression may be exerted through specific DNA sequences in the CG-β gene which, during development, respond to the induction of specific factors in the trophoblast. For example, attenuation of CG synthesis after 12–14 weeks may not be due to a depletion of a particular cellular intermediate but rather to the elaboration of trans factors that act in concert at negative or positive elements in the CG-β gene.

Although the organization and structure of the CG-β gene cluster (there are 6 homologous sequences) have been studied in some detail (Boorstein *et al.*, 1982; Policastro *et al.*, 1983, 1986; Graham *et al.*, 1987), the *cis*-acting control elements, including promoter sequences, associated with their regulation and tissue-specific expression, have not been identified due to a lack of expression of the β promoter when these genes are transfected into homologous cells. Talmadge *et al.* (1984b) inserted 5 of the 6 hCG-β genes into SV40-derived vectors and transfected them into SV40-transformed COS cells; they suggested that at least 2 genes are functional. However, expression of these genes may have been influenced by SV40 sequences.

Defining the promoter region for the hCG-β gene has been difficult since there is no consensus TATAA box in front of the cap site, nor are there other recognizable canonical sequences within 200 base pairs (bp) of the 5′ end of the cap site. Location of the promoter region in the CG-β genes therefore cannot be inferred from previously reported promoter sequences.

Much of the data on the structure of the CG-β genes are from λ clones bearing single and some overlapping CG-β genes (Boorstein *et al.*, 1982; Policastro *et al.*, 1983). As a result, portions of the intragenic regions were not included in these clones; extended regions corresponding to the 5′-flanking sequences were not represented. However, we have isolated a cosmid clone containing the entire CG-β cluster (Graham *et al.*, 1987), and thus the uncloned portions are now available. Here we describe expression of cloned CG-β genes in cultured cells. Using fragments derived from the hCG-β cosmid, we have defined an hCG-β promoter region and possibly other regulatory sequences as well.

Materials and Methods

Construction of hCG-β subclones. Throughout this paper we will refer to the CG-β genes according to the number of assignments of Boorstein *et al.* (1982). Individual CG-β genes were isolated by digesting a cosmid clone (βcos) containing the hCG-β gene cluster (Graham *et al.*, 1987) with *KpnI*. The fragments were ligated to a derivative of pTCF (Grosveld *et al.*, 1982) containing an artificial *KpnI* site at the original *BamHI* site. DH5α (Bethesda Research Laboratories, MD, U.S.A.) transformants were screened for clones bearing each of the 6 genes by determining the insert size (Graham *et al.*, 1987) on a 0·8% agarose gel in 1 × TBE (89 mM-Tris, 89 mM-boric acid, 2 mM-EDTA). Since βcos is bounded by genomic *BamHI* sites, the 5′-flanking sequence of the CG-β7 gene is much shorter than the other genes (see map in Fig. 1a). Therefore, we used a *KpnI* fragment of CG-β7 from a λ subclone (kindly provided by Dr John Fiddes, California, Biotechnology, San Francisco, CA, U.S.A.) which has 5′-flanking sequences comparable in length to those of the other subcloned genes. The clones obtained were designated as pCG-β1 through pCG-β8; CG-β4 which corresponds to LH-β (Talmadge *et al.*, 1983) is not in the cosmid since the cosmid was prepared with BamHI. The previously described CG-β6 gene is not a component of the cluster but arose apparently artefactually during the early cloning of these genes in λ libraries (Policastro *et al.*, 1986; Graham *et al.*, 1987). Construction of truncated CG-β subclones and deletion mutants have been described previously (Otani *et al.*, 1988).

Construction of pCAT NEO. A vector containing both the chloramphenicol acetyltransferase and neomycin resistance (neo) genes was constructed by ligating the chloramphenicol acetyltransferase gene from pSVOCAT (Gorman *et al.*, 1982) to a pTCF fragment containing the origin of replication (ori) and neo gene. pSVOCAT was digested with HindIII and AhaII, and the fragment containing the chloramphenicol acetyltransferase gene was purified. pTCF was digested with BamHI, filled in with Klenow and ligated to a HindIII linker. After digestion with HindIII and ClaI, the fragment containing the neo gene and ori was isolated. The two fragments were ligated with T4 ligase taking advantage of compatible ends created by AhaII and ClaI. This resulted in a vector containing a promoterless chloramphenicol acetyltransferase gene preceded by a HindIII-cloning site and the neo gene in the same plasmid (pCAT NEO). One additional derivative of pCAT NEO was created by inserting XbaI linker to the HindIII site (pCAT NEO ΔX) to facilitate insertion of SalI–SpeI fragment (SalI site of pTCF is conserved just 5′ of the HindIII site and XbaI is compatible with SpeI).

CG-β5-flanking sequences were isolated by digesting pCG-β5ΔK, pCG-β7ΔK, or deletion mutants of pCG-β5ΔK with SalI and SpeI (for map see Fig. 2). This digest was resolved on a 0·8% agarose gel and fragments corresponding to the 5′ region of the gene were isolated. This fragment was ligated to SalI- and XbaI-digested pCAT NEO ΔX. Since this created only clones having the promoter region in correct orientation with the chloramphenicol acetyltransferase gene, additional clones having the promoter region in reverse orientation were created by adding a HindIII linker to the isolated fragment and inserting it into HindIII-digested pCAT NEO.

Transfection of cultured cells. Mouse Y1 and human JAr choriocarcinoma cells were maintained in culture and transfected according to Otani *et al.* (1988). Labelling and immunoprecipitation of transfected Y1 cells and determination of chloramphenicol acetyltransferase activity (CAT) were as described previously (Otani *et al.*, 1988).

Results

Previous experiments to assess the presence of promoter regions in the 5′-flanking sequence by using chloramphenicol acetyltransferase as a reporter gene and transfecting transiently in choriocarcinoma cells were unsuccessful (Policastro, 1984; Jameson *et al.*, 1986a). We attributed this to an insufficient number of cells expressing CG-β in the total population of choriocarcinoma cells (see below and 'Discussion'). However, it was also possible that a critical sequence was lacking the individual genes for expression; there are no obvious canonical sequences in the CG-β genes in positions that resemble common promoters. Since we isolated the complete CG-β gene family in a single cosmid clone (Graham *et al.*, 1987), including sequences which were not available previously, we screened a variety of cell lines for their ability to express CG-β after transfection. We screened both for transient and stable transformants. The mouse cell line, Y1, which is derived from the adrenal cortex (Schimmer, 1981) and is known to act as an efficient recipient for transfected genes (Chaplin *et al.*, 1986), synthesized significant amounts of CG-β protein after transfection of the cosmid clone (data not shown). This result indicated that the $\simeq 40$ kb insert of the CG-β cosmid contained sufficient information for CG-β expression in these stable transformed cells. To define in greater detail (a) the promoter, and (b) the active genes of the cluster, structure–function studies were performed on restriction fragments generated from the CG-β cosmid. Our first approach was to digest the cosmid with *KpnI* since each of the CG-β genes is bounded by a *KpnI* site resulting in the collection of genes each containing $\simeq 3$ kb of the 5′-flanking sequence (see map in Fig. 1). The *KpnI* fragments were subcloned and transfected into Y1 cells. When the stable transformants were labelled with [^{35}S]cysteine, clones bearing CG-β genes 5, 3, and 8 expressed significant amounts of CG-β protein; gene 5 was the most actively expressed (Fig. 1). The migration of the transfected β subunits was comparable to the mobility of CG-β subunit synthesized in choriocarcinoma cells, although in many experiments the CG-β synthesized in Y1 cells migrates slightly faster than the β subunit derived from the hCG dimer. We attribute this difference to post-translational changes of the oligosaccharides in the free versus the dimer forms of the β subunit (Corless *et al.*, 1987). Little, if any, CG-β synthesis was seen for CG-β7 and CG-β genes 1 and 2 were inactive. These data therefore imply that, in transfected Y1 cells, CG-β genes 5, 3 and 8 were driven by CG-β promoters present in the transfected fragments.

Successive deletion of 5′ sequence upstream of CG-β5

To determine the location of the functional promoter region in the 5′-flanking sequence of the *KpnI* fragment, we created several clones which contained variable lengths of 5′-flanking sequence. From a 5–3′ direction, fragments were generated by digests of pCG-β5ΔK with *XbaI*, *AccI*, *MstII*, and *SpeI* (Fig. 2a) and subcloned. When they were transfected into Y1 cells, all but the *SpeI* subclone expressed CG-β at levels comparable to those seen for the *KpnI* fragment (Fig. 3a). Thus, critical promoter sequences are located between the *MstII* site (188 bp upstream from the cap site (Jameson *et al.*, 1986b)) and the *SpeI* site (103 bp downstream from the cap site). To define the activity of this region further, a series of progressive exonuclease III deletion clones was constructed extending from the *AccI* site (-634) to the *SpeI* site (Fig. 2b). The shortest deletion mutant expressing CG-β contained 78 bp of 5′ sequence upstream from the cap site (Fig. 3b). A smaller deletion mutant bearing 20 bp was inactive. The level of CG-β expression was greater in cells

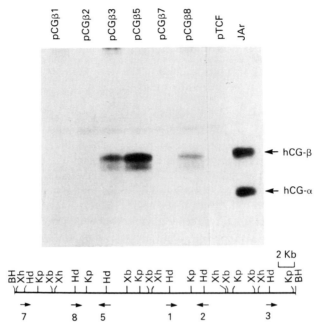

Fig. 1. Synthesis of hCG-β in Y1 cells transfected with individual genes. KpnI subclones containing each of the CG-β genes were transfected into Y1 cells (see map of parent cosmid at bottom). The resulting stable integrants were labelled with [^{35}S]cysteine, immuno-precipitated with hCG-β antiserum, and the proteins resolved on a sodium dodecyl sulphate-polyacrylamide gel. For a standard, labelled hCG was immunoprecipitated from medium of JAr choriocarcinoma cells metabolically labelled with [^{35}S]cysteine. The migrations of the α- and β-subunits are shown. The arrows indicate the direction of transcription and the numbers the CG-β gene assignments according to Boorstein *et al.* (1982).

transfected with the CG-β5 gene containing 249 bp of sequence 5′ of the cap site compared to a construct containing 279 bp of upstream sequence, which may suggest the existence of an additional regulatory element in this region. These data suggest that at least one element promoting the basal expression of the CG-β5 gene is located between −20 and −78.

The above experiments were performed in non-trophoblast cells. It is therefore likely that some regulatory sequences will not be expressed in such heterologous cells. Our initial attempts to express the chloramphenicol acetyltransferase (CAT) gene by transient expression in chorio-carcinoma cells using vectors containing β genomic 5′-flanking sequences were inconclusive. However, based on the predictions from the Y1 data, we re-evaluated this by engineering a con-struct containing CG-β sequences and both the neo and CAT genes in the same plasmid so that cells expressing CAT could be enriched. Stable clones selected for G418 resistance will contain primarily mononucleated progenitor trophoblast cells which do not express CG-β. However, a fraction of the cells will differentiate to the multinucleated β subunit synthesizing cells (Hoshina *et al.*, 1983; McQueen *et al.*, 1987). Each of these β-producing intermediates should contain the CAT gene and the neo gene, and thus an enrichment of cells containing the CAT gene driven by β subunit promoter sequence should be achieved. Experiments were performed with at least two independent pools of at least 50 clones. CG-β5 5′ fragments extending from the *KpnI* site, or *MstII* site to the *SpeI* site (+103 bp downstream from the cap site), in correct and reverse orientations were placed in front of the CAT gene. These plasmids were then transfected into JAr chorio-carcinoma cells (Fig. 4a). Only cells transfected with constructs bearing fragments in the correct

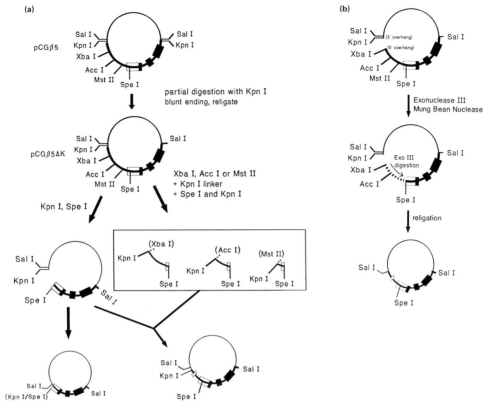

Fig. 2. Construction of CG-β gene 5 subclones containing truncated 5′ sequences. (a) Restriction enzyme digests. The 3′-ward KpnI site of pCG-β5 was deleted to form pCG-β5ΔK, which was digested with KpnI and SpeI to generate a vector for shuttling several fragments containing various lengths of the 5′-flanking region. The 5′-flanking fragments were formed by digesting pCG-β5ΔK with XbaI, AccI, MstII, and then attaching a KpnI linker at the cleavage site, and finally digesting with SpeI. The resulting KpnI–SpeI fragments were then inserted into the shuttle. (b) Exonuclease III deletion mutants. After CG-β5ΔK was digested with KpnI (−3·5 kb from the cap site) and XbaI (−1·7 kb), plasmids were treated with exonuclease III for various times to create a series of deletion mutants. The mutants were self-ligated to create various 5′ deletion clones.

orientation expressed CAT. To define the promoter region recognized in homologous cells in more detail, exonuclease III deletion fragments of CG-β5 were cloned in front of the CAT gene in pCAT NEO and transfected into JAr cells (Fig. 4b). Similar to the Y1 cell data, clones extending to −78 bp from the cap site expressed detectable CAT activity while fragments having −41 or −20 bp were inactive. Clones including various amounts of 5′ sequence up to −634 bp showed a complex pattern of CAT activity suggesting the existence of regulatory elements in this region. Sequence data of this region including a previously uncloned portion is shown. There was a sharp drop in activity between −361 and −279. The clone extending to the *KpnI* site (−3·5 kb) had stronger expression than one extending to the *AccI* site (−634 bp) suggesting additional upstream element(s) regulating CG-β expression. Our results suggest that this element is between the *KpnI* (−3·5 kb) and the *XbaI* (−1·7 kb) site (data not shown). In any case, these data support the conclusions from the Y1 experiments that a basal promoter element lies within 188 bp of the cap site and, importantly, show that it is recognized in homologous cells.

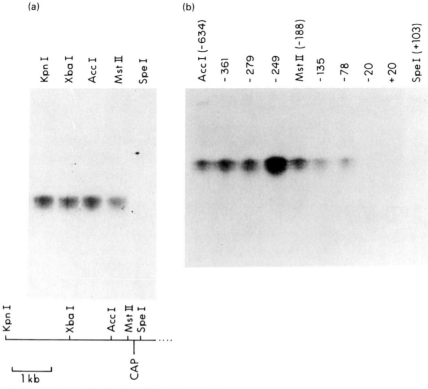

Fig. 3. Expression of hCG-β in Y1 cells transfected with CG-β5 subclones with truncated 5′ ends. The plasmid pCG-β5ΔK was digested with a series of restriction enzymes (a, see inset) or exonuclease III (b) resulting in progressively shortened 5′ ends (see Fig. 2). These clones were transfected into Y1 cells, and [^{35}S]cysteine-labelled proteins were immunoprecipitated from the medium and resolved on a sodium dodecyl sulphate gel. The numbers at the top of (b) correspond to the length of 5′ sequences from the CAP site determined by dideoxy sequencing.

Discussion

Little success has been achieved in expressing the CG-β genes in transfected cell systems. Talmadge *et al.* (1984b) expressed some of the cloned genes using an SV40-derived vector and transfecting into SV40-transformed COS cells, although the possibility that expression was dependent on an SV40 promoter was not excluded.

We have now developed a system using mouse Y1 cells which allowed us to express the CG-β genes. That expression was dependent on a promoter sequence contained in the CG-β gene was based on the following. (1) Adequate information for expression was contained in each KpnI fragment and expression was dependent on the 78 bp upstream from the CAP site. (2) Activity of the transfected genes varied. CG-β5 was the strongest expressor amongst the 6 genes, and the start site of the CG-β transcripts in the transfected cells was the same as in the placenta (Otani *et al.*, 1988). The sequence 200 bp upstream from the CAP site reveals no obvious homology to known promoter regions, e.g. CAAT, TATAA boxes seen in most eukaryotic promoters, although there are several examples of genes whose promoters lack such sequences (Reynolds *et al.*, 1984; Melton *et al.*, 1984; Valerio *et al.*, 1985; McGorgan *et al.*, 1985; Dynan *et al.*, 1986; Yamaguchi *et al.*, 1987).

It is unclear why this heterologous mouse cell line supports transcription of the transfected CG-β genes. The adrenal cells do not share an embryological relationship to trophoblast cells, and

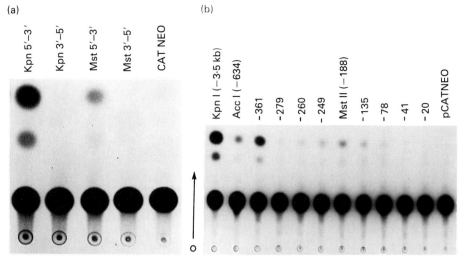

Fig. 4. Expression of the chloramphenicol acetyltransferase gene in JAr choriocarcinoma cells stably transfected with chloramphenicol acetyltransferase NEO constructs linked to 5' regions of CG-β gene 5. [^{14}C]Chloramphenicol (0·1 μCi) was incubated with 20 μg of cell extracts. The ○ and arrow indicate the origin and direction of chromatography, respectively. (a) Clones generated by restriction endonuclease digestion of CG-β5. β5/Kpn 5–3' represents cells transfected with constructs containing the 5' region of CG-β5 extending to the KpnI site. This corresponds to a distance of 3·5 kb from the CAP site and represents the correct orientation in front of the chloramphenicol acetyltransferase gene; β5/Kpn 3–5' designates the reverse orientation of the CG-β upstream sequences. Others are similarly indicated. (b) Exonuclease III-generated CG-β5 deletion clones. The numbers at the top of the panel indicate the number of nucleotides upstream from the cap site. The lane marked pCAT NEO shows cells transfected with that vector.

they do not synthesize endogenous proteins that cross-react with CG subunit-specific antisera. There may be inhibitory factors in human cells which act in transfections to regulate negatively the CG-β genes and such a factor may absent in Y1 cells. CG-β was expressed, albeit weakly, in another cell line, mouse L cells, when a cosmid containing CG-β cluster was transfected (data not shown).

It also appears that the Y1 cells are not simply permissive for all genes since the transfected LH-β gene is inactive. Figure 5 reveals striking similarities between the 5' region of CG-β5 and the LH-β genes. While CG-β apparently evolved from the LH-β gene (Talmadge *et al.*, 1984a), they utilize different transcription initiation sites. LH-β transcription starts just 9 bp upstream of the ATG translation initiation codon and is preceded by a TATAA sequence 38 bp upstream (Virgin *et al.*, 1985; Jameson *et al.*, 1986b). CG-β transcription starts 360–366 bp from the ATG (Policastro *et al.*, 1983; Talmadge *et al.*, 1984a; Jameson *et al.*, 1986b). However, for both CG-β5 and LH-β the first 200 bp upstream from their respective CAP sites are very similar. LH-β may therefore be inactive due to scattered differences in the promoter sequence. Alternatively, there may be inhibitory sequences acting in cis that prevent expression of the LH-β gene in Y1 cells and/or a factor from the gonadotrophs that is required for LH-β expression. In any event, while it is difficult to make inferences regarding tissue-specific regulation of the gonadotropin β subunits, the use of Y1 cells has identified the basal promoter of the CG-β subunit.

As discussed above, previous attempts to express the CG-β promoter in trophoblast-derived cells using constructs containing several hundred base pairs of the 5'-flanking sequence fused to the CAT gene were unsuccessful. Not all trophoblasts synthesize the β subunit and its expression is dependent on the formation of cell intermediates during the differentiation of cytotrophoblasts to

I. Boime et al.

```
       AccI  -630        -620       -610       -600       -590
CGβ5   CTACAGAAGGCCTTTCAGTATCTGGGAGCTGGGGTTCAAATGAGAAATCT

       -580        -570       -560       -550       -540
CGβ5   TACTTGGTGAGAGCGGGCAGGGGTCGGCTTAGAATATTTTGTTTTGAGAT

       -530        -520       -510       -500       -490
CGβ5   AATGAGCTACCGATCACAGGGGGAGTTTAAGCAAGGTTCAATGAGAAGCG

       -480        -470       -460       -450       -440
CGβ5   ATCAAGATGCTGCACAGTTCAGCCCTGGGTGGGGAGCTCAAGTCAGGTTT

       -430        -420       -410       -400       -390
CGβ5   CTAGCCCTCTTCCCTGTGCCAACCTATACCCTACATTGGGAAAGAAACAG

       -380        -370       -360       -350       -340
CGβ5   ACCTTAAAATTGTCCAGCTTGATGGCATCGCGGGGAAGGGACTAAGTCCA

       -330        -320       -310       -300       -290
CGβ5   GATAATGTCCTCTGAGGCTTCGGCCCCGTGGGCAGGACACACCTCCTGCG

       -280        -270       -260       -250       -240
CGβ5   GGCCTATTCAATAATCAGTTAAATCACCTGAAGCACACGCATTTCCGGGG

       -230        -220       -210       -200      MstII
CGβ5   ACCGCTCCGGGCATCCTGGCTTGAGGGTAGAGTGGGCGGAGGTTCCTAAG

       -180        -170       -160       -150       -140
CGβ5   GGGAGAGGTGGG▮GCTCGGGCTGAATCCCTCGTTGGGGGGGCATCTGGGTCA
CGβ3   ...... ........................................
CGβ7   ...........T.................................
LHβ    ..........▮.........T........C.......▮..........

       -130        -120       -110       -100       -90
CGβ5   AGTGGCTTCCCTGGCAGCACAGTCACGGGGAGGCCCTCTCTCATTGGGCA
CGβ3   ..........................A...........C.....
CGβ7   ..........................A...........C.....
LHβ    ............................................

       -80         -70        -60        -50        -40
CGβ5   GAAGCTAAGTCCGAAGCCGCGCCCCTCCTGGGAGGTTGAACTGTGGTGCA
CGβ3   .....................................G..........
CGβ7   ................................TT......G.......
LHβ    ..................A.............TT......G.......

                                            CGβCAP
       -30         -20        -10          ↓        10
CGβ5   GGAAAGCCTCAAGTAGAGGAGGGTTGAGGCTTCAATCCAGCACTTTGCTC
CGβ3   ...................................G...........
CGβ7   ....T.G...........................G....C..T...
LHβ    ..............▮▮▮.................G...........C...

       20          30         40         50         60
CGβ5   GGGTCACGGCCTCCTCCTGGCTCCCAGGACCCCACCATAGGCAGAGGCAG
CGβ3   ..................▮....T...A....................
CGβ7   ................G...T...A....................
LHβ    .....T...........A........A...A..T..........

       70          80         90         100     SpeI
CGβ5   GCCTTCCTACACCCTACTCCCTGTGCCTCCAGGCTCGACTAGTCCCTAGC
CGβ3   ....................................C...........
CGβ7   .................T.............C...........
LHβ    ...............T....C...............

       120         130        140        150        160
CGβ5   ACTCGACGACTGAGTCTCTGAGGTCACTTCACCGTGGTCTCCGCCTCACC
LHβ    .......A................................T.....

       170         180        190        200        210
CGβ5   CTTGGCGCTGGACCAGTGAGAGGAGAGGGCTGGGCGGCTCCGCTGAGCCA
LHβ    TC.......A....C.....G...............A...T.......

       220         230        240        250        260
CGβ5   CTCCTGCGCCCCCCTGGCCTTGTCTACCTCTTGCCCCCGAAGGGTTAGTG
LHβ    ..........T.......A...GC......C.......GG..A......

       270         280        290        300        310
CGβ5   TCGAGCTCACCCCAG▮CATCCTACAACCTCCTGGTGGCCTTGCCGCCCCC
LHβ    ..C..G.T.......G.......TC...................

                                         LHβCAP
       320         330        340        350     ↓
CGβ5   ACAACCCCGAGGTATAAAGCCAGGTACACCAGGCAGGGGACGCACCAAGG
LHβ    ....................................A....G.......T......

       MetGluMetPheGln
       370         380        390        400        410
CGβ5   ATGGAGATGTTCCAGGTAAGACTGCAGGGCCCCTGGGCACCTTCCACCTC
LHβ    ........C.................................
       Leu
```

Fig. 5. Sequence of the CG-β5′ region. Numbers indicate base pairs from the cap site. The sequence upstream of −276 bp from the cap site was sequenced from our βcos subclone while the remainder was from Talmadge *et al.* (1984a, b) and Policastro *et al.* (1986).

syncytium (Hoshina *et al.*, 1983; McQueen *et al.*, 1987). The CG-β-producing cells represent only a minor fraction of the total cellular population and, given the relatively low transfection efficiencies with such transient systems the expression of CAT driven by CG-β promoter would fall below the limits of detection. However, by engineering constructs containing CG-β sequences, a selectable marker and the CAT gene on the same plasmid and selecting stable transfectant clones, a population of trophoblast-derived cells that co-integrated the CG-β–CAT fusion and marker genes could be obtained. While most such stable clones will be mononucleated cells not producing

CG-β, some will differentiate into intermediates expressing CG-β. Each of these intermediates should contain the CAT gene driven by a CG-β promoter. We prepared constructs bearing various CG-β5 5′ fragments. The data show that the basal promoter element of CG-β5 recognized in Y1 cells was also active in homologous trophoblast cells transfected with CAT constructs containing a set of deleted 5′-flanking sequences in length from -634 to -78 bp from the cap site and suggests that there are additional regulatory elements upstream of the basal promoter region. According to this sequence of events, the intermediate cell types are associated with the activation of one or more cellular genes that encode a trans-activating factor. The decrease in CG during gestation may result from depletion of the activator. Alternatively, the presence of possible inhibitory sequences suggests that loss of CG synthesis can be attributed to induction of inhibitory factors that attenuate expression of the CG-β genes.

In conclusion, these systems have identified a promoter region for the CG-β gene and will be useful for providing a known sequence for identifying the trans-acting proteins in normal and tumour-derived trophoblast cells that are associated with the regulated expression of this multigene family.

We thank Dr Maynard Olson for helpful discussions during the course of this study; and Dr John Majors for critical review of the manuscript. Supported by a grant from the Monsanto Co.

References

Boorstein, W.R., Vamvakopoulos, N.C. & Fiddes, J.C. (1982) Human chorionic gonadotropin is encoded by at least eight genes arranged in tandem and inverted pairs. *Nature, Lond.* **300**, 419–422.

Boothby, M., Kukowska, J. & Boime, I. (1983) Imbalanced synthesis of human chorionic gonadotropin α and β subunits reflects the steady-state levels of the corresponding mRNAs. *J. biol. Chem.* **258**, 9250–9254.

Chaplin, D.D., Galbraith, L.G., Seidman, J.G., White, P.C. & Parker, K.L. (1986) Nucleotide sequence analysis of murine 21-hydroxylase genes: mutations affecting gene expression. *Proc. natn. Acad. Sci. U.S.A.* **83**, 9601–9605.

Corless, C.L., Bielinska, M., Ramabhadran, T.V., McQueen, S.D., Otani, T., Reitz, B.A., Tiemeier, D.C. & Boime, I. (1987) Gonadotropin α subunit: differential processing of free and combined forms in human trophoblast and transfected mouse cells. *J. biol. Chem.* **262**, 14197–14203.

Dynan, W.S., Sazer, S., Tijian, R. & Schimke, R.T. (1986) Transcription factor Sp1 recognizes a DNA sequence in the mouse dihydrofolate reductase promoter. *Nature, Lond.* **319**, 246–248.

Gorman, C., Moffat, L. & Howard, B. (1982) Recombinant genomes which express chloramphenicol acetyl transferase in mammalian cells. *Molec. cell. Biol.* **2**, 1044–1057.

Graham, M.Y., Otani, T., Boime, I., Olson, M.V., Carle, G.F. & Chaplin, D.D. (1987) Cosmid mapping of the human chorionic gonadotropin β subunit genes by field-inversion gel electrophoresis. *Nucleic Acids Res.* **15**, 4437–4448.

Grosveld, F.G., Lund, T., Murray, E.J., Mellor, A.L., Dahl, H.H.M. & Flavell, R.A. (1982) The construction of cosmid libraries which can be used to transform eukaryotic cells. *Nucleic Acids Res.* **10**, 6715–6732.

Hoshina, M., Boothby, M. & Boime, I. (1982) Cytological localization of chorionic gonadotropin α and placental lactogen mRNAs during development of human placenta. *J. Cell Biol.* **93**, 193–198.

Hoshina, M., Hussa, R., Patillo, R. & Boime, I. (1983) Cytological distribution of chorionic gonadotropin subunit and placental lactogen mRNAs in neoplasms derived from human placenta. *J. Cell Biol.* **97**, 1200–1206.

Hoshina, M., Boothby, M., Hussa, R., Pattillo, R., Camel, M. & Boime, I. (1985) Linkage of human chorionic gonadotropin and placental lactogen biosynthesis to trophoblast differentiation and tumorigenesis. *Placenta* **6**, 163–172.

Jameson, L.J., Lindell, C.M. & Habener, J.F. (1986a) Evolution of different transcriptional start sites in the human luteinizing hormone and chorionic gonadotropin β-subunit genes. *DNA* **5**, 227–234.

Jameson, L.J., Jaffe, R.C., Gleason, S.L. & Habener, J.F. (1986b) Transcriptional regulation of chorionic gonadotropin α- and β-subunit gene expression by bromoadenosine 3′,5′-monophosphate. *Endocrinology* **119**, 2560–2567.

McGorgan, M., Simonsen, C.C., Smouse, D.T., Farnham, P.J. & Schimke, R.T. (1985) Heterogeneity at the 5′ termini of mouse dihydrofolate reductase mRNAs. *J. biol. Chem.* **260**, 2307–2314.

McQueen, S.D., Krichevsky, A. & Boime, I. (1987) Isolation and characterization of human cytotrophoblast cells. In *Trophoblast Research*, Vol. II, pp. 423–445. Plenum, New York.

Melton, D.W., Konecki, D.S., Brennand, J. & Caskey, T. (1984) Structure, expression, and mutation of the hypoxanthine phosphoribosyltransferase gene. *Proc. natn. Acad. Sci. U.S.A.* **81**, 2147–2151.

Otani, T., Otani, F., Krych, M. & Chaplin, D. (1988) Identification of a promoter region in the CGβ gene cluster. *J. biol. Chem.* **263**, 7322–7329.

Policastro, P.F. (1984) *A map of the hCGβ-LHβ gene cluster*. Ph.D. thesis dissertation, Washington University, St Louis, MO.

Policastro, P.F., Ovitt, C.E., Hoshina, M., Fukuoka, H., Boothby, M.R. & Boime, I. (1983) The β-subunit of human chorionic gonadotropin is encoded by multiple genes. *J. biol. Chem.* **258**, 11 492–11 499.

Policastro, P.F., McQueen, S.D., Carle, G. & Boime, I. (1986) A map of the hCGβ-LHβ gene cluster. *J. biol. Chem.* **261**, 5907–5916.

Reynolds, G.A., Basu, S.K., Osborne, T.F., Chin, D.J., Gil, G., Brown, M.S., Goldstein, J.L. & Luskey, K.L. (1984) HMG CoA reductase: a negatively regulated gene with unusual promoter and 5′ untranslated regions. *Cell* **38**, 275–285.

Schimmer, P. (1981) Functionally differentiated cell lines. In *The Adenocortical Cell Line*, Y1, pp. 61–92. Alan R. Liss, Inc., New York.

Talmadge, K., Boorstein, W.R. & Fiddes, J.C. (1983) The human genome contains seven genes for the β-subunit of chorionic gonadotropin and only one gene for the β-subunit of LH. *DNA* **2**, 281–289.

Talmadge, K., Vamvakopoulos, N.C. & Fiddes, J.C. (1984a) Evolution of human chorionic beta subunit: gene sequence comparison with human luteinizing hormone beta-subunit. *Nature, Lond.* **307**, 37–40.

Talmadge, K., Boorstein, W.R., Vamvakopoulos, N.C., Gething, M.J. & Fiddes, J.C. (1984b) Only 3 of the 7 human chorionic gonadotropin beta subunit genes can be expressed in the placenta. *Nucleic Acids Res.* **12**, 8415–8436.

Valerio, D., Duyvesteyn, M.G.C., Dekker, B.M., Weeda, G., Berkvens, T.M., Voorn, L., Ormondt, H. & Eb, J. (1985) Adenosine deaminase: Characterization and expression of a gene with a remarkable promoter. *EMBO J.* **4**, 437–443.

Virgin, J.B., Silver, B.J., Thomason, A.R. & Nilson, J.H. (1985) The gene for the β subunit of bovine luteinizing hormone encodes a gonadotropin mRNA with an unusually short 5′-untranslated region. *J. biol. Chem.* **260**, 7072–7077.

Yamaguchi, M., Hirose, F., Hayashi, Y., Nishimoto, Y. & Matsukage, A. (1987) Murine DNA polymerase β gene mapping of transcription initiation sites and the nucleotide sequence of the putative promoter region. *Molec. cell. Biol.* **7**, 2012–2018.

J. Reprod. Fert., Suppl. **37** (1989), 11–17

Low molecular weight lipid-soluble luteotrophic factor(s) produced by conceptuses in cows

W. Hansel, Angelika Stock and P. J. Battista

Department of Physiology, New York State College of Veterinary Medicine and Division of Biological Sciences, Cornell University, Ithaca, NY 14853, U.S.A.

Keywords: early pregnancy recognition; progesterone; platelet-activating factor; serotonin; platelet-derived growth factor; prostaglandins

Introduction

Day 16 is generally considered as the day of maternal recognition of pregnancy in cattle. Betteridge *et al.* (1980) showed that transfer of viable Day-16 conceptuses into suitable recipients up to and including Day 16 after ovulation can result in maintenance of the corpus luteum and normal pregnancy. Similarly, Northey & French (1980) showed that removal of embryos at Days 17–19 resulted in a prolongation of luteal lifespan, compared to unmated controls or animals from which embryos were removed at Days 13–15. Intrauterine infusion of homogenates of Day 17 or 18 embryos caused a slight delay in luteal regression and lengthened the cycle by 2·9 days.

However, there was no evidence in these experiments, or in those of Thatcher *et al.* (1985), who infused 'conceptus secretory proteins' from cultures of Day 17–18 bovine conceptuses into the uteri of cyclic cattle, that these preparations caused an increase in plasma progesterone concentrations, such as occurs in normal animals during early pregnancy (Fig. 1). Lukaszewska & Hansel (1980) measured jugular vein plasma progesterone and oestradiol concentrations in 18 pregnant, 17 cyclic and 12 inseminated but non-pregnant Holstein heifers and found higher ($P < 0·05$) progesterone concentrations in pregnant than in non-pregnant or cyclic animals between Days 10 and 18. Jugular oestradiol concentrations were also higher in pregnant than in cyclic animals between Days 6 and 16. Studies of ovarian and uterine vein progesterone concentrations in these animals suggested that the increased values in pregnant animals were due mainly to ovarian production.

Evidence for production of a low molecular weight, lipid-soluble luteotrophin(s) by early embryos of cows

In our first experiment in this area (Beal *et al.*, 1981), homogenates and aqueous extracts of homogenates of Day 18 blastocysts were tested for their abilities to stimulate net progesterone production in bovine luteal cells dispersed and incubated as described by Hixon & Hansel (1979). Both the homogenates and their aqueous extracts stimulated net progesterone synthesis. The activity was lost after dialysis under conditions that removed compounds of $M_r < 12\,000$.

More recently, Hickey & Hansel (1987) developed culture systems for maintenance of Day 13–18 conceptus tissue and assayed the harvested culture media for luteotrophic activity. The luteotrophic effects of the harvested culture media were tested in the dispersed bovine luteal cell incubation system described by Hixon & Hansel (1979) and progesterone concentrations were measured as described by Beal *et al.* (1980).

Significant ($P < 0·05$) luteotrophic activity was present during the first 5 days of culture in 80% of the 31 conceptus tissue cultures studied, and the activity did not depend on the presence of fetal calf serum in the media. The active material did not appear to be a protein, since neither 20 nor 60% $(NH_4)_2SO_4$ precipitates of the culture media contained activity. Maintenance of the culture

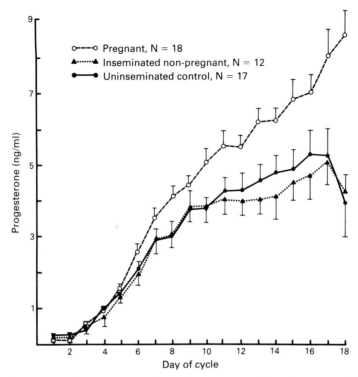

Fig. 1. Jugular venous plasma concentrations of progesterone in cyclic, pregnant, and inseminated but non-pregnant heifers during the first 18 days after oestrus. Values are mean ± s.e.m.
(From Lukaszewska & Hansel, 1980.)

media at 60°C for 30 min resulted in a significant loss of the stimulatory activity (progesterone,
ng/10^6 cells/2 h; control 86 ± 1·7; culture medium 131 ± 5·5; culture medium after heat treatment
77 ± 45; $P < 0.05$).

Conceptus culture media harvested on Days 4 and 7, which contained significant luteotrophic
activity, were pooled and separated into fractions of $M_r < 10\,000$ and $M_r > 10\,000$ using an
Amicon C Centricon filter (Amicon Corp., Danvers, MA, U.S.A.). Testing these fractions showed
that the activity was present only in the $M_r < 10\,000$ fraction (Fig. 2). Furthermore, a lipid extract
of the fraction of $M_r < 10\,000$ (Fig. 2) contained all of the activity. Dextran-coated charcoal, which
has the ability to bind steroids and other small molecules in solution was added to the $M_r < 10\,000$
fraction and after 15 min at 4°C was removed by centrifugation at 2000 *g* for 15 min. This treatment
removed the luteotrophic activity from the culture media ($P < 0.05$).

These results show that cultured Day 13–18 bovine conceptuses produce a low molecular
weight ($M_r < 10\,000$), lipid-soluble, heat-labile luteotrophin(s) that binds to dextran-coated
charcoal. The results suggest that the active principle could be a steroid. Bovine blastocysts are
known to produce oestradiol, progesterone and testosterone (Shemesh *et al.*, 1979) and there is
extensive metabolism of androstenedione to 5β-reduced compounds by the bovine conceptus
during early pregnancy (Thatcher *et al.*, 1984).

It seems unlikely that either oestradiol or progesterone of conceptus origin could exert a luteotrophic effect *in vivo*, since both have been shown to inhibit corpus luteum development when
administered intramuscularly during the oestrous cycle (Ray *et al.*, 1961; Wiltbank *et al.*, 1961).
However, Reynolds *et al.* (1983) found that intrauterine infusion of 150 ng oestradiol-17β plus
250 µg PGE-2 at 6-h intervals from Day 13 of the oestrous cycle to the day of subsequent oestrus

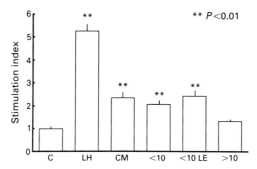

Fig. 2. Net progesterone synthesis (mean ± s.e.) by bovine luteal cells (ng/10^6 cells/2 h) in response to Medium 199 (C), 5 ng LH (LH), culture medium (CM), fractions of culture medium of $M_r < 10\,000$ (<10) or $> 10\,000$ (>10), or lipid extracts of the $M_r < 10\,000$ fractions (<10 LE). Results are expressed as units of stimulation index (progesterone treated/progesterone control). (From Hickey & Hansel, 1987.)

(or Day 21) resulted in a remarkable maintenance of functional corpora lutea. Neither the oestradiol nor the PGE-2 given alone was effective.

There are abundant data to show that early cow embryos (Days 16–18) produce a number of prostanoids, including the known luteotrophins PGE-2 and PGI-2 (Shemesh *et al.*, 1984). PGE-2 and PGI-2 have often been cited as possible luteotrophic signals from the conceptus to the dam to invoke maternal recognition of pregnancy in the cow and the ewe (Pratt *et al.*, 1977; Silvia *et al.*, 1984).

Luteotrophic effects of platelet-derived compounds

There is increasing evidence for the existence of an early pregnancy recognition factor in a number of species (Morton, 1985), and Orozco *et al.* (1986) have shown that injection of synthesized platelet-activating factor (PAF) into mature female mice induces expression of serum early pregnancy factor. Thrombocytopenia is an initial response to pregnancy in mice, marmosets, women, and possibly in other species (O'Neill, 1985a). The thrombocytopenia of early pregnancy is dependent on the presence of fertilized ova in the reproductive tract and is due to the production of PAF by the embryo (O'Neill, 1985b, c). In mice, platelet activation appears to be necessary for implantation. Embryo-derived platelet-activating factor, like PAF from other sources, for example equine leucocytes, has been characterized and appears to be 1-0-alkyl-2-acetyl-sn-glyceryl-3-phosphocholine, or PAF-acether (Wimberly *et al.*, 1985; O'Neill, 1985d).

Upon activation by PAF, platelets release histamine, serotonin, arachidonic acid derivatives, growth factors and other factors that have roles in cellular attachment and adhesion (O'Neill, 1985b). Platelet-derived growth factor was purified by Antoniades *et al.* in 1979 and Raines & Ross (1982) described a high-yield purification procedure and presented evidence for multiple forms of the factor. Human platelet-derived growth factor increases synthesis of products of the cyclooxygenase pathway of arachidonic acid metabolism, particularly PGI-2 and PGE (Habenicht *et al.*, 1985), both of which are known to have luteotrophic effects on bovine luteal cells (Hansel & Dowd, 1986). Furthermore, serotonin, released from platelets by PAF, has been shown to increase progesterone secretion by bovine luteal cells (Battista & Condon, 1986).

In view of these facts, we have initiated a number of in-vitro and in-vivo experiments to determine whether platelets, or the products of platelet activation, might be involved in early pregnancy recognition in cattle. The preliminary results cited below are compatible with such a concept.

O'Neill (1987) reported that PAF, at concentrations of $0.1-1\,\mu g/ml$, enhanced the production of progesterone in human granulosa cell cultures. To test the hypothesis that PAF has a direct luteo-trophic effect on bovine luteal cells, several dose levels $(0.001-10\,\mu g/ml)$ of synthetic PAF (Boehringer Mannheim Biochemicals, Indianapolis, IN, U.S.A.) were added, in the presence and absence of LH, to dispersed bovine luteal cells prepared as described by Hixon & Hansel (1979). Net progesterone production during incubation for 2 h was measured as described by Beal *et al.* (1980). Low concentrations of PAF $(0.001-1\,\mu g/ml)$ had no effect on basal or LH-stimulated progesterone synthesis (P. J. Battista & W. Hansel, unpublished observations). A high concentration $(10\,\mu g/ml)$, which appeared to be cytotoxic, inhibited both basal and LH-stimulated progesterone synthesis. It therefore appears that the low molecular weight lipid-soluble luteotrophin(s) extracted from the media harvested from the cultures of early bovine embryos described above is not PAF.

However, further studies revealed that co-incubation of platelets with dispersed luteal cells resulted in a marked stimulation of basal progesterone synthesis. Platelets obtained from normal Holstein heifers during Days 10–12 (oestrus = Day 0) of the oestrous cycle were processed as described by Liggitt *et al.* (1984) and re-suspended in Tyrode's buffer at a final concentration of 1×10^8 platelets/0.5 mg. To examine the effects of platelet-derived compounds on luteal progesterone production, luteal cells $(2.5 \times 10^5$ cells/0.25 ml) were co-incubated with unactivated or PAF-activated platelets at platelet concentrations of $1 \times 10^7 - 4 \times 10^8$. Pre-activated platelets were prepared by incubating with PAF (20 ng) for 3 min at $37°C$.

The results (Fig. 3) show that co-incubation of luteal cells with platelets increases progesterone synthesis ($P < 0.05$) over a concentration range of 1×10^7 to 4×10^8 platelets. No difference was observed between the abilities of pre-activated and unactivated platelets to stimulate progesterone synthesis. The results indicate that platelets were aggregated *in vitro*, without the addition of PAF, under the conditions of these experiments.

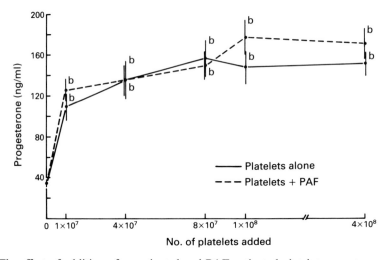

Fig. 3. The effect of addition of unactivated and PAF-activated platelets on net progesterone production by dispersed bovine luteal (Days 10–12) cells (means $\pm$ s.e.m., $n = 6$). Means with different superscripts differ ($P < 0.05$) from control level (no platelets added) of 36.3 ± 4.86 ng/ml.

Subsequent experiments utilizing the 5-hydroxytryptamine (serotinin) receptor antagonist, mianserin (data not shown) indicated that serotonin is the major platelet-derived compound responsible for the platelet-induced stimulation of luteal progesterone synthesis. However, platelet-derived growth hormone was also shown to have a luteotrophic effect on bovine luteal cells *in vitro*. Blockage of the cyclo-oxygenase pathway of arachidonic acid metabolism by addition of indomethacin did not diminish the ability of platelets to stimulate progesterone synthesis by bovine luteal cells *in vitro*.

In view of the report of O'Neill (1985c) that early pregnancy-associated thrombocytopenia in mice was caused by PAF produced by early embryos, we carried out an experiment to determine whether thrombocytopenia during early pregnancy could be demonstrated in cattle. The oestrous cycles of 10 normal regularly cycling Holstein heifers, housed, fed and managed under identical conditions were synchronized by the PRID (progesterone-releasing intravaginal device)–PGF-2α method described by Smith *et al.* (1984). This method entails insertion of PRIDs for 7 days and single injections of PGF-2α (25 mg) on the 6th day of PRID treatment. All animals were artificially inseminated 12 h after the onset of oestrus. Daily blood samples were collected from the tail vein and platelet counts were carried out from 2 days before insemination through Day 19 after insemination. Whole blood was diluted 1:100 with ammonium oxalate (Unopette Microcollection System, Becton Dickson Co., Rutherford, NJ, U.S.A.) and allowed to stand for 10 min to lyse erythrocytes. Platelets were counted in a haemocytometer. The results were analysed by the split-plot method of Gill & Hafs (1971).

Rectal palpations at 7 weeks after insemination revealed that 5 of the 10 inseminated heifers became pregnant. Platelet counts (Fig. 4) were significantly lower ($P < 0.05$) in the pregnant than in the non-pregnant animals between Days 7 and 16 (A. Stock & W. Hansel, unpublished observations).

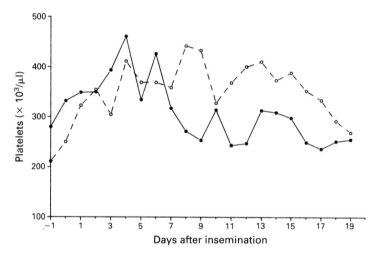

Fig. 4. Mean platelet counts in pregnant (●——●, N = 5) and inseminated non-pregnant (○ – – ○, N = 5) heifers during the first 19 days after insemination.

In other experiments, the effects of infusing PAF into the uteri of normal cycling heifers on plasma progesterone concentrations and oestrous cycle lengths are being studied (A. Stock & W. Hansel, unpublished observations). Infusions are being carried out in 5 treated and 5 control animals each at Days 9–11, 14–16 and 16–18. Preliminary results suggest that plasma progesterone concentrations may be elevated after intrauterine infusions and cycle lengths may be increased in some animals.

These in-vivo and in-vitro results, although limited in scope, are compatible with the idea that the release of platelet-derived products, perhaps under the influence of an embryo-derived platelet activator, play a role in stimulating progesterone synthesis by the corpus luteum of early pregnancy.

Although there is no direct evidence that the early bovine embryo produces PAF, the occurrence of thrombocytopenia during early pregnancy suggests that such may be the case.

The in-vitro data cited above suggest that serotonin may be the major luteotrophin produced by the platelets. However, platelet-derived growth factor was also shown to stimulate luteal progesterone production in these studies. In rat granulosa cells, platelet-derived growth factor facilitates follicle-stimulating hormone-dependent LH receptor induction and progestagen production (Mondschein & Schomberg, 1981). Platelet-derived growth factor may exert its luteotrophic effect in bovine luteal cells through the Ca^{2+}-polyphosphoinositol–protein kinase C second messenger system, activation of which is known to stimulate progesterone synthesis in the small theca-derived luteal cells (Alila *et al.*, 1988). Platelet-derived growth factor stimulates polyphosphoinositol hydrolysis and Ca^{2+} mobilization in Swiss 3T3 cells (Berridge *et al.* , 1984).

Summary and Conclusion

Peripheral plasma progesterone concentrations are higher ($P < 0.05$) in pregnant than in inseminated non-pregnant or cyclic heifers between Days 10 and 18 after insemination. In several experiments, it has been demonstrated that bovine conceptuses produce a low molecular weight (M_r $< 10\,000$), lipid-soluble, heat-labile, dextran-coated charcoal-adsorbable luteotrophic substance(s) that has the ability to stimulate progesterone synthesis in dispersed bovine luteal cells. This substance does not appear to be PAF, since addition of PAF to dispersed luteal cells at several dose levels failed to affect either basal or LH-stimulated progesterone synthesis. However, results of in-vitro and in-vivo experiments suggest that platelet-derived products are luteotrophic. In in-vitro experiments it was shown that co-incubation of dispersed bovine luteal cells with bovine platelets augments basal progesterone synthesis. Serotonin and platelet-derived growth factor appear to be the major products of platelet activation responsible for the luteotrophic activity of platelets. Products of the arachidonic acid cascade do not appear to be important, since addition of the cyclo-oxygenase blocker indomethacin did not reduce the luteotrophic activity of platelets. In in-vivo experiments, it has been possible to demonstrate a significant thrombocytopenia in pregnant heifers between Days 7 and 16 after insemination. These results are compatible with the concept that release of platelet-derived products under the influence of factors produced by the early embryo play a role in stimulating progesterone synthesis by the corpus luteum during early pregnancy.

References

Alila, H.W., Dowd, J.P., Corradino, R.A., Harris, W.V. & Hansel, W. (1988) Control of progesterone production in small and large bovine luteal cells separated by flow cytometry. *J. Reprod. Fert.* **82**, 645–655.

Antoniades, H.N., Scher, C.B. & Stiles, A.D. (1979) Purification of platelet derived growth factor. *Proc. natn. Acad. Sci. U.S.A.* **76**, 1809–1813.

Battista, P.J. & Condon, W.A. (1986) Serotonin-induced stimulation of progesterone production by cow luteal cells *in vitro*. *J. Reprod. Fert.* **76**, 231–238.

Beal, W.E., Milvae, R.A. & Hansel, W. (1980) Oestrous cycle length and plasma progesterone concentrations following administration of prostaglandin F-2α early in the bovine oestrous cycle. *J. Reprod. Fert.* **59**, 393–396.

Beal, W.E., Lukaszewska, J. H. & Hansel, W. (1981) Luteotropic effects of bovine blastocysts. *J. Anim. Sci.* **52**, 567–574.

Berridge, M.J., Heslop, J.P., Irvine, R.G. & Brown, K.D.

(1984) Inositol triphosphate formation and calcium mobilization in Swiss 3T3 cells in response to platelet-derived growth factor. *Biochem. J.* **222**, 195–201.

Betteridge, K.J., Eaglesome, M.D., Randall, G.C.B. & Mitchell, D. (1980) Collection, description and transfer of embryos from cattle 10–16 days after oestrus. *J. Reprod. Fert.* **59**, 205–216.

Gill, J.L. & Hafs, H.D. (1971) Analysis of repeated measurements in animals. *J. Anim. Sci.* **33**, 331–336.

Habenicht, A.J., Goerig, R.M., Grulich, J., Rothe, D., Gronwald, R., Loth, U., Schettler, G., Kommerell, B. & Ross, R. (1985) Human platelet derived growth factor stimulates prostaglandin synthesis by activation and by rapid de novo synthesis of cyclooxygenase. *J. clin. Invest.* **75**, 1381–1387.

Hansel, W. & Dowd, J.P. (1986) New concepts of the control of corpus luteum function. *J. Reprod. Fert.* **78**, 755–768.

Hickey, G.J. & Hansel, W. (1987) In-vitro synthesis of a low molecular weight lipid-soluble luteotropic factor by conceptuses of cows at Day 13–18 of pregnancy. *J. Reprod. Fert.* **80**, 569–576.

Hixon, J.E. & Hansel, W. (1979) Effects of prostaglandin F-2α, estradiol and luteinizing hormone in dispersed cell preparations of bovine corpora lutea. In *Ovarian Follicular and Corpus Luteum Function*, pp. 613–620. Eds C. P. Channing, J. M. Marsh & W. A. Sadler. Plenum Publishing, New York.

Liggitt, H.D., Leid, R.W. & Huston, L. (1984) Aggregation of bovine platelets by acetyl glyceryl ether phosphorylcholine (platelet activating factor). *Vet. Immunol. Immunopath.* **7**, 81–87.

Lukaszewska, J. & Hansel, W. (1980) Corpus luteum maintenance during early pregnancy in the cow. *J. Reprod. Fert.* **59**, 485–493.

Mondschein, J.S. & Schomberg, D.W. (1981) Platelet-derived growth factor enhances granulosa cell luteinizing hormone receptor induction by follicle stimulating hormone. *Endocrinology* **109**, 325–327.

Morton, H. (1985) EPF as a pregnancy protein. In *Early Pregnancy Factors*, pp. 53–64. Eds F. Ellendorff & E. Koch. Perinatology Press, Ithaca.

Northey, D.L. & French, L.R. (1980) Effect of embryo removal and intrauterine infusion of embryonic homogenates on the lifespan of the bovine corpus luteum. *J. Anim. Sci.* **50**, 298–302.

O'Neill, C. (1985a) Embryo derived platelet activating factor. In *Early Pregnancy Factors*, pp. 261–266. Eds F. Ellendorff & E. Koch. Perinatology Press, Ithaca.

O'Neill, C. (1986b) Thrombocytopenia is an initial response to fertilization in mice. *J. Reprod. Fert.* **73**, 559–566.

O'Neill, C. (1985c) Examination of the causes of early pregnancy associated thrombocytopenia in mice. *J. Reprod. Fert.* **73**, 567–577.

O'Neill, C. (1985d) Partial characterization of embryo derived platelet activating factor in mice. *J. Reprod. Fert.* **75**, 375–380.

O'Neill, C. (1987) Embryo derived platelet activating factor: a preimplantation embryo mediator of maternal recognition of pregnancy. *Dom. Anim. Endocr.* **4**, 69–75.

Orozco, C., Perkins, T. & Clarke, F.M. (1986). Platelet-activating factor induces the expression of early pregnancy factor activity in female mice. *J. Reprod. Fert.* **78**, 549–555.

Pratt, B.R., Butcher, R.L. & Inskeep, E.K. (1977) Antiluteolytic effect of the conceptus and of prostaglandin E-2 in ewes. *J. Anim. Sci.* **46**, 784–791.

Ray, D.E., Emmerson, M.A. & Melampy, R.M. (1961) Effect of exogenous progesterone on reproductive activity in the beef heifer. *J. Anim. Sci.* **20**, 373–379.

Raines, E.W. & Ross, R. (1982) Platelet derived growth factor. I. High yield purification and evidence of multiple forms. *J. biol. Chem.* **257**, 5154–5160.

Reynolds, L.P., Robertson, D.A. & Ford, S.P. (1983) Effects of intrauterine infusion of oestradiol-17β and prostaglandin E-2 on luteal function in non-pregnant heifers. *J. Reprod. Fert.* **69**, 703–709.

Shemesh, M., Mileguir, F., Ayalon, N. & Hansel, W. (1979) Steroidogenesis and prostaglandin synthesis by cultured bovine blastocysts. *J. Reprod. Fert.* **56**, 181–185.

Shemesh, M., Hansel, W., Strauss, J., III, Raefaeli, A., Lavi, S. & Mileguir, F. (1984) Control of prostanoid synthesis in bovine trophoblast and placentome. *Anim. Reprod. Sci.* **7**, 177–194.

Silvia, W.J., Ottobre, J.S. & Inskeep, E.K. (1984) Concentrations of prostaglandin E-2, F-2α and 6-keto-prostaglandin F-1α in the utero-ovarian venous plasma of non-pregnant and early pregnant ewes. *Biol. Reprod.* **30**, 936–944.

Smith, R.D., Pomerantz, A.J., Beal, W.E. McCann, J.P., Pilbeam, T.E. & Hansel, W. (1984) Insemination of Holstein heifers at a preset time after estrous cycle synchronization using progesterone and prostaglandin. *J. Anim. Sci.* **58**, 792–800.

Thatcher, W.W., Bartol, F.F., Knickerbocker, J.J., Curl, J.S., Wolfenson, D., Bazer, F.W. & Roberts, S.M. (1984) Maternal recognition of pregnancy in cattle. *J. Dairy Sci.* **67**, 2797–2811.

Thatcher, W.W., Knickerbocker, J.J., Helmer, S.D., Hansen, P.J., Bartol, F.F., Roberts, R.M. & Bazer, F.W. (1985) Characteristics of conceptus secretory proteins and their effect on PGF-2α secretion by maternal endometrium in cattle. In *Early Pregnancy Factors*, pp. 25–28. Eds F. Ellendorff & E. Koch. Perinatology Press, Ithaca.

Wiltbank, J.N., Ingalls, J.E. & Rowden, W.W. (1961) Effects of various forms and levels of estrogens alone or in combinations with gonadotrophins on the estrous cycle of beef heifers. *J. Anim. Sci.* **20**, 341–346.

Wimberly, H.C., Slauson, R.O. & Neilsen, N.R. (1985) Functional and biochemical characterization of immunologically derived equine platelet activating factor. *Vet. Pathol.* **22**, 375–386.

J. Reprod. Fert., Suppl. **37** (1989), 19–27

Embryo-derived platelet-activating factor

C. O'Neill, M. Collier, J. P. Ryan and N. R. Spinks

*Human Reproduction Unit, Royal North Shore Hospital of Sydney, St Leonards,
New South Wales 2065, Australia*

Keywords: PAF; embryo; implantation; PAF antagonist; autocrine control

Introduction

Maternal recognition of pregnancy can be defined as alterations to maternal physiology that are a consequence of the presence of the embryo and which are necessary for the establishment and/or maintenance of pregnancy. Until recently the earliest expression of maternal recognition of pregnancy was thought to be the prolongation of the life-span of the corpus luteum by the presence of the embryo. In some species (e.g. sheep and cow), the rescue of the corpus luteum occurs before the completion of implantation (Basu, 1985) and can therefore be considered to be an example of preimplantation-stage maternal recognition of pregnancy. In others (e.g. man and rodents), the rescue of the corpus luteum occurs some time after implantation and it seems less likely that potential preimplantation embryonic signals in these species would be primarily involved in the rescue of the corpus luteum.

O'Neill (1985c, 1987) has reported that the preimplantation embryo of a number of species produces and secretes the very potent ether phospholipid, 1-0-alkyl-2-acetyl-*sn*-glyceryl-3-phosphocholine (variously known as platelet-activating factor, PAF, PAF-acether, AGEPC) (Fig. 1). This paper reviews the current state of our knowledge on embryo-derived PAF, discusses general aspects of its chemistry and physiology and considers the evidence for PAF acting as a mediator of maternal recognition of pregnancy during the preimplantation phase of pregnancy.

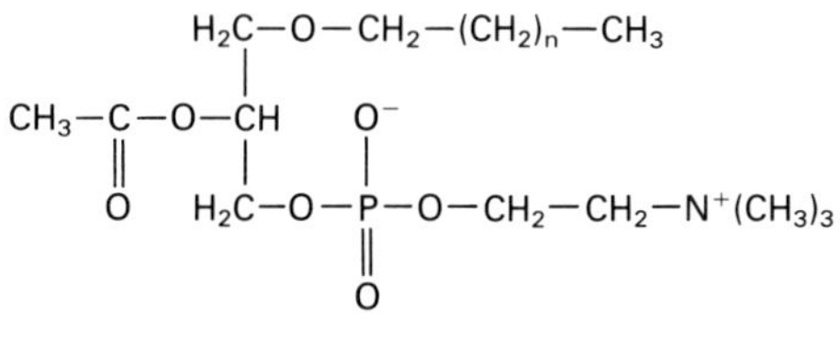

$$H_2C-O-CH_2-(CH_2)_n-CH_3$$
$$CH_3-C-O-CH$$
$$\underset{O}{\overset{\parallel}{}} \quad H_2C-O-\underset{O}{\overset{O^-}{\underset{\parallel}{P}}}-O-CH_2-CH_2-N^+(CH_3)_3$$

Fig. 1. The structure of synthetic PAF. Embryo-derived PAF from the 2-cell human (Collier *et al.*, 1988) and mouse (O'Neill, 1985c) embryo has been shown to be homologous with this structure. In the biologically active molecules examined N = 12 or 14.

PAF as a mediator of maternal recognition of pregnancy

O'Neill (1985a) reported that an initial maternal response to conception in mice was thrombocytopenia which was accompanied by splenic contraction. This was due to platelet consumption but was not caused by intravascular coagulation or activation of the immune system (O'Neill, 1985b). A soluble platelet-activating factor produced by the embryo was reported (O'Neill 1985b) which was homologous with 1-0-alkyl-2-acetyl-*sn*-glyceryl-3-phosphocholine (O'Neill, 1985c; Collier *et al.*, 1988).

The production of PAF by human embryos, derived from in-vitro fertilization, was correlated with their pregnancy potential (O'Neill & Saunders, 1984; O'Neill *et al.*, 1987). A causal relationship was supported by the observation that the platelet-activation inhibitor, iloprost (ZK 36374, a PGI-2 analogue; Schering AG, Berlin, F.R.G.), was able to inhibit implantation in mice, as was a PAF receptor antagonist, SRI 63-441 (Sandoz Research Institute, East Hanover, NJ, U.S.A.) (Spinks & O'Neill, 1987). Further, this inhibition could be reversed by the addition of exogenous PAF (Spinks & O'Neill, 1987).

To determine the action of PAF on embryos, culture was performed *in vitro* in the presence of PAF (Ryan *et al.*, 1987a). PAF induced a dose-dependent enhancement of the utilization of lactate, with 1·0 μg PAF/ml medium causing a 20% increase in the production of CO_2 from lactate. When embryos grown for 72 h in 0·1 or 1·0 μg PAF/ml were transferred to Day-3-pseudopregnant females a significant increase in the implantation rate occurred (Ryan *et al.*, 1987b). PAF therefore appears to be an embryonic autacoid which promotes implantation.

The maternal requirements for PAF are less clear. The PAF antagonist SRI 63-441 did not significantly affect the luteal function of mice throughout the peri-implantation period (Spinks & O'Neill, 1988). Smith & Kelly (1988) showed that PAF enhanced PGE-2 synthesis but had no effect on production of PGF-2α by human endometrial tissue *in vitro* and speculated that this may implicate a role for PAF in the proinflammatory response of implantation. In mice, however, SRI 63-441 had no effect on the decidual reaction induced by intraluminal oil injection (N. R. Spinks & C. O'Neill, unpublished data). Angle *et al.* (1985) have demonstrated that the rabbit endometrium contains significant levels of PAF which decreased around the time of implantation in pregnant but not pseudopregnant does. It is not clear whether this PAF was strictly cell-associated or was also released and what role it may play in pregnancy. It is possible, however, that PAF antagonists could disrupt the activity of this source of PAF as well as embryo-derived PAF.

In mice, there is no clear evidence for a luteotrophic role for PAF. The PAF antagonist SRI 63-441 had no significant effect on progesterone production throughout the luteal phase in mice at doses which caused significant inhibition of implantation (Spinks & O'Neill, 1988). *In vitro*, however, PAF did enhance progesterone production by human granulosa cells in the early luteal phase (O'Neill, 1987). In mice, administration of oestradiol in the peri-implantation phase (Spinks & O'Neill, 1988) did not prevent the contragestational action of PAF antagonists, suggesting that it did not influence the nidatory oestrogen surge necessary for implantation in these animals.

The essential role for PAF may well be more indirect. O'Neill (1986) has shown that blastocyst outgrowth *in vitro* was supported by whole serum but not by serum derived from platelet-depleted plasma. If platelet-derived trophic factors are required for blastocyst outgrowth then the provision of these may occur by localized PAF-induced platelet activation. A further maternal response to the production of PAF is the production of early pregnancy factor (EPF) (Orozco *et al.*, 1986). The role of EPF in pregnancy is not clear. It is claimed to be immunosuppressive (Morton *et al.*, 1976). PAF also has immunosuppressive actions (Braquet *et al.*, 1987); it reduces proliferation of lymphocytes, decreases interleukin-2 production and increases suppressor cell activity. In contrast to this, however, it enhanced responsiveness of lymphocytes to interleukin-2 and increased natural killer activity. Therefore, while PAF and EPF appear to be related, the significance of modulation of the maternal immune response has yet to be clarified. Conceivably, such modulation may perform some immuno-protective function for the embryo, but its importance up until the implantation stage is not clear since morphologically normal blastocysts were collected from the uteri of mice treated with PAF antagonists throughout the preimplantation stage (Spinks & O'Neill, 1988).

The action of PAF in the establishment of pregnancy in mice appears to be at multiple levels. At the embryonic level, it acts as an autacoid (Ryan *et al.*, 1987a, b) whereas its maternal actions on the establishment of pregnancy are less clearly defined. The fact that marmoset and human embryos also produce PAF throughout early pregnancy, and that these species share broadly similar reproductive patterns with mice, suggests that PAF may have similar actions in maternal recognition of pregnancy in these species. The production of PAF in other species, particularly in those in which implantation occurs after the rescue of the corpus luteum, has yet to be studied. The possibility that in such animals embryo-derived PAF has luteotrophic or antiluteolytic actions is currently being investigated.

The evidence for considerable variability in PAF production (O'Neill & Saunders, 1984; O'Neill *et al.*, 1987; Spinks *et al.*, 1986) together with its implication as a mediator of maternal recognition of preg iancy suggests that an understanding of PAF metabolism is essential for further significant progress in the definition and manipulation of the role of PAF in pregnancy.

Biosynthesis of PAF

The biosynthetic pathways of PAF in some cell types are now becoming well defined. A recent review (Snyder, 1987) provides a sound description of the pathways, their control and the enzymes involved. The following is an overview of the current knowledge based on this review and examines the likely potential of the early embryo to produce PAF.

Current evidence indicates that there are two pathways of PAF production (Fig. 2): (1) the conversion of 1-0-alkyl-2-acyl-*sn*-glyceryl-3-phosphocholine to the corresponding lyso-lipid by a deacylation reaction followed by its acetylation to create the active PAF (acetyltransferase pathway), and (2) the alternative pathway involves the transfer of phosphocholine to 1-0-alkyl-2-acetyl-*sn*-glycerol to produce PAF (cholinephosphotransferase pathway). The acetyltransferase pathway appears to require metabolic activation of cells while the cholinephosphotransferease pathway appears active at basal metabolic conditions in a number of cell types.

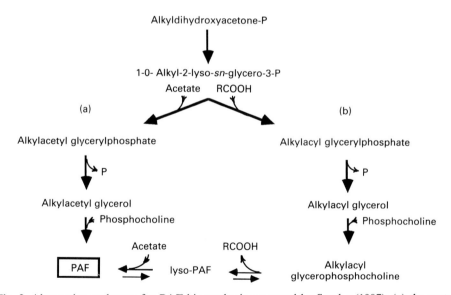

Fig. 2. Alternative pathways for PAF biosynthesis proposed by Snyder (1987): (a) the acetyltransferase pathway and (b) the phosphocholine transferase pathway. RCOOH is long-chain free fatty acids and P is phosphate.

A precursor for both pathways is dihydroxyacetone phosphate, an intermediate of glycolysis. This is then converted to acyldihydroxyacetone phosphate, which also commonly forms the precursors of the esterified phospholipids. For ether phospholipids, including PAF, the acyl chain is replaced by a long-chain fatty alcohol to form alkyldihydroxyacetone phosphate. This is reduced by an NADPH-dependent oxidoreductase to form 1-0-alkyl-2-lyso-*sn*-glyceryl-3-phosphate. This compound marks the bifurcation of the two pathways. The pentose phosphate pathway, which is highly active in early embryo (O'Fallon & Wright, 1986), is also a potential supply of dihydroxy-acetone phosphate, while the NADPH produced is an important co-factor in PAF production.

Acetylation of the second carbon of the glyceryl backbone commits the compound to the phos-phocholinetransferase pathway while acylation leads to the acetyltransferase pathway. PAF is produced via the cholinephosphotransferase pathway by dephosphorylation of 1-0-alkyl-2-acetyl-*sn*-glyceryl-3-phosphate to form 1-0-alkyl-2-acetyl-*sn*-glycerol. This is the substrate of CDP-choline cholinephosphotransferase (EC 2.7.8.16), resulting in the production of PAF. The acetyltransferase pathway is somewhat longer: 1-0-alkyl-2-acyl-*sn*-glyceryl-3-phosphate is also dephosphorylated followed by addition of cholinephosphate. The 1-0-alkyl-2-acyl-*sn*-glyceryl-3-phosphocholine is deacylated by phospholipase A_2 to form 1-0-alkyl-2-lyso-*sn*-glyceryl-3-phosphocholine (lyso-PAF). This is acetylated by an acetyl-CoA-dependent acetyltransferase to give PAF.

In principle, PAF can be produced *de novo* by either of these two pathways. In reality however, it appears that de-novo synthesis primarily occurs via the cholinephosphate pathway (Snyder, 1987). The acetyltransferase pathway generally appears to act via the utilization of the stored precursor 1-0-alkyl-2-acyl-*sn*-glyceryl-3-phosphocholine (Snyder, 1987). PAF is also readily con-verted back to the alkylacyl glycerophosphocholine precursor, providing a futile PAF metabolic cycle (see below).

PAF production by the preimplantation embryo throughout the preimplantation phase appears to be relatively high (Spinks *et al.*, 1986) and, in view of the known phospholipid composition of the mouse embryo (Pratt, 1980), it would seem unlikely that significant reserves of 1-0-alkyl-2-acyl-*sn*-glyceryl-3-phosphocholine precursor would be available to the embryo. In such a case, de-novo synthesis seems most probable. The carbohydrate substrate requirements of most embryo culture media would be sufficient to provide the material for the hydrocarbon components of PAF. Phosphate is a common component of all media, but the available choline may be limiting. The early work of Cholewa & Whitten (1970) suggested that a nitrogen source was not required for preimplantation embryo development and hence most embryo media in common use do not have a defined nitrogen source. Little is known of the endogenous pool size of choline in preimplantation mammalian embryos (Pratt, 1980) but early sea urchin embryos have a significant pool of choline (Pasternak, 1973). If this is also true for mammalian oocytes, choline may well be a source for PAF production. It would seem likely, however, that this pool would be rapidly depleted *in vitro*, result-ing in reduced PAF production. This may well explain the reduced PAF production observed *in vitro* with time (Spinks *et al.*, 1986). A possible pathway for de-novo synthesis of PAF by the early embryo is shown in Fig. 3.

The enzymes involved in the synthesis of PAF appear to be associated with intracellular membranes, most likely the endoplasmic reticulum. PAF may remain associated with the cell or be secreted (Lynch & Henson, 1986). There is considerable variability between cell types as to the fate of newly synthesized PAF. The majority of cells producing PAF appear to retain most of it within the cell, while relatively few cells secrete a significant amount of PAF. Cells secreting PAF include the inflammatory cells, and the preimplantation embryo. The extensive amount of retained, cell-associated PAF in many cells suggests that PAF may play an intracellular as well as extracellular role. For preimplantation embryos, the relative amounts of synthesized PAF secreted compared to that retained is currently not known.

After its production within cells, PAF is transferred to the plasma membrane whence it can be secreted. Extracellular protein is required for retrieval of PAF and albumin appears to serve this role well (Ludwig *et al.*, 1985). The hydrophobic regions of PAF have a high affinity for this protein. In the absence of extracellular protein, PAF secretion is reduced. The secretion of PAF means that this cell activator can potentially exert autocrine, paracrine or endocrine effects. The relative contribution to these physiological processes depends largely on the metabolic fate of PAF.

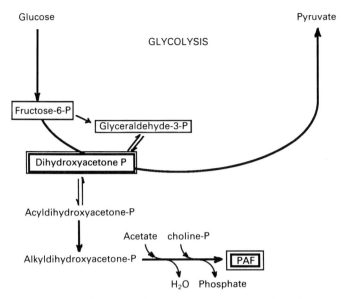

Fig. 3. This represents a possible source of dihydroxyacetone phosphate for use by the embryo in production of alkyldihydroxyacetone-phosphate (principal precursor of PAF production by either pathway). The diversion of dihydroxyacetone-phosphate from glycolysis to PAF production may explain the apparent block to glycolysis in the early embryo.

Catabolism of PAF

The key intermediate of PAF catabolism is 1-0-alkyl-2-lyso-*sn*-glyceryl-3-phosphocholine (lyso-PAF) (Snyder, 1987). The enzyme responsible, acetylhydrolase (Blank *et al.*, 1981) appears to be ubiquitous. It is found intracellularly and in serum and plasma. Cell-associated acetylhydrolase, unlike serum acetylhydrolase, is inhibited by phenylmethylsulphonylfluoride. This enzyme has a high affinity for PAF but not for the alkylacyl derivative. The specificity of the enzyme is demonstrated by its inability to hydrolyse the biologically active PAF analogue 1-0-alkyl-2-*N*-methylcarbamyl-*sn*-glyceryl-3-phosphocholine (O'Flaherty *et al.*, 1987).

In human plasma/serum acetylhydrolase activity is associated with low and very low-density lipoproteins (Osterman *et al.*, 1986; Stafforini *et al.*, 1987). Its activity is positively correlated with the concentration of low-density lipoproteins while being negatively correlated with the concentration of high density lipoproteins. The concentrations of low-density lipoproteins in blood probably therefore influence the half-life and hence concentration of PAF *in situ*. The sex steroids influence lipoprotein profiles and long-term oestrogen treatment is known to cause elevated high-density lipoproteins and reduced low-density lipoproteins levels (Tikkanen & Nikkila, 1987). This might be expected to be correlated with reduced acetylhydrolase activity. The possible influence of the maternal hormonal milieu on PAF catabolism warrants investigation.

The rapid degradation of PAF in the various pools limits its activity and hence its range of action to the immediate locality of its production. An endocrine role for PAF, as might be required for it to have luteotrophic actions, would be dependent on the presentation of PAF in a less labile form. Tissue culture experiments have shown that albumin is very effective in lifting PAF from the plasma membrane and acting as a carrier in the fluid phase (Ludwig *et al.*, 1985). There have been several reports of PAF binding to other serum proteins. PAF binds with high affinity to alpha-1-

acid glycoprotein (McNamara *et al.*, 1986). Another serum protein of molecular weight 16 000–18 000 also binds to PAF (Matsumoto & Miwa, 1985). It has a higher affinity for PAF than does albumin and offers protection from acetylhydrolase activity (Matsumoto & Miwa, 1985). Erythrocytes have been shown to bind a spin-labelled analogue of PAF and thus, by shear weight of numbers, may act as a major receptor (Bette-Bobillo *et al.*, 1986). The relatively slow transmembrane flux of PAF (Lachachi *et al.*, 1985) would result in a slower rate of degradation by intracellular acetylhydrolase compared with that in plasma. The potential of these mechanisms for transport of PAF, which could allow it to fulfil an endocrine role, has yet to be fully investigated.

The lyso-PAF produced by acetylhydrolase is potentially cytotoxic (Hoffman *et al.*, 1984). Rapid further processing of lyso-PAF is required to avoid cell and tissue damage. The most well defined catabolic fate is that of its re-acylation by an acyltransferase to form 1-0-alkyl-2-acyl-*sn*-glyceryl-3-phosphocholine (alkylacyl glycerophosphocholine). In most cells studied to date, the fatty acid used in this esterification step is preferentially but not specifically arachidonic acid (Ramesha & Pickett, 1986; Kumar *et al.*, 1987). The alkylacyl glycerophosphocholine may then be inserted into the membranes or undergo conversion to phosphatidylcholine (Kumar *et al.*, 1987). The stored alkylacyl glycerophosphocholine may then serve as a substrate for the acetyltransferase pathway, thus creating a PAF cycle (Osterman *et al.*, 1986).

Alternative pathways for handling lyso-PAF also exist. Cells of the rabbit renal medulla contain a lysophospholipase D which is capable of converting lyso-PAF to 1-0-alkyl-2-lyso-*sn*-glyceryl-3-phosphate and, contrary to the case of acyltransferase, is Ca^{2+}-dependent (Kawasaki & Snyder, 1987). The liver may also process the material in a different manner since hepatocytes *in vitro* have been shown to contain a lyso-PAF:phospholipase C which converted PAF to 1-0-alkyl-2-lyso-*sn*-glycerol. This was then degraded by an alkyl mono-oxygenase, giving fatty aldehydes (Okayasu *et al.*, 1986).

Catobolism of PAF by the reproductive tract and embryo is an area which remains to be adequately investigated.

Cellular actions

While PAF is an extremely potent activator of blood platelets, it also stimulates a wide variety of other cells (Snyder, 1985; Hanahan, 1986). The ability of cells to respond to PAF appears to be dependent upon the presence of membrane receptors. The presence of a receptor was first demonstrated by the saturatable binding of [^{3}H]PAF to blood platelets (Valone & Ruis, 1986). The plasma membrane binding protein can be extracted from platelets with detergents, it appears to have a molecular weight of around 160 000 and pI 8·0 (Nishihira *et al.*, 1985). It is not yet clear whether receptors on various tissue and cell types differ. There is, however, considerable variation in responses of cells to various PAF receptor antagonists, suggesting that some differences may exist.

The binding of PAF to its receptor is dependent upon monovalent and divalent ions; K^+, Cs^+, Rb^+ Mg^{2+} Ca^{2+}, Mn^{2+} enhance binding, while Na^+ and to a lesser degree Li^+ depress binding by increasing the equilibrium dissociation constant (Hwang *et al.*, 1986).

Guanosine triphosphate (GTP) (10^{-7}–10^{-3} M) depressed PAF binding to neutrophils (Ng & Wong, 1986) and this, together with the observation that PAF enhanced GTP hydrolysis by cells (Avdonin *et al.*, 1985; Haslam *et al.*, 1985), has prompted the suggestion that the receptor is coupled to a guanosine nucleotide-binding protein (G protein) (Ng & Wong, 1986). While PAF has been demonstrated to cause elevated cytoplasmic Ca^{2+} through the polyinositolphosphate pathway (Lapetina, 1982), there remains some discussion as to whether the receptor is coupled primarily to an adenylate cyclase through an inhibitory G protein or to a phosphatidylinositol: phospholipase C. The mechanism of signal transduction may well vary between different tissue types.

Physiology and pathology

In general the physiological and pathological responses are governed by: (1) the site of production and concentration of PAF; (2) the rate of PAF degradation and hence its half-life; (3) the presence of endogenous inhibitors (Nakayama *et al.*, 1987); (4) the types and numbers of cells in the vicinity with PAF receptors; and (5) the programmed genetic response of these cells, including their further modulation by autocrine, paracrine and endocrine interactions with other cells. These factors can lead to generalized systemic responses or very specific localized reactions. Thus, PAF can play a central role in mediating a vast range of pathological and physiological responses. It activates a variety of inflammatory cells including platelets and polymorphonuclear leucocytes (Halohen *et al.*, 1985; Braquet & Róla-Pleszazynski, 1987). It is also a potent vasodilator and enhances vaso-permeability by platelet-dependent and -independent mechanisms. Thus PAF is a potent mediator of localized inflammation. In contrast to these actions, PAF has been shown (Braquet & Róla-Pleszazynski, 1987) to elicit immunosuppressive actions by suppressing interleukin-2 production and causes constriction of the coronary artery, resulting in reduced cardiac performance (Montrucchio *et al.*, 1986). Its renal effects are to reduce blood flow and glomerular filtration, resulting in reduced fluid and electrolyte excretion (Schlondorff & Neuwirth, 1986). PAF mediates prolonged non-specific increase in bronchial hyperreactivity (Page, 1987). These adverse affects of PAF mean that, at sufficient doses, PAF is a very potent mediator of shock. PAF antagonists have been shown to be effective in reducing the symptoms of septic/endotoxic and anaphylactic shock. There has been extensive study of these pathological and physiological actions of PAF, with the hope that the recent development of PAF antagonists may prove to be of therapeutic benefit. PAF antagonists could therefore be used in treatment of endotoxic and anaphylactic shock, in asthma and may have a role in the control of hypertension and immunosuppression. The observation that PAF antagonists could inhibit implantation in rodents (Spinks & O'Neill, 1987, 1988) suggests a potential contraindication for their use in early pregnancy.

Conclusions

In rodents, at least, embryo-derived PAF clearly fulfils the requirements of a mediator of pre-implantation maternal recognition of pregnancy. Its production causes significant alterations to maternal physiology and is necessary for the establishment of pregnancy. It appears to exert its effects primarily by supporting implantation, although it has a variety of other actions. Whether a single action or the cumulative effect of all its actions is essential for the support of pregnancy is yet to be defined. The fact that PAF is also produced by the human and marmoset monkey embryos suggests that it is also likely to be a mediator of maternal recognition of pregnancy in these species.

We thank D. Gillespie for typing the manuscript; M. Beuk for assistance in its preparation; and K. Battye for discussion. Some of the studies described herein were supported by the Australian NH and MRC.

References

Angle, M.Y., Jones, M.A., Pinckard, R.N., McManus, L.M. & Harper, M.J.K. (1985) Platelet activating factor in the rabbit uterus during early pregnancy. *Biol. Reprod.* **32**, (Suppl. 1), 212, Abstr.

Avdonin, P.V., Svitina-Ulitina, I.V. & Kulikov, V.I. (1985) Stimulation of high-affinity hormone sensitive GTPase of human platelets by 1-0-alkyl-2-acetyl-sn-glyceryl-3-phosphocholine. *Biochem. Biophys. Res. Commun.* **731**, 307–313.

Basu, S. (1985) Maternal recognition of pregnancy. A review of the literature. *Nord. VetMed.* **37**, 57–79.

Bette-Bobillo, P., Luxembourg, A. & Bienvenue, A. (1986) Interaction between blood components and a spin-labelled analogue of PAF-acether. *Biochim. Biophys. Acta* **860,** 194–200.

Blank, M.L., Lee, T., Fitzgerald, V. & Snyder, F. (1981) A specific acetylhydrolase for 1-alkyl-2-acetyl-sn-gylcero-3-phosphocholine (a hypotensive and platelet activating lipid). *J. biol. Chem.* **256,** 175–178.

Braquet, P. & Rola-Pleszazynski, M. (1987) Platelet activating factor and cellular immune responses. *Immunology Today* **8,** 345–352.

Cholewa, J.A. & Whitten, W.K. (1970) Development of two-cell mouse embryos in the absence of a fixed nitrogen source. *J. Reprod. Fert.* **22,** 553–555.

Collier, M., O'Neill, C., Ammit, A.J. & Saunders, D.M. (1988) Biochemical and pharmacological characterisation of human embryo-derived platelet-activating factor. *Human Reproduction* (in press).

Halohen, M., Lohman, I.C., Dunn, A.M., McManus, L.M. & Palmer, J.D. (1985) Participation of platelets in physiological alterations of the AGEPC response and of IGE anaphylaxis in the rabbit. Effects of PGI$_2$ inhibition of platelet function. *Am. Rev. Respir. Dis.* **131,** 11–17.

Hanahan, D.J. (1986) Platelet activating factor: a biologically active phosphoglyceride. *Ann. Rev. Biochem.* **55,** 483–509.

Haslam, R.J., Williams, K.A. & Davidson, M.M. (1985) Receptor-effector coupling in platelets: roles of guanine nucleotides. *Adv. exp. Med. Biol.* **192,** 265–280.

Hoffman, D.R., Hajdu, J. & Snyder, F. (1984) Cytotoxicity of platelet activating factor and related alkyl-phospholipid analogs in human leukemia cells, polymorphonuclear neutrophils, and skin fibroblasts. *Blood* **63,** 545–552.

Hwang, S.B., Lam, M.H. & Pong, S.S. (1986) Ionic and GTP regulation of binding of platelet-activating factor to receptors and platelet-activating factor induced activation of GTPase in rabbit platelet membranes. *J. biol. Chem.* **261,** 532–537.

Kawasaki, T. & Snyder, F. (1987) The metabolism of lyso-platelet (1-0-alkyl-2-lyso-sn-glycero-3-phosphocholine) by a calcium-dependent lysophospholipase D in rabbit medulla. *Biochim. Biophys. Acta* **920,** 85–93.

Kumar, R., King, R.J., Martin, H.M. & Hanahan, D.J. (1987) Metabolism of platelet activating factor by type-II epithelial cells and fibroblasts from rat lung. *Biochim. Biophys. Acta* **917,** 33–41.

Lachachi, H., Plantavid, M., Simon, M.F., Chap, H., Braquet, P. & Douste-Blazy, L. (1985) Inhibition of transmembrane movement and metabolism of platelet activating factor (PAF-acether) by a specific antagonist, BN 52021. *Biochim. Biophys. Res. Commun.* **132,** 460–466.

Lapetina, E.G. (1982) Platelet-activating factor stimulates the phosphatidylinositol cycle. *J. biol. Chem.* **257,** 7314–7317.

Ludwig, J.C., Hoppens, C.L., McManus, L.M., Mott, G.E. & Pinckard, R.N. (1985) Modulation of platelet activating factor synthesis and release from human polymorphonuclear leukocytes (PMN)—role of extra cellular albumin. *Archs Biochem. Biophys.* **241,** 337–347.

Lynch, J.M. & Henson, P.M. (1986) The intracellular retention of newly synthesized platelet activating factor. *J. Immunol.* **137,** 2653–2661.

Matsumoto, M. & Miwa, M. (1985) Platelet activating factor-binding protein in human serum. *Adv. Prost. Thromb. Leuk. Res.* **15,** 705–706.

McNamara, P.H., Brouwer, K.R. & Gillespie, M.N. (1986) Autacoid binding to serum proteins. Interactions of platelet activating factor (PAF) with human serum alpha-1-acid-glycoprotein. *Biochem. Pharmacol.* **35,** 621–624.

Montrucchio, G., Alloatti, G., Mariano, F., Tetta, C., Emannelli, G. & Camussi, G. (1986) Cardiovascular alteration in the rabbit infused with platelet activating factor (PAF): effect of kadsurenone, a PAF receptor antagonist. *Int. J. Tissue React.* **8,** 497–504.

Morton, H., Hegh, V. & Clunie, G.J.A. (1976) Studies of the rosette inhibition test in pregnant mice: evidence of immunosuppression. *Proc. R. Soc. B.* **193,** 413–419.

Nakayama, R., Yasuda, K. & Saito, K. (1987). Existence of endogenous inhibitors of platelet activating factor (PAF) in rat uterus. *J. biol. Chem.* **262,** 13174–13179.

Ng, D.S. & Wong, K. (1986) GTP regulation of platelet activating factor binding to human neutrophil membranes. *Biochem. Biophys. Res. Commun.* **141,** 353–359.

Nishihira, J., Ishibashi, T., Imai, Y. & Muramatsu, T. (1985) Purification and characterization of the specific binding protein for platelet activating factor (1-0-alkyl-2-acetyl-sn-glycero-3-phosphocholine) from human platelets. *Tohuku J. exp. Med.* **147,** 145–152.

O'Fallon, J.V. & Wright, R., Jr (1986) Quantitative determination of the pentose phosphate pathway in preimplantation mouse embryos. *Biol. Reprod.* **34,** 58–64.

O'Flaherty, J.T., Redman, J.F., Jr, Schmitt, J.D., Ellis, J.M., Surles, J.R., Marx, M.H., Piantadosi, C. & Wykle, R.L. (1987) 1-0-alkyl-2-N-methylcarbanyl-glycerophosphocholine: a biologically, potent, non-metabolizable analog of platelet activating factor. *Biochem. Biophys. Res. Commun.* **147,** 18–24.

Okayasu, T., Hoshii, K., Seyama, K., Ishibashi, T. & Imai, Y. (1986) Metabolism of platelet activating factor in primary cultured adult rat hepatocytes by a new pathway involving phospholipase C and alkyl mono-oxygenase. *Biochim. Biophys. Acta* **876,** 58–64.

O'Neill, C. (1985a) Thrombocytopenia is an initial maternal response to fertilization in mice. *J. Reprod. Fert.* **73,** 567–577.

O'Neill, C. (1985b) Examination of the causes of early pregnancy associated thrombocytopenia in mice. *J. Reprod. Fert.* **73,** 578–585.

O'Neill, C. (1985c) Partial characterization of the embryo-derived platelet-activating factor in mice. *J. Reprod. Fert.* **75,** 375–380.

O'Neill, C. (1986) The role of blood platelets in the establishment of pregnancy. In *Pregnancy Proteins in Animals*, pp. 261–266. Ed. J. Hau. Walter de Gruyter, Berlin.

O'Neill, C. (1987) Embryo-derived platelet-activating factor: a pre-implantation embryo mediator of maternal recognition of pregnancy. *Dom. Anim. Endocrinol.* **4,** 69–86.

O'Neill, C. & Saunders, D.M. (1984) Assessment of embryo quality. *Lancet* ii, 1035.

O'Neill, C., Gidley-Baird, A.A., Pike, I.L. & Saunders, D.M. (1987) A bio-assay for embryo-derived platelet-activating factor as a means of assessing quality and pregnancy potential of human embryos. *Fert. Steril.* 47, 969–975.

Orozco, C., Perkins, F. & Clarke, F.M. (1986) Platelet activating factor induces the expression of early pregnancy factor activity in female mice. *J. Reprod. Fert.* 78, 549–555.

Osterman, G., Kertscher, H.P., Winkler, L., Schlag, B., Rushling, K. & Till, U.C. (1986) The role of lipoproteins in the degradation of platelet activating factor. *Throm. Res.* 44, 503–514.

Page, C.P. (1987) A role for platelet activating factor and platelets in the induction of bronchial hyperreactivity. *Int. J. Tissue. React.* 9, 27–32.

Pasternak, C.A. (1973) Phospholipid synthesis in cleaving sea urchin eggs. Model for specific membrane assembly. *Devl Biol.* 30, 403–410.

Pratt, H.P.M. (1980) Phospholipid synthesis in the preimplantation mouse embryo. *J. Reprod. Fert.* 58, 237–248.

Ramesha, C.S. & Pickett, W.C. (1986) Metabolism of platelet-activating factor by arachidonic acid-depleted rat polymorphonuclear leukocytes. *J. biol. Chem.* 261, 519–523.

Ryan, J.P., Wiegand, M.H., O'Neill, C. & Wales, R.G. (1987a) In vitro development and metabolism of lactate by mouse embryos in the presence of platelet activating factor (PAF). *Proc. Aust. Soc. Reprod. Biol.* 19, 47, Abstr.

Ryan, J.P., Spinks, N.R., O'Neill, C., Saunders, D.M. & Wales, R.G. (1987b) Enhanced rates of implantation and increased metabolism of mouse embryos cultured in the presence of platelet activating factor. *Proc. Fertil. Soc. Aust.* 6, 47, Abstr.

Schlondorff, D. & Neuwirth, R. (1986) Platelet-activating factor and the kidney. *Am. J. Physiol.* 211, F1–11.

Smith, S.K. & Kelly, R.W. (1988) Effect of platelet-activating factor on the release of PGF-2α and PGE-2 by separated cells of human endometrium. *J. Reprod. Fert.* 82, 271–276.

Snyder, F. (1985) Chemical and biochemical aspects of platelet activating factor: A novel class of acetylated ether linked choline phospholipids. *Med. Res. Rev.* 5, 107–140.

Snyder, F. (1987) The significance of dual pathways for the biosynthesis of platelet activating factor: 1-alkyl-2-lyso-sn-glycero-3-phosphate as a branch point. In *New Horizons in Platelet Activating Factor Research*, pp. 13–26. Eds C. M. Winslow & M. Lee. John Wiley and Sons, Chichester.

Spinks, N.R. & O'Neill, C. (1987) Embryo-derived platelet-activating factor is essential for establishment of pregnancy in the mouse. *Lancet* i, 106–107.

Spinks, N. & O'Neill, C. (1988) Antagonists of embryo-derived platelet-activating factor prevent implantation of mouse embryos. *J. Reprod. Fert.* 84, 89–98.

Spinks, N.R., Ammit, A.J., Saunders, D.M. & O'Neill, C. (1986) Embryo-derived platelet-activating factor (PAF): Kinetics of its production in vitro. *Proc. Aust. Soc. Reprod. Biol.* 18, 1, Abstr.

Stafforini, D.M., McIntyre, T.M., Carter, M.E. & Prescott, S.M. (1987). Human plasma activating factor acetylhydrolase. Association with lipoprotein particles and role in the degradation of platelet-activating factor. *J. biol. Chem.* 262, 4215–4222.

Tikkanen, M.J. & Nikkila, E.A. (1987) Regulation of hepatic lipase and serum lipoproteins by sex steroids. *Am. Heart. J.* 113, 562–567.

Valone, F.H. & Ruis, N.M. (1986) Platelet-activating factor binding to human platelet membranes. *Biotechnol. appl. Biochem.* 8, 465–470.

J. Reprod. Fert., Suppl. 37 (1989), 29–35

Printed in Great Britain
© 1989 Journals of Reproduction & Fertility Ltd

Identification of a luteotrophic protein in bovine allantoic fluid

G. J. Hickey*†, J. S. Walton‡ and W. Hansel†

†*Department of Physiology, New York State College of Veterinary Medicine, Cornell University, Ithaca, New York 14853, U.S.A.; and* ‡*Department of Animal and Poultry Science, University of Guelph, Guelph, Ontario, Canada N1G 2W1*

Summary. Allantoic fluids ($n = 65$) of Day 24–37 bovine conceptuses were collected and assayed for luteotrophic activity *in vitro* with dispersed bovine luteal cells. Significant luteotrophic activity was found in 41% of the samples, with the highest percentage occurring between Days 25 and 28. The activity is ammonium sulphate-precipitable, heat-labile and inactivated by trypsin and chymotrypsin. Gel filtration column chromatography identified one peak of luteotrophic activity with a molecular weight of 68 000. Concanavalin A bound the luteotrophic activity, thus allowing rapid and substantial purification from a major protein of M_r 68 000 which was concanavalin A non-reactive. The results of one- and two-dimensional SDS–PAGE of concanavalin A-reactive fractions containing activity suggest that the luteotrophic activity present in allantoic fluid is associated with a glycoprotein of M_r 68 000 present in very low concentrations. The active factor does not appear to be α-fetoprotein. This protein may be an important conceptus-derived luteotrophin that stimulates progesterone production by the corpus luteum of cows during pregnancy.

Keywords: pregnancy; luteotrophin; corpus luteum; allantoic fluid; cow

Introduction

In the study of maternal recognition of pregnancy much attention has been given to identifying conceptus-derived luteotrophic and antiluteolytic factors during the peri-implantation period and first missed oestrus. In the ruminant, since implantation does not occur before the period of first missed oestrus (King *et al.*, 1980), harvested media of conceptus tissue cultures and conceptus homogenates have been examined *in vitro* and *in vivo* for their ability to regulate luteal steroidogenesis. In the cow, both luteotrophic (Beal *et al.*, 1981; Hickey & Hansel, 1987) and antiluteolytic (Knickerbocker *et al.*, 1986) factors have been identified and partly characterized. The putative luteotrophic factor(s) has a molecular weight of <12 000 and is lipid soluble, characteristics that would facilitate uptake by the endometrium and transport to the ovary. The antiluteolytic factor(s) identified in conceptus tissue culture is proteinaceous and appears to block normal luteolysis by inhibiting prostaglandin synthesis by the endometrium. A chorionic gonadotrophin-like (CG-like) protein was identified in homogenates of bovine placentomes during the first third of pregnancy by Ailenberg & Shemesh (1983). Since chorionic gonadotrophins identified in primates and equids are synthesized by fetal trophoblast cells after these cells have implanted into the maternal endometrium (Allen & Moor, 1982; Hoshina *et al.*, 1985), a bovine chorionic gonadotrophin, if synthesized, could be expected at the 4th week of pregnancy, the period of implantation.

---

*Present address: Department of Cell Biology, Baylor College of Medicine, 1 Baylor Plaza, Houston, TX 77030, U.S.A.

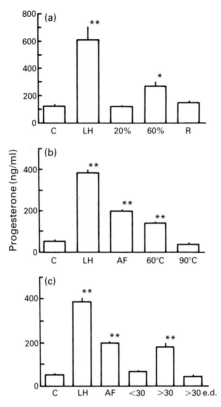

Fig. 1. Net progesterone synthesis during 2 h by bovine luteal cells (10^6) in response to: (a) Medium 199 (C), 5 ng LH (LH), ammonium sulphate precipitates of allantoic fluid (20%, 60%), or the residual fraction of allantoic fluid (R); (b) Medium 199 (C), 5 ng LH (LH) and allantoic fluid before (AF) and after heating at 60°C for 30 min (60°C) or 90°C for 30 min (90°C); and (c) Medium 199 (C), 5 ng LH (LH), allantoic fluid (AF), M_r < 30 000 fraction (< 30) or M_r > 30 000 fraction before (> 30) or after enzymic digestion (> 30 e.d.) with trypsin and chymotrypsin. Values are mean ± s.e. for $n = 4$ (a), 2 (b) and 2 (c). *$P < 0.05$; **$P < 0.01$.

We report in this paper on a luteotrophic glycoprotein present in fetal allantoic fluid of cattle between Days 24 and 37 of gestation. It is during this period that the vascularized allantoic sac fuses with the avascular chorionic membrane to form the fetal chorio-allantoic membrane, the fetal component of the bovine placenta (Perry, 1981).

Luteotrophic activity of allantoic fluid

Sixty-five cross-breed beef cows were slaughtered between 24 and 37 days after insemination. The reproductive tracts were isolated and opened along the antimesometrial border, and fetal allantoic fluids were collected by aspiration. The harvested fluids were stored at −20°C.

Luteotrophic activity of whole or fractionated allantoic fluid was determined by their ability to stimulate progesterone synthesis by dispersed bovine luteal cells incubated for 2 h in tissue culture Medium 199 (Hickey & Hansel, 1987). Net progesterone synthesis for each treatment was determined by subtracting initial progesterone concentration at time zero from the final progesterone concentration at 2 h. For control luteal stimulation, luteal cells were incubated (i) in Medium 199

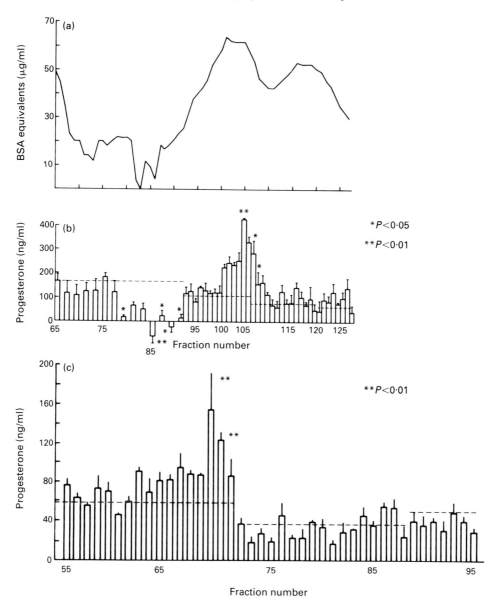

Fig. 2. Net progesterone synthesis during 2 h by bovine luteal cells (10⁶) in response to Medium 199 (broken line) or allantoic fluid after fractionation through: (b) a Sephacryl S-300 column (void volume: fractions 1–64) (protein concentration of the eluate is shown in (a)) and (c) a Sephadex G-100 column (void volume: fractions 1–54). Values are mean ± s.e. for $n = 2$ (b, c).

alone or (ii) in the presence of 5 ng luteinizing hormone (LH). The progesterone concentration of allantoic fluid was ∼70–267 pg/ml. The allantoic fluid volume added in each biassay was 100 μl, and so its contribution to the total progesterone content was negligible.

Of the 65 allantoic fluid samples tested, 28 (41%) had significant luteotrophic activity compared with the control ($P < 0.05$). Of the 31 allantoic fluid samples collected before or on Day 28, 20 contained significant activity compared to 8 of 34 samples harvested between Days 29 and 37.

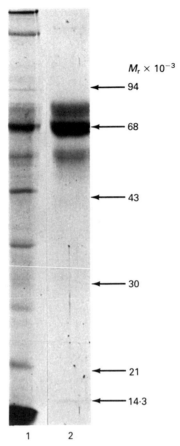

$M_r \times 10^{-3}$

94

68

43

30

21

14·3

1   2

Fig. 3. Analytical SDS–PAGE of allantoic fluid of cows. Lane 1: allantoic fluid; Lane 2: fractions 100–106 collected from the Sephacryl S-300 column after addition of allantoic fluid.

Characterization of luteotrophic activity of allantoic fluid

Preliminary characterization indicated that the luteotrophic factor(s) present in allantoic fluid was proteinacous since activity was ammonium sulphate precipitable and inactivated by trypsin and chymotrypsin digestion (Fig. 1). The luteotrophic activity also appeared to be heat labile (Fig. 1). Gel filtration chromatography of allantoic fluid by Sephacryl S-300 (Fig. 2a) or Sephadex G-100 (Fig. 2b) identified only one peak of luteotrophic activity in the eluate. The activity corresponded to a protein of M_r 68 000 as determined from column calibration. One-dimensional sodium dodecyl sulphate–polyacrylamide gel electrophoresis of the pooled active fractions of the Sephacryl S-300 column identified three major protein bands of M_r 55 000–75 000 (Fig. 3). No qualitative differences in protein content of these major proteins were seen between allantoic fluid samples of high and low luteotrophic activity.

Alpha-fetoprotein (M_r ~72 000) was identified in the fetal allantoic fluid by Ouchterlony double-immunodiffusion assay of allantoic fluid against rabbit anti-bovine α-fetoprotein antiserum, as reported by Janzen *et al.* (1982). Purified bovine α-fetoprotein was assayed for luteotrophic activity *in vitro* over a concentration of 1 ng to 1 μg and did not increase progesterone concentrations above control.

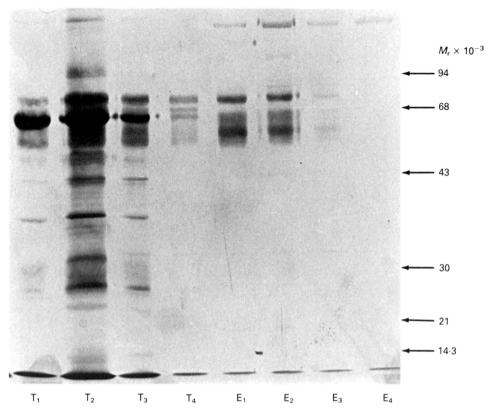

$M_r \times 10^{-3}$

$\longleftarrow$ 94

$\longleftarrow$ 68

$\longleftarrow$ 43

$\longleftarrow$ 30

$\longleftarrow$ 21

$\longleftarrow$ 14·3

T₁   T₂   T₃   T₄   E₁   E₂   E₃   E₄

Fig. 4. Analytical SDS–PAGE of allantoic fluid of cows after separation into Con-A non-reactive (lanes T_1–T_4) and Con A-reactive (lanes E_1–E_4) fractions.

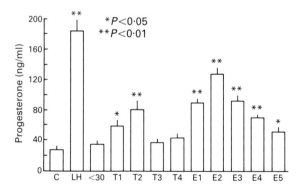

Fig. 5. Net progesterone synthesis during 2 h by bovine luteal cells (10^6) in response to Dulbecco's PBS + 0·5 M-NaCl (C), Dulbecco's PBS + 0·5 M-NaCl + 5 ng LH (LH), an M_r < 30 000 fraction (< 30), and an M_r > 30 000 fraction of allantoic fluid after fractionation into Con-A non-reactive (T_1–T_4) and Con A-reactive fractions (E_1–E_5). Values are mean ± s.e. for $n = 5$.

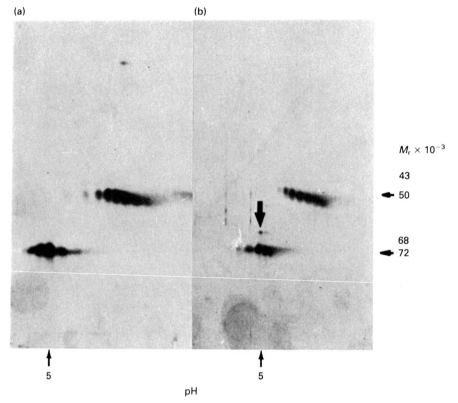

Fig. 6. Analytical two-dimensional SDS–PAGE of the Con A-reactive fractions of allantoic fluid with low (a) or high (b) luteotrophic activity. The protein with M_r 68 000 and pI $\sim 5 \cdot 0$ that is present only in allantoic fluid containing high luteotrophic activity is indicated by the arrow.

A Concanavalin A (Con A) chromatographic affinity column was used to isolate the glyco-proteins of allantoic fluid that were Con-A reactive. After collection of the non-reactive proteins which passed through the affinity column, the Con A-reactive proteins were eluted with α-manno-side. One-dimensional SDS–PAGE of both fractions showed that the major allantoic fluid protein of M_r 68 000 was not reactive to Con A, but the proteins of M_r 55 000 and 72 000 were both Con-A reactive (Fig. 4). Significant luteotrophic activity ($P < 0 \cdot 01$) was partitioned predominantly in the Con A-reactive fractions (Fig. 5). Protein determinations of both fractions showed that $< 1 \cdot 0\%$ of the allantoic fluid protein content was Con-A reactive.

Two-dimensional SDS–PAGE was carried out on Con A-reactive fractions of allantoic fluid that contained either significant or no luteotrophic activity before and after fractionation. In both samples, the proteins of M_r 55 000 and 72 000 were clearly detectable. However, a low abundance protein of M_r 68 000 with an isoelectric point of $\sim 5 \cdot 0$ was present in the Con A-reactive fraction containing high luteotrophic activity but undetectable in the Con A-reactive fraction with no luteotrophic activity (Fig. 6). Both gels were loaded with the same protein concentration.

We are now trying to purify the low abundance glycoprotein of M_r 68 000 and to make mono-clonal antibody against this putative luteotrophin. This should allow a rapid one-step isolation from whole allantoic fluid by affinity chromatography. The purified protein will then be assayed for luteotrophic activity both *in vitro* and *in vivo*. The monoclonal antibodies and, at a later stage, polyclonal antibodies will be used to screen a bovine cDNA expression library made from placental membranes of cows in the first third of pregnancy. The positive cDNA clones isolated, together with the specific antibodies, will allow us to study the expression and regulation of this putative luteotrophin.

Discussion

We have identified and characterized a luteotrophic glycoprotein of M_r 68 000 in allantoic fluids of Day 24–37 bovine conceptuses. The glycoprotein is present in small amount, and at a higher frequency in those samples harvested up to and including Day 28 than from Days 29–37. The luteotrophic protein is similar in approximate molecular size and functional activity to the 'CG'-like protein described by Ailenberg & Shemesh (1983). A bovine pregnancy-specific, Con A-reactive glycoprotein of M_r 70 000 has been reported by Klima *et al.* (1987). It remains to be determined whether either or both of these proteins is or are the same as that described in these studies.

The functional role of luteotrophic glycoproteins in allantoic fluid, if any, is unknown. However, the presence of a luteotrophin is not remarkable if one considers the synthesis of the known chorionic gonadotrophins, the dynamics of chorio-allantoic membrane formation and implantation, along with the earlier report of a 'CG'-like protein identified in bovine placentomes in early pregnancy (Ailenberg & Shemesh, 1983). The CG proteins of the horse and primate are synthesized by the fetal trophoblast cells after they have implanted into the maternal endometrium. If the fetal trophoblast cells of the chorion of the cow synthesize such a protein, then fusion of allantoic and chorionic membranes in the 4th week of pregnancy would facilitate its diffusion into the adjacent allantoic fluid. The decreasing frequency of luteotrophic activity in allantoic fluid seen with increasing gestational age may be due to dilution with the expanding allantoic fluid volume, along with a more complete attachment between fetal and maternal placental units allowing more rapid transfer of macromolecules. Final and definitive evidence concerning the functional role and transfer of this protein to the allantoic fluid and to the corpus luteum must await its purification.

References

Ailenberg, M. & Shemesh, M. (1983) Partial purification of a chorionic gonadotropin-like protein from bovine cotyledons. *Biol. Reprod.* **28**, 517–522.

Allen, W.R. & Moor, R.M. (1972) The origin of the equine endometrial cups 1. Production of PMSG by fetal trophoblast cells. *J. Reprod. Fert.* **29**, 313–316.

Beal, W.E., Lukaszewska, J.H. & Hansel, W. (1981) Luteotropic effects of bovine blastocysts. *J. Anim. Sci.* **52**, 567–574.

Hickey, G.J. & Hansel, W. (1987) *In vitro* synthesis of a low molecular weight lipid-soluble luteotrophic factor by conceptuses of cows at Day 13–18 of pregnancy. *J. Reprod. Fert.* **80**, 569–576.

Hoshina, M., Boothby, M., Hussa, R., Pattillo, R., Camel, H.M. & Boime, I. (1985) Linkage of human chorionic gonadotrophin and placental lactogen biosynthesis to trophoblast differentiation and tumorigenesis. *Placenta* **6**, 163–172.

Janzen, R.G., Malby, E.R., Tamaoki, T., Church, R.B. &

Lorscheider, F.L. (1982) Synthesis of alpha-fetoprotein by the pre-implantation and post-implantation bovine embryo. *J. Reprod. Fert.* **65**, 105–110.

King, G.J., Atkinson, B.A. & Robertson, H.A. (1980) Development of the bovine placentome from Days 20 to 29 of gestation. *J. Reprod. Fert.* **59**, 95–100.

Klima, F., Tiemann, U., Pitra, C. & Kauffold, P. (1987) Serological detection of early pregnancy in cattle and partial characterization of a serum glycoprotein associated with early pregnancy. *J. Reprod. Immunol.* **11**, 31–39.

Knickerbocker, J.J., Thatcher, W.W., Bazer, F.W., Barron, D.H. & Roberts, R.M. (1986) Inhibition of uterine prostaglandin-F2α production by bovine conceptus secretory proteins. *Prostaglandins* **31**, 777–793.

Perry, J.S. (1981) The mammalian fetal membranes. *J. Reprod. Fert.* **62**, 321–335.

J. Reprod. Fert., Suppl. **37** (1989), 37–44

Partial purification of a luteotrophic substance from bovine fetal cotyledon granules

M. Izhar and M. Shemesh

Department of Hormone Research, Kimron Veterinary Institute, Bet Dagan, P.O.B. 12, Israel 50200

Summary. To determine whether luteotrophic activity is present in the bovine placental granules, fetal cotyledons from fetuses of 50–100 days of gestation were used. Enriched granules were prepared using a Percoll gradient. Active substances were obtained from the granules by freeze–thawing. The extracts thus obtained were then eluted on a Sephacryl S-300 column. The resultant fractions were then analysed by (1) a radio-receptor assay for hCG-like substances and (2) a bioassay using progesterone production by bovine luteal cells. There were two peaks of activity, one indicative of a high molecular weight substance and the second of a low molecular weight substance. Higher molecular weight substances were eliminated by using acidic extracts. The low molecular weight fraction was further analysed using reverse phase h.p.l.c. (acetonitrile:water gradient). The elution of this substance at 45% acetonitrile resulted in a 100-fold increase in luteotrophic activity in the bioassay compared to the Sephacryl fraction. The small molecular weight substance is heat-stable and not extracted to the organic phase when partitioned between methanol and chloroform.

Keywords: cattle; luteotrophin; progesterone; cotyledon; placenta

Introduction

Chorionic gonadotrophins are glycoprotein hormones synthesized by the chorionic cells. In humans and other primates during early pregnancy stages chorionic gonadotrophins convey a signal from the placenta to the corpus luteum. This signal results in maintenance of the corpus luteum and progesterone production. This action of placental gonadotrophins is mediated by specific receptors located on the corpus luteum cell surface (Bahl, 1977). Luteal progesterone synthesis is essential for normal development of the fetus during the first third of gestation in most domestic species. Corpus luteum removal in the first third of pregnancy in cattle causes miscarriage which is prevented by progesterone administration (Deanesly, 1966).

Chorionic gonadotrophins have been characterized for man (Saxena *et al.*, 1974), other primates (Hodgen *et al.*, 1974), the mare (Cole & Goss, 1943) and partly purified for cows (Ailenberg & Shemesh, 1983; Hickey & Hansel, 1987). Lunnen & Foote (1967) extracted a substance exhibiting LH-like activity from bovine cotyledons and maternal plasma. Ailenberg & Shemesh (1983) reported the presence of chorionic gonadotrophin-like activity in bovine cotyledons from 50–100 day-old fetuses. This protein, having a molecular weight of ~60 000, significantly increased progesterone and testosterone production by granulosa and Leydig cells in culture, respectively. Hickey *et al.* (1985) extracted a substance with LH-like luteotrophic activity from allantoic fluids of Day 25–37 bovine conceptuses. The substance was found to be a protein of M_r 50 000–70 000.

Bovine trophoblastic protein 1 (bTP-1) is a polypeptide of M_r 22 000–24 000 which prolongs the life-span of the corpora lutea (Thatcher *et al.*, 1985a, b). The administration of bTP-1 has not been shown to lead to luteotrophic activity on the corpus luteum, as indicated by progesterone production (Bazer *et al.*, 1985).

Gadsby & Lancaster (1987) studied a small molecular weight luteotrophic substance, produced by rabbit fetal placenta, which is required to maintain the high progesterone concentration necessary during the second half of pregnancy.

The importance of such substances found in many species, and known to maintain pregnancy, stimulated the present research. Since the bovine chorionic gonadotrophin has been only partly characterized, we conducted further studies to identify and purify such a substance.

Materials and Methods

Animals

Multiparous Holstein–Friesian cows were obtained at a slaughter house. Fetuses at 50–100 days of gestation were collected with their uteri within 20 min of slaughter and placed on ice. Corpora lutea of non-pregnant cows at mid-cycle were collected and placed immediately in Eagle's Minimal Essential Medium (MEM) at 4°C.

Cytosolic preparation

Fetal cotyledons were homogenized in Tris–HCl buffer (50 mM; pH 7·4) and centrifuged at 10 000 g for 10 min. The supernatant was centrifuged at 100 000 g for 60 min and the cytosolic fraction was stored at -20°C.

Granule preparation

Granules were prepared according to Byatt *et al.* (1986) with slight modifications. Briefly, fetal cotyledons were removed from the chorion, the tissue was minced with scissors and granules were released by stirring vigorously for 2 h at 22°C in MEM (1:1; v/v). The material was filtered through two layers of gauze and centrifuged at 350 g for 5 min. The supernatant was further centrifuged at 4800 g for 15 min. The pellet was resuspended in a small volume of MEM and loaded on a discontinuous Percoll gradient (1·03, 1·04, 1·06, 1·06 g/ml). After 15 min centrifugation at 4800 g, the density layer of 1·04 g/ml, which contained the granules, was collected.

Total extract. The granules were lysed by freezing and thawing and membranes were pelleted by centrifugation (100 000 g, 30 min at 4°C). The supernatant was collected and lyophilized.

Acidic extract. Granules were heated to 97°C for 5 min in 2 N-acetic acid immediately after collecting from the Percoll gradient. The granule lysate was centrifuged at 100 000 g for 30 min at 4°C and the supernatant was lyophilized.

Gel filtration

Total granule extracts were fractionated on a Sephacryl S-300 column (100 × 2·5 cm; Pharmacia, Uppsala, Sweden) and eluted, using Tris-buffered saline (0·0137 M-Tris–HCl, 0·012 M-NaCl and 0·005 M-KCl; pH 7·4). Fractions of 4·7 ml were collected and lyophilized.

Reverse-phase chromatography (h.p.l.c.)

The acidic granules extract was fractioned on a C-18 reverse phase column (Econosphere, 5 µm: Alltech, Avondale, PA, U.S.A.) with a linear gradient of 0–80% acetonitrile containing 0·1% trifluoroacetic acid. Fractions of 1 ml were collected and lyophilized.

Chorionic gonadotrophin-like activity

Activity of the various fractions obtained throughout purification procedures was determined by a radioreceptor assay (RRA) for hCG, using rat testicular tissue, and ^{125}I-labelled hCG as described by Catt *et al.* (1972). hCG was radiolabelled with ^{125}I by the Iodo-gen method (Ferguson *et al.*, 1983).

Bovine luteal cells were dispersed with collagenase (Simmons *et al.*, 1976). The trypan blue dye exclusion test indicated that 80% of all cells were viable. The cells (200 000) in 0·5 ml MEM were incubated in 5 replicates with hCG, h.p.l.c. or Sephacryl S-300 chromatographed fractions. After a 2-h incubation at 37°C, in the presence of 5% CO_2, cells were pelleted by centrifugation, and progesterone radioimmunoassay (RIA) was performed as previously described (Shemesh *et al.*, 1979).

Protein determination

Protein was measured by the method of Bradford (1976), with bovine IgG as the standard.

SDS–polyacrylamide gel electrophoresis

Polyacrylamide gel electrophoresis (10%) was performed according to Laemmli (1970), and followed by silver staining (Wray *et al.*, 1981).

RNA extraction and hybridization

Total RNA was extracted from fetal and maternal placenta by the method described by Chirgwin *et al.* (1979). RNA was loaded on nitrocellulose, using the dot-blot technique. The nitrocellulose paper was prehybridized and hybridized at 45°C for 16 h (Melton *et al.*, 1984) with [^{32}P]cDNA probes. (The cDNA probes of α- and β-hCG were kindly donated by Dr J. C. Fiddes, California Biochemistry Inc., Mountain View, CA, U.S.A.) as described by Fiddes & Goodman (1980). The nitrocellulose was treated as described by Izhar *et al.* (1986) and then subjected to autoradiography.

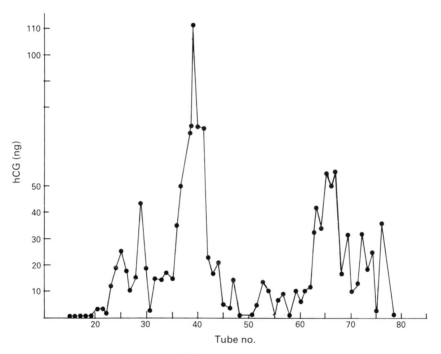

Fig. 1. Relative inhibitory binding of ^{125}I-labelled hCG in a radioreceptor assay by the fractions obtained using Sephacryl S-300. Total granule proteins were fractionated on Sephacryl S-300 column and analysed for displacement of ^{125}I-labelled hCG. The data were calculated from a standard curve for hCG (not shown).

Results

The total extract of the granules was fractionated on a Sephacryl S-300 column, lyophilized and analysed for relative inhibitory binding of ^{125}I-labelled hCG in the radioreceptor assay. Figure 1 shows displacement of iodinated hCG by substances found in the granule fractions (according to a standard curve, not shown). Two main peaks showed displacement of hCG: (a) Fractions 36–41 and (b) Fractions 65–73 of smaller molecular weight. The first peak is equivalent to 110 ng hCG/20 μg protein, as detected by RRA, and the low molecular weight peak is equivalent to 55 ng

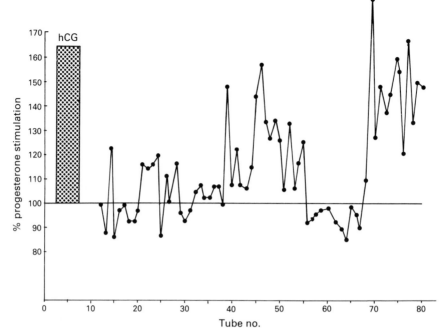

Fig. 2. Progesterone production by bovine luteal cells (2×10^5) treated with granule proteins fractionated on Sephacryl S-300 column. The amount of secreted progesterone was measured using radioimmunoassay. The control group ($4\cdot7$ ng $\pm$ $0\cdot3$ s.e., $n = 10$) is represented as 100%. The stippled bar is the stimulation of progesterone synthesis by 5 ng hCG/ml.

hCG/20 μg protein. Chorionic gonadotrophin activity of the major peak was not stable after 2 days at $-20°C$, but the lower molecular weight peak was stable to freezing for at least 1 month.

Luteal cell cultures were incubated with Sephacryl S-300 fractions and progesterone synthesis was measured by RIA. As can be seen in Fig. 2, hCG (5 ng/ml) increased progesterone synthesis by 65% above control. The low molecular weight fractions (Nos 67–78) increased progesterone synthesis by 85%, and the higher molecular weight peak (Fractions 45–50) increased it by 57%.

Since low molecular weight substances were potent (RRA and RIA), acidic extraction of granules was performed to enrich low molecular weight substances from fetal cotyledons, as described under 'Methods'. Figure 3 shows the results of SDS–polyacrylamide gel electrophoresis: a cytosolic extract of bovine fetal cotyledons (a) was compared to the total granule extract (b) and to the acidic granule extract (c). Different protein profiles were obtained using these purification steps. The total and acidic extracts both showed a larger variety of low molecular weight proteins than did cytosol. In the total extract (b) there was enrichment of the proteins of M_r 29 000 and 35 000, whereas the acidic extract exhibited proteins of M_r 31 000 and 32 000.

The acidic granule extract was fractionated using h.p.l.c. C-18 columns, lyophilized and analysed in the bioassay, i.e. the enhancement of progesterone production by dispersed bovine luteal cells, as described above. Fractions 17–20 enhanced progesterone production $3\cdot4$ times more than in the control (Fig. 4), while hCG by itself increased progesterone secretion 3-fold. None of these fractions replaced binding of ^{125}I-labelled hCG to rat testicular receptors in RRA.

The acidic granule extract ($10\cdot2$ ng progesterone/μg granule protein/200 000 cells/2 h) was 10 times more active than the total granule extract ($0\cdot8$ ng). The Sephacryl S-300 high molecular weight peak produced $3\cdot84$ ng progesterone while the C-18 peak produced 470 ng progesterone/μg granule protein/200 000 cells/2 h.

$M_r \times 10^{-3}$ a   b   c

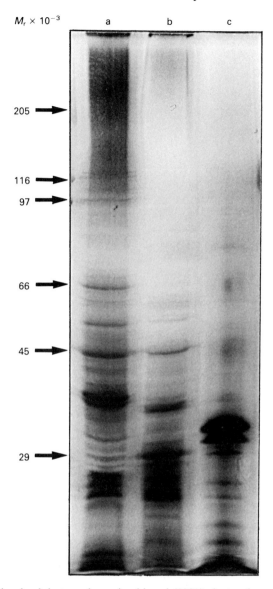

Fig. 3. Sodium dodecyl sulphate–polyacrylamide gel (10%) electrophoresis followed by silver staining. Lane a, cytosol of fetal cotyledons; Lane b, total granule extract; Lane c, acidic granule extract. Number on the left side of the gel shows the migration of molecular weight marker proteins.

The h.p.l.c.-active fractions were extracted by phase partition of methanol:chloroform (2:1, v/v). No biological activity of progesterone enhancement was found in the chloroform phase.

Total RNA extractions of bovine fetal and maternal placenta were analysed using a dot-blot technique. RNAs were hybridized with ^{32}P-radiolabelled α- and β-cDNA of hCG. No hybridization signals were detected (data not shown).

Discussion

Two criteria were used to define luteotrophic activity in this paper: (1) inhibition of the binding of hCG to its receptor and (2) enhancement of progesterone production by dispersed bovine luteal cell

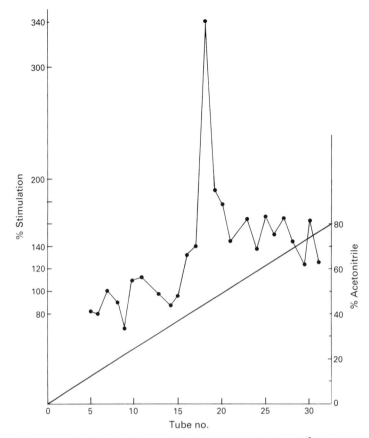

Fig. 4. Progesterone production by dispersed bovine luteal cells (2×10^5) treated with h.p.l.c.-derived fractions of the acidic granule extract. The C-18 reverse-phase column was eluted with a linear gradient of acetonitrile (0–80% in H_2O). Fractions of 1 ml were collected and lyophilized. The amount of secreted progesterone was measured by radioimmunoassay. The control group is represented by 100%.

cultures. The present study describes two luteotrophic substances extracted from bovine cotyledons which fulfil at least one of these criteria: (1) a high molecular weight substance that displaces the binding of ^{125}I-labelled hCG to rat testicular cell membranes, but does not enhance progesterone production by luteal cell preparations; and (2) a low molecular weight substance that enhances progesterone secretion by dispersed bovine luteal cells but does not compete with ^{125}I-labelled hCG in the RRA. The biological activity of the high molecular weight substance was not stable. The biologically active low molecular weight substance was (a) heat stable, (b) soluble in 2 N-acetic acid (96°C for 5 min) and (c) not extracted to the chloroform phase when partitioned against methanol:chloroform. The molecular weight was <40 000. These data suggest that a low molecular weight substance, probably a peptide, is present in the bovine placenta.

The biologically active granule substances studied in this work differ from those previously described by Ailenberg & Shemesh (1983) or Hickey & Hansel (1987) as follows: (1) lower molecular weight (<35 000 according to SDS–PAGE); (2) heat-stable; (3) not competing with ^{125}I-labelled hCG for binding in the radioreceptor assay.

The appearance of proteins of molecular weight ≤ 35 000 in the acidic granules raises the question of whether this substance is identical with the pituitary gonadotrophins of cattle which have subunits of a molecular weight of 15 000–16 000 (Pierce & Parsons, 1981). It is unlikely to be a bovine pituitary gonadotrophin considering (a) the tissue source differs (LH is extracted from pituitary and plasma and the active substance from the placenta); (b) the active substance does not compete with ^{125}I-labelled hCG in the radioreceptor assay; and (c) bovine RNAs extracted from fetal cotyledons do not hybridize with the α- or β-subunits of hCG–cDNA. Ailenberg & Shemesh (1983) described a chorionic gonadotrophin of cattle that did compete with iodinated hCG in a radioreceptor assay, and so the active peptide investigated in this study is probably neither a chorionic gonadotrophin nor LH.

It is possible that the granule active substance of lower molecular weight is a degradation product of a larger unstable molecule which does bind hCG. Alternatively, it may be a novel substance that does not bind the hCG receptor but does enhance progesterone secretion by bovine luteal cells. Therefore it is possible that the granules of the cow placenta contain two different substances with partial luteotrophic activity: (1) a progesterone production enhancer and (2) an hCG receptor binding competitor.

Gadsby & Lancaster (1987) described a small molecular weight peptide (6000–8000) luteotrophin of the rabbit that induced progesterone production in granulosa cells in culture. The presence of small molecular weight substances that enhance progesterone synthesis in another species could mean that there is a different novel group of luteotrophic substances chemically different from the chorionic gonadotrophins.

This work was supported by BARD grant no. I-740-84 and AID grant no. DPE-5544-G-SS-6046.

References

Ailenberg, M. & Shemesh, M. (1983) Partial purification of a chorionic gonadotrophin-like protein from bovine cotyledons. *Biol. Reprod.* **28**, 517–522.

Bahl, O.P. (1977) Human chorionic gonadotrophin, its receptor and mechanism of action. *Fedn Proc. Fedn Am. Socs exp. Biol.* **36**, 2119–2127.

Bazer, F.W., Roberts, R.M., Thatcher, W.W. & Sharp, D.C. (1985) Mechanisms related to establishment of pregnancy. In *Early Pregnancy Factors*, pp. 13–24. Eds F. Ellendorff & E. Koch. Perinatology Press, Ithaca.

Bradford, M.M. (1976) A rapid and sensitive method for the quantitation of microgram quantities of protein utilizing the principle of protein dye binding. *Analyt. Biochem.* **72**, 248–254.

Byatt, J.C., Shimonura, K., Duello, T.M. & Bremel, P.D. (1986) Isolation and characterization of multiple forms of bovine placental lactogen from secretory granules of the fetal cotyledon. *Endocrinology* **119**, 1293–1350.

Catt, K.J., Dufau, M.L. & Tsuruhaara, T. (1972) Radio-ligand-receptor assay of luteinizing hormone and chorionic gonadotropin. *J. clin. Endocr. Metab.* **34**, 123–132.

Chirgwin, J.M., Przybyla, A.E., MacDonald, R.J. & Rutter, W.J. (1979) Isolation of biologically active ribonucleic acid from sources enriched in ribonuclease. *Biochemistry, N.Y.* **18**, 5294–5299.

Cole, H.H. & Goss, H.T. (1943) The source of equine gonadotropin. In *Essays in Biology in Honour of Hebert M. Evans*, pp. 102–109. University of California Press, Berkeley.

Deanesly, R. (1966) The endocrinology of pregnancy and foetal life. In *Marshalls' Physiology of Reproduction*, 3rd edn, Vol. 3, pp. 891–1063. Ed. A. S. Parkes. Longmans, Green & Co., London.

Ferguson, K.M., Hayes, M.M. & Jeffcoate, S.L. (1983) Preparation of tracer LH and FSH for multicenter use. In *Immunoassays for Clinical Chemistry*, pp. 289–294. Eds W. M. Hunter & J. E. Corrie. Churchill-Livingstone, Edinburgh.

Fiddes, J.C. & Goodman, H.M. (1980) The cDNA for the β-subunit of human chorionic gonadotropin suggests evolution of a gene by readthrough into the 3'-untranslated region. *Nature, Lond.* **286**, 684–687.

Gadsby, J. & Lancaster, M. (1987) Effect of rabbit "placental luteotrophin" on granulosa cells in culture: preliminary characterization of "placental luteotrophin". *Biol. Reprod.* **36**, *Suppl.* 2, p. 50, Abstr.

Hickey, G.J. & Hansel, W. (1987) Purification of luteotrophic substances from allantoic fluids of 28–37-day bovine conceptuses. *J. Reprod. Fert.* **80**, 569–576.

Hickey, G.J., Walton, J.S., Harper, H.S. & Hansel, W. (1985) Partial purification of a luteotropic substance from allantoic fluid of 28–37 day bovine conceptuses. *Biol. Reprod.* **32**, *Suppl.* 1, 64, Abstr.

Hodgen, G.D., Tullner, W.W., Vaitukaitis, J.L., Ward, D.N. & Ross, G.T. (1974) Specific radioimmunoassay of chorionic gonadotropin during implantation in rhesus monkeys. *J. clin. Endocr. Metab.* **39**, 457–464.

Izhar, M., Siebert, P.D., Oshima, R.G., DeWolf, W.C. & Fukuda, M.N. (1986) Trophoblastic differentiation of human teratocarcinoma cell line HT-H. *Devl Biol.* **116**. 510–518.

Laemmli, U.K. (1970) Cleavage of structural proteins during assembly of the head of bacteriophage T4. *Nature, Lond.* **227**, 680–685.

Lunnen, J.E. & Foote, W.C. (1967) Gonadotropin activity in bovine serum and placental tissues. *Endocrinology* **81**, 61–66.

Melton, D.A., Krieg, P.A., Rebaglliati, M.R., Maniatis, T., Zinn, K. & Green, M.R. (1984) Efficient *in vitro* synthesis of biologically active RNA and RNA hybridization probes from plasmids containing a bacteriophage SP6 promoter. *Nucleic Acids Res.* **12**, 7035–7056.

Pierce, J.G. & Parsons, T.F. (1981) Glycoprotein hormones: structure and function. *Ann. Rev. Biochem.* **50**, 465–495.

Saxena, B.B., Hasan, S., Haour, F. & Schmidt-Gollwitzer, M. (1974) Radioreceptor assay of human chorionic gonadotrophin detection of early pregnancy. *Science, N.Y.* **184**, 793–795.

Shemesh, M., Mileguir, F., Ayalon, N. & Hansel, W. (1979) Steroidogenesis and prostaglandin synthesis by cultured bovine blastocyst. *J. Reprod. Fert.* **56**, 181–185.

Simmons, K.R., Caffrey, J.L., Phillips, J.L., Abel, J.H. & Niswender, G.D. (1976) A simple method for preparing suspensions of luteal cells. *Proc. Soc. exp. Biol. Med.* **152**, 366–371.

Thatcher, W.W., Knickerbocker, J.J., Bartol, F.F., Bazer, F.W., Roberts, R.M. & Drost, M. (1985a) Maternal recognition of pregnancy in relation to the survival of transferred embryos: endocrine aspects. *Theriogenology* **23**, 129–143.

Thatcher, W.W., Knickerbocker, J.J., Helmer, S.D., Hansen, P.J., Bartol, F.F., Roberts, R.M. & Bazer, F.W. (1985b) Characteristics of conceptus secretory proteins and their affects of $PGF_{2\alpha}$ secretion by maternal endometrium in cattle. In *Early Pregnancy Factors*, pp. 13–24. Eds F. Ellendorff & E. Koch. Perinatology Press, Ithaca.

Wray, W., Boulikas, T., Wray, V.P. & Hancock, R. (1981) Silver staining of protein in polyacrylamide gels. *Analyt. Biochem.* **118**, 197–203.

J. Reprod. Fert., Suppl. **37** (1989), 45–54

Control of corpus luteum function in the pregnant rabbit

J. E. Gadsby

Department of Anatomy, Physiological Sciences and Radiology, College of Veterinary Medicine, North Carolina State University, 4700 Hillsborough St., Raleigh, NC 27606, U.S.A.

Keywords: corpus luteum; pregnancy; rabbit; 'placental luteotrophin'; oestrogen

Introduction

The rabbit is an example of a species in which the corpora lutea are the only significant source of progesterone, which is required throughout gestation for pregnancy maintenance. In fact, as shown in Fig. 1, in order to sustain pregnancy, the functional lifespan (i.e. period of progesterone secretion) of the corpora lutea must be extended to approximately 30–32 days, compared with 17–18 days in pseudopregnant rabbits. As these data show (Fig. 1), there is little evidence of a luteotrophic effect of the blastocyst, in terms of circulating progesterone concentrations, before implantation (~ Day 6–7), and indeed, there is no convincing evidence for the secretion of a chorionic gonadotrophin by the preimplantation rabbit blastocyst (Sundaram *et al.*, 1975; Holt *et al.*, 1976). The earliest time when a difference in serum progesterone concentrations between pregnant and pseudopregnant rabbits could be observed was ~ Day 12 (Fig. 1; Browning *et al.*, 1980). Furthermore, other studies involving conceptus removal have suggested that the maternal recognition of pregnancy in this species occurs after implantation (~ Day 10–12; Browning & Wolf, 1981; Nowak & Bahr, 1983).

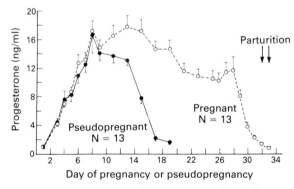

Fig. 1. Serum progesterone concentrations in pregnant and pseudopregnant Dutch rabbits. Pseudopregnancy was induced by mating to a vasectomized male; the day after fertile or sterile mating is designated Day 1. Values are given as mean ± s.e.m. N = number of animals. (From Keyes *et al.*, 1983.)

The factors controlling the extended period of luteal progesterone secretion during pregnancy in the rabbit are not completely understood. There is considerable circumstantial evidence to suggest that the placenta plays an important physiological role in this process (Greep, 1941; Chu *et al.*, 1946; Holt & Ewing, 1974; Lanman & Thau, 1979; Browning & Wolf, 1981; Browning *et al.*, 1982; Nowak & Bahr, 1983; Gadsby & Keyes, 1984), probably via the secretion of a putative 'factor'/'hormone' (called "placental luteotrophin"; Gadsby & Keyes, 1984), about which little is known at present. This 'placental luteotrophin' appears to be a product of trophoblast cells of the fetal placenta rather than the maternal placenta/decidua (Holt & Ewing, 1974). In addition to 'placental luteotrophin', other studies have indicated that oestrogen produced by ovarian follicles also plays an important physiological role in luteal maintenance during pregnancy (Robson, 1939; Keyes & Nalbandov, 1967; Keyes & Armstrong, 1968; Spies *et al.*, 1968; Rippel & Johnson, 1976; Gadsby *et al.*, 1983).

Experiments and Results

Since it appeared that two 'factors'/'hormones' (oestrogen and 'placental luteotrophin') are involved in luteal maintenance during pregnancy, we designed experiments to examine more precisely their luteotrophic roles, and to indicate how they may interact to promote corpus luteum progesterone secretion. Initially, we asked the following questions: (1) can 'placental luteotrophin' maintain luteal function in the absence of oestrogen? and (2) can oestrogen maintain luteal function in the absence of 'placental luteotrophin'?

Can 'placental luteotrophin' maintain luteal function in the absence of oestrogen?

In these experiments we attempted to remove/withdraw oestrogen in pregnant rabbits by using two different approaches: (1) injection of hCG to ovulate follicles and (2) hypophysectomy to remove pituitary support for follicles. In addition, these rabbits were treated with medroxy-progesterone acetate (MPA), which did not cross-react with the progesterone RIA, to ensure fetal/placental viability (and thus 'placental luteotrophin' secretion). Luteal function was monitored by measurement (radioimmunoassay) of serum progesterone concentrations.

In the first experiment, pregnant rabbits were given 5 mg MPA (i.m.) on Day 20 (day of mating = Day 0), and on Day 21 they were given 10 i.u. hCG (i.v.). On Day 22, 24 h after hCG, the rabbits were anaesthetized with xylazine and ketamine and laparotomized, and ovulated follicles were carefully dissected out. Also on Day 22, rabbits were each given an oestradiol-filled (or empty) Silastic implant (Gadsby *et al.*, 1983) s.c., which were found to produce physiological levels (6–7 pg/ml) of oestradiol in serum. The changes in serum progesterone concentrations are shown in Fig. 2. Treatment with hCG initially (within 6 h) appeared to cause an increase (to ~ 27 ng/ml) in serum progesterone concentrations from 16 to 19 ng/ml on Days 20–21, but then there was a dramatic decline to 2 ± 0.5 ng/ml by 24 h (Day 22). This fall in serum progesterone concentrations was associated with a decline in serum oestradiol-17β concentrations (induced by hCG) from ~ 5 pg/ml on Day 20 to 0.8 pg/ml on Day 22. In rabbits given oestradiol implants, progesterone concentrations returned to pre-treatment values (16–22 ng/ml) on Days 24–27. However, in rabbits given empty implants, progesterone concentrations remained low (1–3 ng/ml) up to Day 24, and then gradually increased to ~ 7 ng/ml on Day 27. Pregnancy was maintained in all rabbits as determined by the presence of viable fetuses at autopsy on Day 27.

In the second experiment, hypophysectomy was performed on Day 4 of pregnancy, by the parapharyngeal approach, and all rabbits were given an oestradiol-containing implant (s.c.). On Day 20 of pregnancy, rabbits were treated with MPA and on Day 21, the implant was removed, constituting oestradiol-withdrawal (serum oestradiol concentrations were reduced from 4.7 ± 0.9 pg/ml on Day 20 to 1.6 ± 0.3 pg/ml on Day 22). As shown in Fig. 3, serum progesterone concentrations fell dramatically from 17 ± 3 ng/ml on Day 21 to <1 ng/ml within 24 h (Day 22). Progesterone concentrations remained low (<1 ng/ml) thereafter, up to Day 30. Pregnancy was maintained in all animals throughout this period (up to Day 30).

These results indicated that luteal progesterone secretion dramatically decreased after removal of oestrogen, demonstrating the potent luteotrophic role of oestrogen during pregnancy. Further-more, they indicated that the presence of viable fetuses/placentae (i.e. 'placental luteotrophin'), was

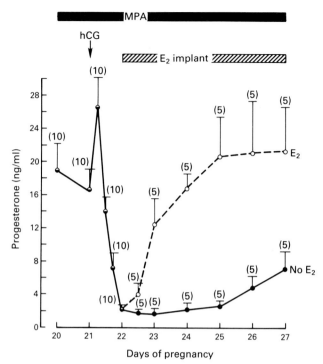

Fig. 2. Effect of hCG-induced ovulation on serum progesterone concentrations in pregnant rabbits. All rabbits were treated with medroxyprogesterone acetate (MPA) on Days 20–27 and hCG (10 i.u./rabbit, i.v.) on Day 21 (arrow). On Day 22, rabbits received either an oestradiol (E_2)-containing or blank (No E_2) Silastic implant s.c. Values are given as mean $\pm$ s.e.m. for the no. of animals in parentheses. (From Gadsby *et al.*, 1983.)

unable to prevent the decline in, or to restore, luteal steroidogenesis, in the absence of oestrogen. The observation that replacement of oestradiol in hCG-treated rabbits was able to restore progesterone concentrations to pre-treatment levels demonstrated that oestrogen was able to maintain luteal function in the presence of viable fetuses/placentae.

Can oestrogen maintain luteal function in the absence of 'placental luteotrophin'?

In these experiments, we used bilateral hysterectomy as a convenient and rapid approach for removing 'placental luteotrophin' during pregnancy (Holt & Ewing, 1974). On Day 21 of pregnancy, rabbits were hysterectomized (or sham-hysterectomized) via a mid-line abdominal incision. Sham-hysterectomy involved manipulation of the uterus without its excision. Some groups of rabbits were given an oestradiol-containing implant (s.c.) either before (Day 20) or after (Day 22) hysterectomy. As before, luteal function was monitored by measurement of serum progesterone concentrations.

As shown in Fig. 4, serum progesterone concentrations in sham-hysterectomized rabbits fluctuated between 9 and 15 ng/ml on Days 20–27, similar to the pattern seen in normal pregnancy (Fig. 1). Pregnancy was maintained in all sham-hysterectomized rabbits up to Day 27. In contrast, serum progesterone concentrations in hysterectomized rabbits declined markedly from ~ 13 ng/ml on Day 21 to 5 ± 2 ng/ml on Day 22, and then continued to decline to 1 ng/ml or less on Days 24–27. Serum oestradiol concentrations measured in these same animals showed that the decline in

48 J. E. Gadsby

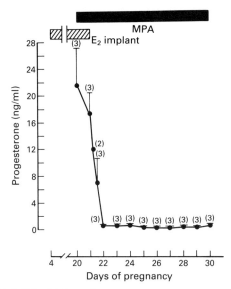

Fig. 3. Effect of oestradiol-17β withdrawal on serum progesterone concentrations in hypophy-sectomized (on Day 4) pregnant rabbits. All rabbits were treated with MPA on Days 20–27. The oestradiol (E_2) implant inserted s.c. on Day 4 was removed on Day 21 of pregnancy. Values are given as mean ± s.e.m. for the no. of animals in parentheses. (From Gadsby *et al.*, 1983.)

luteal progesterone secretion in hysterectomized rabbits was not associated with a fall in circulating oestradiol concentrations (data not shown; Gadsby & Keyes, 1984). Figure 5 shows the serum progesterone concentrations in rabbits which received an oestradiol-containing implant before (Day 20) or after (Day 22) hysterectomy performed on Day 21. In rabbits given oestradiol on Day 22, progesterone levels declined dramatically from ~16 ng/ml on Day 20–21 to 5 ± 1 ng/ml on Day 22, and then more gradually to 2–3 ng/ml on Days 24–27. The fall in serum progesterone concentrations in the 'Hys + E_2, Day 20' group, induced by hysterectomy on Day 21, was more protracted, falling from ~18 ng/ml on Days 20–21 to only 13 ± 1 ng/ml by Day 22. However, progesterone concentrations continued to decline to 1–2 ng/ml on Days 24–27.

The results given in Fig. 4 provide additional evidence of the luteotrophic role of the rabbit placenta ('placental luteotrophin') during pregnancy. In view of the fact that both serum and luteal tissue concentrations of oestradiol were found to be similar in hysterectomized and sham-hysterectomized rabbits (data not shown; Gadsby & Keyes, 1984), it is probable that luteolysis induced by hysterectomy cannot be explained by inadequate (circulating or luteal tissue) levels of oestradiol. Furthermore, treatment with exogenous oestrogen (implants) before or after hysterectomy, was unable to prevent or reverse the decline in serum progesterone concentrations induced by removal of 'placental luteotrophin' (Fig. 5). We concluded from these experiments that oestradiol alone was not sufficient to maintain corpus luteum function in the absence of 'placental luteotrophin'.

It appeared from these experiments that both oestradiol and 'placental luteotrophin' were required for full corpus luteum function in the pregnant rabbit. One hypothesis we proposed which may account for the interaction between these two physiological luteotrophins was that 'placental luteotrophin' may regulate the 'responsiveness' of corpora lutea to oestrogen via an action on the luteal oestrogen receptor, which is known to be present in corpora lutea of pseudopregnant (Lee *et al.*, 1971; Scott & Rennie, 1971; Mills & Osteen, 1977; Drake & Cook, 1979; Yuh & Keyes, 1979) and pregnant (Gadsby, 1981; Keyes & Gadsby, 1987) rabbits.

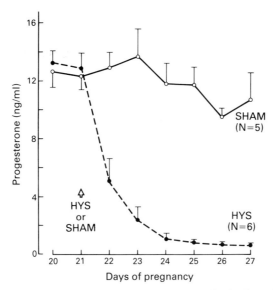

Fig. 4. Effect of hysterectomy (HYS) or sham-hysterectomy (SHAM) performed on Day 21 of pregnancy (arrow) on serum progesterone concentrations in rabbits. Values are given as mean ± s.e.m. for the no. of animals in parentheses. (From Gadsby & Keyes, 1984.)

Does 'placental luteotrophin' regulate the luteal cell oestrogen receptor?

In an attempt to address this question directly, we examined the concentrations and binding characteristics of the luteal oestrogen receptor in corpora lutea removed 24 h (Day 22) after hysterectomy (or sham-hysterectomy), performed on Day 21. Blood samples were taken on Days 21 and 22 to confirm the changes in serum progesterone concentrations observed previously (Fig. 4). After removal of corpora lutea on Day 22, they were homogenized in Tris–HCl/EDTA buffer at 4°C. The homogenate was centrifuged at 800 *g* for 10 min at 4°C to obtain a crude nuclear fraction (800 *g* pellet). The 800 *g* supernatant was then centrifuged at 105 000 *g* for 1 h at 4°C to obtain the cytoplasmic receptor preparation (cytosol; 105 000 *g* supernatant). Specific [³H]oestradiol-17β binding to cytosolic and nuclear fractions was determined by incubating cytosol with 0·6 nM-[³H]oestradiol-17β and the nuclear fraction with 1 nM-[³H]oestradiol-17β, in the presence or absence of a 100-fold excess diethylstilboestrol (DES) at 0–4°C for 2 h (unoccupied cytosol), 0–4°C for 24 h (total cytosol receptor, exchange assay) and 25°C for 2 h (total nuclear receptor, exchange assay). The binding characteristics (dissociation constant and binding capacity) of the cytosol (0–4°C for 24 h) and nuclear (25°C for 2 h) oestrogen receptors were examined by saturation binding analysis, using the method of Scatchard (1949); for these studies a range of tritiated oestradiol concentrations (1×10^{-7}–$2\cdot5 \times 10^{-10}$ M, cytosol; 2×10^{-7}–$7\cdot5 \times 10^{-10}$ M, nuclear) in the presence or absence of a 100-fold excess of DES, were used.

As shown in Fig. 6(a), serum progesterone concentrations fell in hysterectomized rabbits from ∼ 12 ng/ml on Day 21 to ∼ 3 ng/ml on Day 22, whereas progesterone levels remained unchanged in sham-hysterectomized rabbits. However, there were no differences in the concentrations of cytoplasmic or nuclear oestrogen receptors measured in the corpora lutea taken from these two groups of rabbits on Day 22 (Fig. 6b). Table 1 shows the binding characteristics of luteal oestrogen receptors measured on Day 22 in hysterectomized or sham-hysterectomized rabbits. These results also reveal that there were no major differences in dissociation constants or binding capacities of luteal cytosolic or nuclear oestrogen receptors in hysterectomized or sham-hysterectomized rabbits, as determined on Day 22.

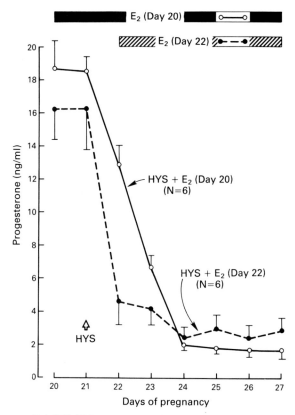

Fig. 5. Effect of oestradiol-17β (E_2) on serum progesterone concentrations (ng/ml) in rabbits hysterectomized (HYS) on Day 21 of pregnancy (arrow). Oestradiol (E_2) implants were inserted s.c. on Day 20 (Hys + E_2, Day 20) or on Day 22 (Hys + E_2, Day 22). Values are given as mean ± s.e.m. for the no. of animals in parentheses. (From Gadsby & Keyes, 1984.)

We concluded from this study that 'placental luteotrophin' probably does not act directly on the luteal oestrogen receptor or its binding characteristics, at least as determined during the 24-h period of its withdrawal by hysterectomy on Day 21, during which there was a dramatic (60–70%) fall in luteal progesterone secretion. However, since the determinations made in this study were static measurements of the oestrogen receptor, we cannot rule out the possibility that 'placental luteotrophin' may act on receptor dynamics (e.g. replenishment or recycling). Furthermore, it is also possible that 'placental luteotrophin' regulates luteal oestrogen responsiveness by acting at a post-receptor site.

What is the identity/nature of 'placental luteotrophin'?

As demonstrated and discussed above, the putative 'placental luteotrophin' plays an important physiological role in corpus luteum maintenance in the pregnant rabbit and yet its identity/nature remains unknown. In some recent experiments, we have used an in-vitro 'bioassay' for fetal placental 'factor(s)/hormone(s)', using granulosa-lutein cells maintained in culture, which we proposed to use in our efforts to isolate, purify and identify 'placental luteotrophin'. These experiments are described below.

Rabbits were superovulated with PMSG/hCG and on Day 1 of pseudopregnancy (~24 h after hCG), granulosa-lutein cell 'cores' were dissected from the corpora lutea (Yuh *et al.*, 1986).

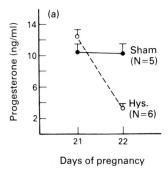
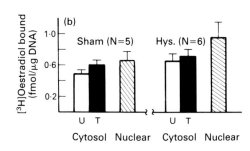

Fig. 6. Serum progesterone concentrations (a) and luteal oestrogen receptor concentrations (b) in rabbits, hysterectomized (Hys) or sham-hysterectomized (Sham) on Day 21 of pregnancy. Blood samples were collected on Days 21 and 22 for measurement of serum progesterone concentrations. On Day 22, corpora lutea were removed, homogenized and cytosol (105 000 g supernatant) and crude nuclear (800 g pellet) fractions were prepared. Unoccupied cytosol (U: 0–4°C for 2 h), total cytosol (T: 0–4°C for 24 h; exchange assay) and total nuclear (25°C for 2 h; exchange assay) oestrogen receptor concentrations were measured (see text for details). Values are mean ± s.e.m. for the no. of animals in parentheses. (From Keyes & Gadsby, 1987.)

Table 1. Scatchard analysis of the luteal oestrogen receptor 24 h after hysterectomy or sham-hysterectomy of pregnant rabbits on Day 21 of pregnancy

		Dissociation constant (M)	Binding capacity (M)
Cytosol	Sham	$5.0\,(\pm1.8)\times10^{-11}$	$2.4\,(\pm0.6)\times10^{-11}$
	Hys	$4.8\,(\pm1.8)\times10^{-11}$	$2.7\,(\pm0.7)\times10^{-11}$
Nuclear	Sham	$1.2\,(\pm0.6)\times10^{-10}$	$0.8\,(\pm0.2)\times10^{-11}$
	Hys	$1.6\,(\pm0.2)\times10^{-10}$	$1.4\,(\pm0.7)\times10^{-11}$

Values are mean ± s.e.m. of 3 independent experiments (pools of tissue); each pool comprised tissue from 5 animals. (From Keyes & Gadsby, 1987.)

The 'cores' were dissociated with collagenase/hyaluronidase, and were plated (Day 0 of culture) in 96-well culture plates ($\sim 50\,000$ cells/well) in Medium 199 (plus antibiotics; M199) containing 5% fetal bovine serum, to form monolayer cultures. After 24 h (Day 1 of culture), the plating medium was removed and fresh M199 (plus 0.1% BSA) containing hormones (e.g. oestradiol, 10^{-8} M; ovine LH, 100 ng/ml) or placenta-conditioned medium (see below) was added. Media were removed and replaced daily for 5 days, and progesterone concentrations were measured in spent medium by radioimmunoassay. Data were expressed as fold stimulation which was calculated as the total progesterone accumulated over 5 days of culture for each hormone/medium treatment, divided by the total progesterone accumulated over 5 days by control cultures. Placenta-conditioned medium was obtained as follows. Fetal–placental tissue was removed on Day 21 of pregnancy and was incubated in M199 for 6 h at 37°C. Fetal placenta-conditioned medium (FPI) was obtained after centrifugation at 800 g for 15 min at 4°C. Aliquots of FPI were subjected to heating (95°C for 1 h), dialysis (using 6000–8000 molecular wt cutoff membrane) and trypsin treatment (incubation with

1 mg trypsin/ml for 1 h at 37°C). All FPI media were filter sterilized and were added to granulosa-lutein cell cultures as 50% (v/v) mixtures in M199 (+0·1% BSA).

Figure 7 shows the effects of oestradiol-17β (10^{-8} M), LH (100 ng/ml) and FPI, with and without oestradiol (10^{-8} M), on progesterone accumulation by granulosa cells in culture. Oestradiol marginally stimulated progesterone accumulation ($\sim 1\cdot5$-fold), whereas LH had a marked stimulatory effect ($11\cdot4 \pm 0\cdot5$-fold) on granulosa-lutein cell progesterone production. FPI alone increased progesterone accumulation ~ 3-fold, but in the presence of oestradiol, this was further elevated to 6-fold (FPI + E$_2$ *vs* FPI; $P < 0\cdot05$, *t*-test). In Fig. 8, data are presented to illustrate the effects of heating, dialysis and trypsin treatment of FPI, all of which were examined in the presence of oestradiol. Untreated and heated FPI stimulated progesterone accumulation ~ 6-fold over controls, and dialysed FPI also retained its 'luteotrophic' bioactivity, giving a 7-fold stimulation over controls. However, the stimulatory effect of FPI on granulosa-lutein cell progesterone accumulation was abolished after trypsin treatment ($0\cdot9 \pm 0\cdot1$-fold).

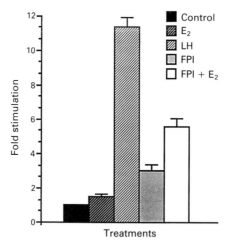

Fig. 7. Effects of oestradiol-17β (E$_2$; 10^{-8} M), LH (100 ng/ml) and fetal placenta-conditioned medium (FPI) on progesterone accumulation (fold stimulation *versus* controls) by cultured rabbit granulosa-lutein cells. Fold stimulation was calculated as the total progesterone accumulation over 5 days of culture for each hormone/conditioned medium treatment, divided by total progesterone accumulated by control cultures, over the same time period. Values are given as mean $\pm$ s.e.m. for 4 replicate culture wells.

These results indicate the presence of 'factor(s)/hormone(s)' in fetal placenta-conditioned medium which was able to increase progesterone accumulation by granulosa-lutein cells in culture ~ 3-fold. Furthermore, this stimulatory effect was enhanced in the presence of oestradiol to about 6-fold, a finding which was of particular interest in view of the involvement of both a fetal placental 'factor/hormone' ('placental luteotrophin') and oestrogen for complete luteal maintenance *in vivo*. In our initial attempts to characterize the bioactive 'luteotrophic' factor/hormone in FPI, we noted that it was remarkably heat-stable (95°C for 1 h), had a molecular weight of > 6000–8000 and was probably a protein or peptide, in view of its sensitivity to trypsin. In other experiments (data not shown), we have shown that the 'luteotrophic' bioactivity found in FPI appears to be tissue specific, since neither media conditioned by incubation of skeletal muscle, heart muscle, liver and uterus, nor 5–10% serum (pseudopregnant or pregnant), exerted a stimulatory effect on granulosa cell progesterone accumulation in culture.

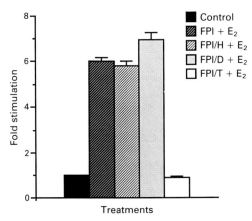

Fig. 8. Effects of heated (FPI/H), dialysed (FPI/D), trypsin-treated (FPI/T) or untreated (FPI), fetal placenta-conditioned media on progesterone accumulation (fold stimulation), by rabbit granulosa-lutein cells during 5 days of culture. All treatments (except controls) contained 10^{-8} M oestradiol (E_2). Values are given as mean $\pm$ s.e.m. for 4 replicate culture wells.

Concluding Remarks

In these studies we have demonstrated physiological roles both for ovarian follicular oestradiol and the putative 'placental luteotrophin' for complete maintenance of luteal function during pregnancy in the rabbit, although the precise mechanism by which these two luteotrophins act to maintain corpus luteum progesterone secretion remains to be elucidated. Among the possible hypotheses which may account for the interaction of these two luteotrophins, we were unable to show that 'placental luteotrophin' exerted a direct, acute (within 24 h) effect upon luteal oestrogen receptor concentrations or affinities, although it is possible that it may influence the dynamics of oestrogen receptor replenishment/recycling, or may have an action at a post-receptor site.

A complete understanding of the mechanism by which 'placental luteotrophin' acts to promote luteal function during pregnancy will require its identification, and the isolation and purification of large quantities of this 'factor'/'hormone' which can be used for studies *in vivo* and *in vitro*. Our initial attempts to determine the identity/nature of 'placental luteotrophin' by using rabbit granulosa-lutein cells in culture as an in-vitro bioassay have indicated the presence of a 'luteotrophic' 'factor'/'hormone' in fetal placenta-conditioned medium which was able to stimulate directly granulosa-lutein cell progesterone secretion, and to synergize with oestradiol in further promoting steroidogenesis. Preliminary fractionation of this conditioned medium has indicated that this 'factor'/'hormone' is probably a protein/peptide of molecular weight >6000–8000. Further studies are in progress to isolate, purify and identify this 'luteotrophic' 'factor'/'hormone' in fetal-placenta conditioned medium, which is a good source for 'placental luteotrophin'.

I thank NATO and the Mellon Foundation for financial support (Research Fellowships). The research was supported in part by funds from the State of North Carolina.

References

Browning, J.Y. & Wolf, R.C. (1981) Maternal recognition of pregnancy in the rabbit: effect of conceptus removal. *Biol. Reprod.* **24**, 293–297.

Browning, J.Y., Keyes, P.L. & Wolf, R.C. (1980) Comparison of serum progesterone, 20α-dihydroprogesterone and estradiol-17β in pregnant and pseudopregnant rabbits: Evidence for post-implantation recognition of pregnancy. *Biol. Reprod.* **23**, 1014–1019.

Browning, J.Y., Amis, M.M., Meller, P.A., Bridson, W.E. & Wolf, R.C. (1982) Luteotrophic and antiluteolytic activities of the rabbit conceptus. *Biol. Reprod.* **27**, 665–672.

Chu, J.P., Le, C.C. & You, S.S. (1946) Functional relation between the uterus and the corpus luteum. *J. Endocr.* **4**, 392–398.

Drake, R.G. & Cook, B. (1979) The estrogen receptor of rabbit corpus luteum: Binding, dissociation and stability characteristics. *Endocrinology* **105**, 561–569.

Gadsby, J.E. (1981) Does the rabbit placenta control the luteal estrogen receptor during pregnancy? *Biol. Reprod.* **24** (Suppl. 1), 30A, Abstr.

Gadsby, J.E. & Keyes, P.L. (1984) Control of corpus luteum function in the pregnant rabbit: Role of the placenta ("placental luteotropin") in regulating responsiveness of corpora lutea to estrogen. *Biol. Reprod.* **31**, 16–24.

Gadsby, J.E., Keyes, P.L. & Bill, C.H., II (1983) Control of corpus luteum function in the pregnant rabbit: Role of estrogen and lack of a direct luteotropic role of the placenta. *Endocrinology* **113**, 2255–2262.

Greep, R.O. (1941) Effects of hysterectomy and of estrogen treatment on volume changes in the corpora lutea of pregnant rabbits. *Anat. Rec.* **80**, 465–477.

Holt, J.A. & Ewing, L.L. (1974) Acute dependence of ovarian progesterone output on the presence of placentas in 21-day pregnant rabbits. *Endocrinology* **94**, 1438–1444.

Holt, J.A., Heise, W.F., Wilson, S.M. & Keyes, P.L. (1976) Lack of gonadotropic activity in the rabbit blastocyst prior to implantation. *Endocrinology* **98**, 904–909.

Keyes, P.L. & Armstrong, D.T. (1968) Endocrine role of follicles in the regulation of corpus luteum function in the rabbit. *Endocrinology* **83**, 509–515.

Keyes, P.L. & Gadsby, J.E. (1987) Role of estrogen and the placenta in the maintenance of the rabbit corpus luteum. In *Regulation of Ovarian and Testicular Function*, pp. 361–378. Eds V. B. Mahesh, D. S. Dhindsa, E. Anderson & S. P. Kalra. Plenum, New York.

Keyes, P.L. & Nalbandov, A.V. (1967) Maintenance and function of corpora lutea in rabbits depend on estrogen. *Endocrinology* **80**, 938–946.

Keyes, P.L., Gadsby, J.E., Yuh, K-C.M. & Bill, C.H. (1983) The corpus luteum. In *Reproductive Physiology IV. International Review of Physiology*, pp. 57–97. Ed. R. O. Greep. University Park Press, Baltimore.

Lanman, J.T. & Thau, R.B. (1979) Effect of the fetal placenta and of a pituitary extract on plasma progesterone in fetectomized rabbits. *J. Reprod. Fert.* **57**, 341–344.

Lee, C., Keyes, P.L. & Jacobson, H.I. (1971) Estrogen receptor in the rabbit corpus luteum. *Science, N.Y.* **173**, 1032–1033.

Mills, T.M. & Osteen, K.G. (1977) 17β-Estradiol receptor and progesterone and 20α-hydroxy-4-pregnen-3-one content of the developing corpus luteum of the rabbit. *Endocrinology* **101**, 1744–1750.

Nowak, R.A. & Bahr, J.M. (1983) Maternal recognition of pregnancy in the rabbit. *J. Reprod. Fert.* **69**, 623–627.

Rippel, R.H. & Johnson, E.S. (1976) Regression of corpora lutea in the rabbit after injection of a gonadotropin-releasing peptide (39320). *Proc. Soc. exp. Biol. Med.* **152**, 29–32.

Robson, J.M. (1939) Maintenance of pregnancy in the hypophysectomized rabbit by the administration of oestrin. *J. Physiol. Lond.* **95**, 83–91.

Scatchard, G. (1949) The attractions of proteins for small molecules and ions. *Ann. N.Y. Acad. Sci.* **51**, 660–672.

Scott, R.S. & Rennie, P.I.C. (1971) An estrogen receptor in the corpora lutea of the pseudopregnant rabbit. *Endocrinology* **89**, 297–301.

Spies, H.G., Hilliard, J. & Sawyer, C.H. (1968) Maintenance of corpora lutea and pregnancy in hypophysectomized rabbits. *Endocrinology* **83**, 354–367.

Sundaram, K., Connell, K.G. & Passantino, T. (1975) Implication of absence of hCG-like gonadotropin in the blastocyst for control of corpus luteum function in pregnant rabbits. *Nature, Lond.* **256**, 739–741.

Yuh, K-C.M. & Keyes, P.L. (1979) Properties of nuclear and cytoplasmic estrogen receptor in the rabbit corpus luteum: Evidence for translocation. *Endocrinology* **105**, 690–696.

Yuh, K-C.M., Possley, R.M., Brabec, R.K. & Keyes, P.L. (1986) Steroidogenic and morphological characteristics of granulosa and thecal compartments of the differentiating rabbit corpus luteum in culture. *J. Reprod. Fert.* **76**, 267–277.

IMMUNOLOGY OF PREGNANCY

Chairmen

M. Sela
K. Perk

J. Reprod. Fert., Suppl. **37** (1989), 55–61

Modification of immune function during pregnancy by products of the sheep uterus and conceptus

P. J. Hansen, D. C. Stephenson, B. G. Low and G. R. Newton

Dairy Science Department, University of Florida, Gainesville, Florida 32611-0701, U.S.A.

Summary. The preimplantation sheep conceptus produces several molecules that inhibit lymphocyte responses *in vitro* to mitogens or allogeneic cells, including prostaglandin E-2 and a lactosaminoglycan-containing glycoprotein of M_r 800 000–900 000. Additionally, the definitive placenta releases immunosuppressive factors when placed in culture. One of these is a heat- and protease-stable, carbohydrate-containing molecule released by explants of cultured fetal cotyledons. The pregnant uterus also produces molecules that alter lymphocyte responsiveness *in vitro*, including a dialysable, heat- and trypsin-stable factor and a high-molecular weight factor (M_r $>4 \times 10^6$). An important regulator of uterine immune function is progesterone. This hormone can induce the production of uterine immunosuppressants such as seen during pregnancy and prolong the life of skin allografts placed *in utero*. Taken together, results suggest that the conceptus resides in an immunosuppressive environment throughout most of gestation, a situation that may be critical to maintenance of pregnancy.

Keywords: immunosuppression; pregnancy; uterus; conceptus; placenta; sheep

Introduction

The fetal placenta expresses transplantation antigens (Clark *et al.*, 1986) and is therefore at risk of being destroyed by the maternal immune system. While expression of transplantation antigens on the sheep placenta has not been characterized, the conceptus of this species probably suffers the same immunological problem as for more well-studied species. The sheep uterus possesses an immune system capable of rejecting tissue grafts (Reimers & Dziuk, 1974; Hansen *et al.*, 1986) and antibodies against the conceptus can be found in maternal blood (Ford & Elves, 1974). Given this immunological predicament, the fact that the sheep conceptus is usually not immunologically rejected by its mother is a testament to the existence of one or more immunological adjustments to protect the conceptus.

A host of theories has arisen to explain survival of the 'fetal allograft' and at least some evidence is available to support each (Head & Billingham, 1984; Clark *et al.*, 1986). One of these theories states that rejection of the conceptus is avoided because of local production of non-specific immunosuppressive factors by the conceptus and uterus. These immunosuppressants are believed to block the maternal immune response at the fetal–maternal interface, thus preventing tissue rejection. The most commonly used approach to testing this hypothesis has been to identify molecules produced during pregnancy that depress in-vitro proliferative responses of lymphocytes to allogeneic cells or mitogens. While in-vitro tests cannot be conclusive, these experiments have led to the identification of several putative immunosuppressive molecules that could exert regulatory effects in the uterus during pregnancy. The properties of such molecules produced in sheep will be reviewed in this paper.

Immunoregulatory products of the conceptus

The sheep conceptus produces several molecules that inhibit lymphocytes *in vitro*. One of these is prostaglandin (PG) E-2, which is produced by the preimplantation conceptus, cotyledons and chorioallantois (Hyland *et al.*, 1982; Evans *et al.*, 1982; Risbridger *et al.*, 1985). This prostaglandin is immunosuppressive at concentrations as low as 10^{-8} M (Fig. 1) and is found in placental tissue during late pregnancy at concentrations as high as 10^{-6}M (Evans *et al.*, 1982).

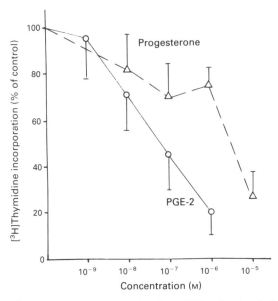

Fig. 1. Inhibition of [^{3}H]thymidine incorporation into PHA-stimulated sheep lymphocytes by progesterone and PGE-2. Data on thymidine incorporation are expressed as a percentage of values for control lymphocytes cultured without exogenous hormone. Note the greater immunosuppressive activity of PGE-2. Neither PGE-2 nor progesterone exerted their inhibitory effects by causing cytotoxicity since cell viabilities were unaffected by either hormone. B. G. Low & P. J. Hansen (unpublished observations).

The peri-implantation conceptus also secretes proteins that display immunoregulatory properties. At Day 16–17 of pregnancy, a lactosaminoglycan-containing glycoprotein of M_r 800 000–900 000 is secreted (Masters *et al.*, 1982; Newton & Hansen, 1988) that inhibits mixed lymphocyte reactions and phytohaemagglutinin (PHA)-induced lymphocyte proliferation (Murray *et al.*, 1987; Newton *et al.*, 1988; see Fig. 2). Another immunosuppressive protein may be ovine trophoblast protein-1 (oTP-1), an antiluteolytic polypeptide of M_r 17 000 secreted from about Days 13–21 of pregnancy (Godkin *et al.*, 1982; Hansen *et al.*, 1985). There is a strong degree of sequence homology between oTP-1 and the alpha interferons (Imakawa *et al.*, 1987), which are themselves immunosuppressive (Bielefeldt Ohmann *et al.*, 1987). Inhibition of mitogen-stimulated lymphocytes has been associated with fractions of Day-16 conceptus secretory proteins enriched in oTP-1 (Wallace *et al.*, 1984; Newton *et al.*, 1988).

The definitive placenta also produces molecules that inhibit lymphocyte responses *in vitro*. Besides PGE-2, the cotyledonary placenta releases non-dialysable products into culture that inhibit PHA-stimulated lymphocytes (Low *et al.*, 1988; see Fig. 3). The major factor having immunosuppressive activity in cotyledon-conditioned culture medium is a large (M_r >4 × 10^6), heat- and

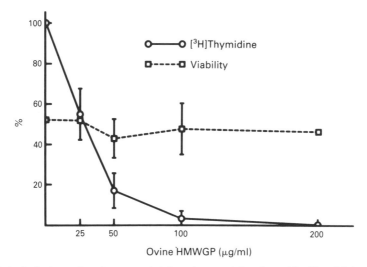

Ovine HMWGP (µg/ml)

Fig. 2. Effect of a lactosaminoglycan-containing glycoprotein released by Day-16 sheep conceptuses on lymphocyte blastogenesis in response to PHA (from Murray *et al.*, 1987). Incorporation of [³H]thymidine is shown in the solid line and is expressed as a percentage of values for control lymphocytes cultured without the glycoprotein. Cell viability (% live after 60 h of culture) as determined by trypan blue staining is shown by the broken line. The immunosuppressive activity of this molecule has been further studied by Newton *et al.* (1988). The molecule was shown to inhibit both early and late events in the proliferative response since inhibitory activity of the glycoprotein could only be partly reversed by delaying addition until 24 h after addition of PHA. In addition, the glycoprotein blocked proliferation induced by interleukin-2, and suppression of PHA-stimulated cells could not be removed by adding exogenous interleukin-2.

protease-stable molecule (Fig. 4). Activity can be destroyed by periodate, suggesting that carbohydrate is a crucial component of the molecule. Staples & Heap (1984) have suggested that ovine pregnancy-associated antigen, a protein existing at molecular weights of 17 000 and 43 000 and which may be of endometrial or placental origin, is an immunosuppressant because it inhibited thymidine incorporation into mitogen-stimulated lymphocytes.

Endometrium-derived immunosuppressive molecules

The endometrium also contributes to local regulation of the immune system. Segerson & Libby (1984) found that lymphocytes derived from curettage of the endometrium at oestrus or Day 14 of the oestrous cycle had lower reactivity towards PHA than did lymphocytes derived from jugular and uterine venous blood. This difference was not observed in ovariectomized ewes, suggesting ovarian regulation of uterine immune function. Uterine flushings obtained during the oestrous cycle can inhibit PHA-induced proliferation and mixed lymphocyte reaction, with activity being greater at Day 14 of the cycle than at Days 4 and 9 (Segerson, 1981).

The presence of uterine immunosuppressants has been studied during mid- and late gestation by creating unilaterally pregnant ewes in which a ligature is placed around the uterine horn contralateral to the side of ovulation early in pregnancy (Bazer *et al.*, 1979). The fluid that collects in this non-pregnant uterine horn at Days 60, 100 and 140 of pregnancy has been found to inhibit mitogen-induced blastogenesis of lymphocytes (Hansen *et al.*, 1987; Stephenson *et al.*, 1988). Most of the immunosuppressive activity is heat- and protease-stable and 50–80% can be removed by dialysis. Some activity can also be seen in the non-dialysable portion of the fluid (Hansen *et al.*, 1987; Stephenson *et al.*, 1988) which elutes at the void volume of a Sepharose CL-6B column (Fig. 5).

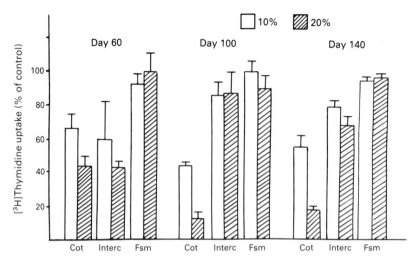

Fig. 3. Immunosuppressive activity in conditioned culture medium from explant cultures of fetal cotyledons (Cot), intercotyledonary chorioallantois (Interc) and fetal skeletal muscle (Fsm) from Days 60, 100 and 140 of pregnancy. Explants were cultured for 24 h and then medium was harvested, dialysed (M_r exclusion limit = 1000) and tested for immunosuppressive activity. Data shown are incorporation of [³H]thymidine of PHA-stimulated lymphocytes cultured with 10 or 20% placenta-conditioned medium. Data are expressed as a percentage of incorporation of control cultures performed without conditioned medium. The most inhibitory material was cotyledon-conditioned medium. This medium was further examined and also inhibited mixed lymphocyte cultures. The medium was not cytotoxic. Activity was stable to heat and proteases but could be destroyed by periodate treatment. (Data are from Low *et al.*, 1988.)

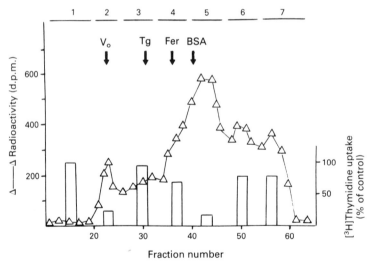

Fig. 4. Resolution of immunosuppressants in conditioned-medium from explant cultures of Day-100 fetal cotyledons using gel filtration. Cotyledonary cultures were performed in the presence of [³H]leucine to label newly synthesized secretory protein (d.p.m.). Conditioned medium was dialysed (M_r exclusion limit = 6000–8000) and separated by gel filtration using Sepharose CL-6B. Fractions were pooled as indicated (1–7) and tested for ability to inhibit thymidine incorporation by PHA-stimulated lymphocytes. A peak of immunosuppressive activity could always be found at the void volume (V_o) (pool 2) and a second peak could sometimes be detected that eluted at M_r = 60 000 (pool 5). Tg = thyroglobulin; Fer = ferritin; BSA = bovine serum albumin. Data for this figure are from Low *et al.* (1988).

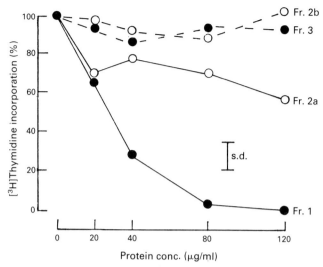

Fig. 5. Resolution of the immunosuppressive molecules in the basic protein fraction of uterine fluid from the non-pregnant uterine horn of unilaterally pregnant ewes at Days 136–140 of pregnancy. Pooled, dialysed (M_r exclusion limit = 12 000–14 000) uterine fluid was separated by cation-exchange chromatography and the basic-protein fraction resolved by gel filtration using Sepharose CL-6B. Data presented are [^{3}H]thymidine incorporation by PHA-stimulated lymphocytes cultured with various protein concentrations of the fractions resolved by gel filtration. Data are expressed as a percentage of values for control lymphocytes cultured without uterine protein fractions. Immunosuppressive activity was present primarily in the fraction that eluted at the void volume of the column (Fr. 1). Data are reproduced from Hansen *et al.* (1987). In other experiments, a similar high-molecular weight immunosuppressant was found in the acidic fraction of uterine fluid (Stephenson *et al.*, 1988).

Because this non-dialysable immunosuppressive factor is of such large molecular weight ($>4 \times 10^6$), we have termed it 'megasuppressin'. While originally described as being in the basic-protein fraction of uterine fluid resolved by cation exchange chromatography (Hansen *et al.*, 1987), a megasuppressin-like material has also been observed in the acidic fraction (Stephenson *et al.*, 1988).

Involvement of progesterone

Progesterone is an important regulator of uterine immune function that may cause production of uterine immunosuppressants during pregnancy. The immunosuppressive actions of progesterone were demonstrated in an experiment showing that administration of this steroid can delay skin graft rejection in the uterine lumen. Hansen *et al.* (1986) placed an autograft and allograft of skin into the uterine lumen of anoestrous sheep that received 0, 50 or 200 mg progesterone/day from 30 days before graft placement until 30 days after. Regardless of treatment, autografts were present in the uterine lumen 30 days after placement. In contrast, allografts placed in the uterine lumen of vehicle-treated ewes were completely resorbed within the lumen. Although in a necrotic condition, all allografts from progesterone-treated ewes were present within the uterus. In contrast, Reimers & Dziuk (1974) were unable to affect allograft rejection in the uterus when lower doses of progesterone were given for a shorter time and in combination with oestrogen.

Progesterone probably altered skin-graft survival by inducing secretion of uterine immunosuppressants: uterine flushings from progesterone-treated ewes have an enhanced ability to inhibit

PHA-stimulated lymphocytes (Hansen *et al.*, 1986; Stephenson & Hansen, 1987). The chemical properties of these immunosuppressants in uterine secretions have been partly characterized (D. C. Stephenson & P. J. Hansen, unpublished observations). The immunosuppressants are very similar to those present in uterine fluids of unilaterally pregnant animals; a dialysable, heat- and protease-stable component and a megasuppressin-like fraction can both be identified. Progesterone is probably not affecting skin-graft survival by acting directly on uterine lymphocytes. Progesterone can directly inhibit lymphocyte proliferation at micromolar concentrations (Staples *et al.*, 1983; see also Fig. 1) but injection of progesterone at 100 mg/day resulted in average serum progesterone concentrations of only 20 ng/ml (i.e. 10^{-8} M; Stephenson & Hansen, 1987).

Are immunosuppressive factors relevant to pregnancy?

Head & Billingham (1984) have called into question the existence of so many immunosuppressants associated with pregnancy. If all these are active, they argue, mammals would have been so susceptible to pathogens during pregnancy that they could not have survived as a group. It should be pointed out, however, that the existence of immunosuppressive molecules in the uterus will not necessarily result in systemic immunosuppression of the pregnant female as long as the molecules remain primarily in the uterus. Also, it is not inconceivable that pregnancy might be associated with some adverse immunological consequences as occurs for other aspects of physiological function.

Whether systemic immunosuppression occurs during gestation in the sheep is controversial (Miyasaka & McCullagh, 1981; Rai-el-Balhaa *et al.*, 1987). Regardless, Head & Billingham's (1984) reservation is a pertinent one because of the apparent ease at which pregnancy-associated immunosuppressants can be discovered. Anyone who has performed cell culture knows that cellular function can be inadvertently inhibited. Consequently, use of the lymphocyte proliferation test to identify immunosuppressants must be done with proper controls and with physiological concentrations of test substances so as to allow one to distinguish artefacts from molecules likely to play an immunological role in pregnancy. In addition, immunosuppressive molecules identified *in vitro* should also be tested for a similar function *in vivo*. When this has been done, as for the effects of progesterone on skin-graft survival (Hansen *et al.*, 1986), the proposed function of the molecule is strengthened.

We thank F. W. Bazer and E. C. Segerson, who made important contributions to several of the experiments described in this paper. Research performed by the authors was supported by NIH (HD 20671).

References

Bazer, F.W., Roberts, R.M., Basha, S.M.M., Zavy, M.T., Caton, D. & Barron, D.H. (1979) Method for obtaining ovine uterine secretions from unilaterally pregnant ewes. *J. Anim. Sci.* **49**, 1522–1527.

Bielefeldt Ohmann, H., Lawman, M.J.P. & Babiuk, L.A. (1987) Bovine interferon: its biology and application in veterinary medicine. *Antiviral Res.* **7**, 187–210.

Clark, D.A., Slapsys, R., Chaput, A., Walker, C., Brierley, J., Daya, S. & Rosenthal, K.L. (1986) Immunoregulatory molecules of trophoblast and decidual suppressor cell origin at the maternofetal interface. *Am. J. reprod. Immun. Microb.* **10**, 100–104.

Evans, C.A., Kennedy, T.G. & Challis, J.R.G. (1982) Gestational changes in prostanoid concentrations in intrauterine tissues and fetal fluids from pregnant sheep, and the relation to prostanoid output in vitro. *Biol. Reprod.* **27**, 1–11.

Ford, C.H.J. & Elves, M.W. (1974) The production of cytotoxic anti-leucocyte antibodies by parous sheep. *J. Immunogenet.* **1**, 259–264.

Godkin, J.D., Bazer, F.W., Moffatt, J., Sessions, F. & Roberts, R.M. (1982) Purification and properties of a major, low molecular weight protein released by the trophoblast of sheep blastocysts at Day 13–21. *J. Reprod. Fert.* **65**, 141–150.

Hansen, P.J., Anthony, R.V., Bazer, F.W., Baumbach, G.A. & Roberts, R.M. (1985) *In vitro* synthesis and secretion of ovine trophoblast protein-1 during the period of maternal recognition of pregnancy. *Endocrinology* **117**, 1424–1430.

Hansen, P.J., Bazer, F.W. & Segerson, E.C. (1986) Skin graft survival in the uterine lumen of ewes treated with progesterone. *Am J. reprod. Immun. Microb.* **12**, 48–54.

Hansen, P.J., Segerson, E.C. & Bazer, F.W. (1987) Characterization of immunosuppressive substances in the basic protein fraction of uterine secretions from pregnant ewes. *Biol. Reprod.* **36**, 393–403.

Head, J.R. & Billingham, R.E. (1984) Mechanisms of non-rejection of the feto-placental allograft. In *Immunological Aspects of Reproduction in Mammals*, pp. 133–152. Ed. D. B. Crighton. Butterworths, London.

Hyland, J.H., Manns, J.G. & Humphrey, W.D. (1982) Prostaglandin production by ovine embryo and endometrium *in vitro. J. Reprod. Fert.* **65**, 299–304.

Imakawa, K., Anthony, R.V., Kazemi, M., Marotti, K.R., Polites, H.G. & Roberts, R.M. (1987) Interferon-like sequence of ovine trophoblast protein secreted by embryonic trophectoderm. *Nature, Lond.* **330**, 377–379.

Low, B.G., Hansen, P.J. & Newton, G.R. (1988) Inhibition of in vitro lymphocyte proliferation by ovine-placenta conditioned culture medium. *J. Anim. Sci.* **66**, (Suppl. 1), 423, Abstr.

Masters, R.A., Roberts, R.M., Lewis, G.S., Thatcher, W.W., Bazer, F.W. & Godkin, J.D. (1982) High molecular weight glycoproteins released by expanding, pre-attachment sheep, pig and cow blastocysts in culture. *J. Reprod. Fert.* **66**, 571–583.

Miyasaka, M. & McCullagh, P. (1981) Immunological responsiveness of maternal and foetal lymphocytes during normal pregnancy in the ewe. *J. reprod. Immun.* **3**, 15–27.

Murray, M.K., Segerson, E.C., Hansen, P.J., Bazer, F.W. & Roberts, R.M. (1987) Suppression of lymphocyte activation by a high-molecular-weight glycoprotein released from preimplantation ovine and porcine conceptuses. *Am. J. reprod. Immun. Microb.* **14**, 38–44.

Newton, G.R. & Hansen, P.J. (1988) Classification of the saccharide portion of a high-molecular-weight glycoprotein secreted by day 16 sheep conceptuses. *J. Anim. Sci.* **66** (Suppl. 1), 74–75, Abstr.

Newton, G.R., Vallet, J.L., Hansen, P.J. & Bazer, F.W. (1988) A high-molecular-weight glycoprotein (HMWG) secreted by the Day 16–17 sheep conceptus inhibits both early and late events in mitogen-induced proliferation of lymphocytes. *J. Anim. Sci.* **66** (Suppl. 1), 424, Abstr.

Rai-el-Balhaa, G., Abdullah, A., Pellerin, J.L., Thibaud, D. & Bodin, G. (1987) Blastogenic response of peripheral blood lymphocytes from multiparous pregnant ewes. *Am. J. reprod. Immun. Microb.* **14**, 110–114.

Reimers, T.J. & Dziuk, P.J. (1974) The survival of intrauterine skin autografts and allografts in sheep. *J. Reprod. Fert.* **38**, 465–467.

Risbridger, G.P., Leach Harper, C.M., Wong, M.H. & Thorburn, G.D. (1985) Gestational changes in prostaglandin production by fetal trophoblast cells. *Placenta* **6**, 117–126.

Segerson, E.C. (1981) Immunosuppressive effect of ovine uterine secretory protein upon lymphocytes in vitro. *Biol. Reprod.* **25**, 77–84.

Segerson, E.C. & Libby, D.W. (1984) Mitogenic response of lymphocytes collected from jugular and uterine veins and the uterine lumen of estrous, day 14 and ovariectomized ewes. *Biol. Reprod.* **30**, 126–133.

Staples, L.D. & Heap, R.B. (1984) Studies of steroids and proteins in relation to the immunology of pregnancy in the sheep. In *Immunological Aspects of Reproduction in Mammals*, pp. 195–218. Ed. D. B. Crighton. Butterworths, London.

Staples, L.D., Binns, R.M. & Heap, R.B. (1983) Influence of certain steroids on lymphocyte transformation in sheep and goats studied *in vitro. J. Endocr.* **98**, 55–69.

Stephenson, D.C. & Hansen, P.J. (1987) Progesterone alters protein secretion and induces immunosuppressants in the uterine lumen of ewes. *J. Anim. Sci.* **65** (Suppl. 1), 413, Abstr.

Stephenson, D.C., Hansen, P.J. & Newton, G.R. (1988) Immunosuppressive properties of uterine fluid from pregnant ewes. *J. Anim. Sci.* **66** (Suppl. 1), 420–421, Abstr.

Wallace, A.L.C., Nancarrow, C.D. & Sutton, R. (1984) Proteins secreted by the 16-day-old sheep blastocyst have immunosuppressive properties. In *Reproduction in Sheep*, pp. 118–120. Eds D. R. Lindsay & D. T. Pearce. Cambridge University Press, Cambridge.

J. Reprod. Fert., Suppl. **37** (1989), 63–68

Printed in Great Britain
© 1989 Journals of Reproduction & Fertility Ltd

Role of macrophages in the maternal recognition of pregnancy

C. Tachi and S. Tachi*

*Zoological Institute, Faculty of Science, University of Tokyo, Hongo, Bunkyo-ku, Tokyo 113, Japan and *Department of Anatomy, Tokyo Women's Medical College, Kawada-cho, Shinjuku-ku, Tokyo 162, Japan*

Keywords: macrophages; blastocysts; implantation; decidua; leukotriene C_4

There is a crucial absence of knowledge concerning the precise nature of the local immune responses elicited in the endometrium by the blastocysts during the early phase of implantation, despite the possible importance of such responses in the early recognition of pregnancy by the maternal immune system. As an approach to the problem, we have been attempting to determine the roles played by macrophages in the immunological recognition of the conceptuses during the peri-implantation period of gestation in the rat and mouse (Tachi, C. *et al.*, 1981; Tachi, C., 1985; Tachi, S. *et al.*, 1985; Tachi, C. & Tachi, 1986). Surprisingly little attention had been paid until relatively recently (Tachi, C. *et al.*, 1981) to this aspect of embryo–maternal relationships in the enigmatic conditions of true viviparity.

Macrophages in the uterus of the rat after implantation

Nicol (1935) histologically analysed the distribution of cells vitally stained with trypan blue in the post-implantation endometrium of the early invasion stage of gestation in guinea-pigs; this dye had been used as a means to demonstrate macrophages in animal tissues (Cappell, 1929).

Curiously, no report dealing with macrophages in the uterus about the time of implantation was published until 1981 when Tachi, C. *et al.* (1981) suggested a possible involvement of macrophages in the early embryo–maternal interactions during implantation.

We demonstrated, at histological as well as ultrastructural levels, that in the rat numerous macrophages appear around the implantation site shortly after the onset of implantation, and that these phagocytes were not present within the decidua (Tachi, C. *et al.*, 1981; Tachi, C. & Tachi, 1986). We inferred from the results that the mobilization of macrophages might be an essential part of the early endometrial responses to implantation and that the decidua might serve as a block regulating the flow of immunological information in the afferent arm of the maternal immune system.

We also analysed quantitatively the distribution of immunocytes which carry IgG, IgA or IgE as a marker on their surfaces, in the uterus of the mouse after implantation, by using FITC-labelled antibodies raised against the respective immunoglobulins (Tachi, C., 1983, 1985; Tachi, C. & Tachi, 1986). One of the salient observations made in this series of the experiments was the lack of FITC-labelled cells within the decidua, regardless of the immunoglobulin classes examined. Rachman *et al.* (1984) and Parr & Parr (1985) analysed the localization of IgA, IgG and IgM in the endo-metrium of pregnant rats. However, no detailed analyses of the distribution of the immunocytes in the endometrium near the implantation chambers were attempted by these authors.

The distribution of FITC-labelled cells in the cross-section of a Day 7 uterus is presented quan-titatively in Fig. 1. In this specimen, <3% of the entire FITC-labelled cell population were found in the decidua. It also can be seen in the figure that more labelled cells were present in the anti-mesometrial area than in the mesometrial area, i.e. ∼48% in the antimesometrial and 22% in the mesometrial region (Tachi, C. 1985). The patterns of the distribution of cells which bind anti-IgA or anti-IgE in the implantation sites closely resembled those obtained for the anti-IgG binding cells (Tachi, C. & Tachi, 1986); the FITC-labelled cells were found at the periphery of the decidua and in the myometrium, but only a few were in the decidua.

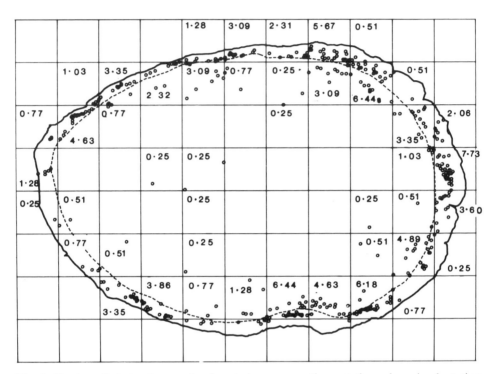

Fig. 1. Tracing of photomicrograph of a uterine cross-section cut through an implantation chamber of a mouse on Day 7 of pregnancy illustrates the distribution of FITC-labelled cells in the area. Each circle indicates the location of a labelled cell. The number in each square indicates the relative number (%) of the labelled cells found within the area. One division of the grid corresponds to ∼600 μm. The tracing was made by means of a microcomputer-based image analysis system developed in our laboratory. (From Tachi, C., 1985.)

These results, taken together, strongly indicated that the decidua indeed functions as an immunological barrier during the peri-implantation period of gestation by preventing the access of not only the macrophages but also other immunocytes to the embryos (Tachi, C. et al., 1981; Tachi, C. & Tachi, 1986).

Although the possible presence of an immunological barrier blocking the afferent arm of the maternal immune system in the endometrium during gestation has been suggested (Beer et al., 1971), the cellular basis of the putative barrier has never been clarified adequately.

Propositions have been made indicating that the decidual cells in the mouse might be ultimate descendants of the bone marrow cells (Kearns & Lala, 1982; Lala et al., 1983) and the decidua does contain several different types of immunocytes which might be responsible for the successful maintenance of the hemi-allogeneic pregnancy (Lala et al., 1986). However, the topographical distribution of immunocytes in the endometrium located near the implantation chamber was not examined by these authors.

Cells which suppressed maternal immune responses against paternal antigens have been isolated from the decidua of the mouse in the advanced stages of gestation (Slapsys & Clark, 1982). The uterine suppressor cells were identified as small lymphocytes (Slapsys & Clark, 1982; Tawfik *et al.*, 1986) and macrophages (Hunt *et al.*, 1984, 1985; Tawfik *et al.*, 1986). No similar studies, however, have been done using the decidua of the early post-implantation period.

Blastocyst–macrophage interactions *in vitro*

A question arises concerning the possible mode of interactions between trophoblast cells and macrophages when they are allowed to come directly in contact with each other. Glass *et al.* (1980) examined, in the mouse, interactions between the trophoblast cells cultured *in vitro* and the macro-phages layered onto them. No detailed analysis of such interactions, however, was attempted by Glass *et al.* (1980). We therefore investigated cell-to-cell interactions between mouse blastocysts and macrophages of allogeneic origin cultured together *in vitro*, at both light and electron microscopic levels (Tachi, S. & Tachi, 1981; Tachi, S. *et al.*, 1985). The results we obtained are summarized below.

In our system, the blastocysts had started trophoblast spreading about 48 h after the start of culture. At the interface between the macrophages and the trophoblast cells, no evidence for either the accumulation or the repulsion of macrophages was clearly recognized. Some of the macro-phages were seen adhering to the trophoblast cell layer during this period; they tended to be localized around the inner cell mass (ICM).

Table 1. Effect of calcium ionophore, cytochalasin B and colchi-cine upon the rate of production of leukotriene C_4 and cellular shape of the purified peritoneal macrophages of the mouse

Additions	Leukotriene production (ng/10^6 cells per h)	Relative proportion of elongated cells (%)
None	1·3	45·5
A23187 (0·5 µg/ml)	112·5	97·5
Cytochalasin B (0·5 µg/ml)	1·18	94·0
Colchicine (0·5 µg/ml)	1·8	83·5

Electron microscopic studies of the periphery of the spread trophoblast revealed that thin cytoplasmic processes were extended from the cells and that such processes were often in contact with the macrophages which appeared as if they were pushed aside by a physical force. No signs of cytotoxicity directed either from the macrophages towards the trophoblast cells or *vice versa* were detected.

Macrophages were found both on the surface of and within the embryos about the 72nd hour of co-culture. No specialized junctions were formed between the macrophages and the embryonic cells. It was not possible, during this series of experiments, to ascertain definitely whether the macrophages were cytotoxic to the ICM cells or not.

In the macrophages co-cultured with blastocysts, cells with distinctly different cellular morphology were present, i.e. those that were rounded, and the rest which were either elongated or spread (unpublished observations).

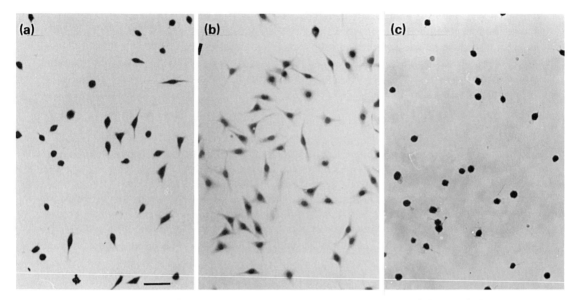

Fig. 2. Photomicrographs showing the light microscopic appearance of the purified macrophages (a) without treatment with drugs, (b) after addition of calcium ionophore (0·5 µg/ml), and (c) after addition of cytochalasin B (0·5 µg/ml). The cells were incubated in MEM containing cysteine (4 mM) but no FCS for 2 h under an atmosphere of 3% CO_2 and 97% air. The cells were fixed with 3·5% formaldehyde in phosphate buffer (pH 7·2) and stained with Giemsa. Scale indicates 10 µm.

To try to answer the question of whether the two macrophage populations of different morphology also differ in their functions we chose leukotriene C_4, which is known to be synthesized by macrophages and released into the medium, as a biochemical marker of macrophage activity, and attempted to correlate the changes in cellular shape with those in the rate of leukotriene C_4 production.

Highly purified macrophages used in this series of experiments (Tachi, C., 1988; Tachi, C. & Zor, 1986; C. Tachi & U. Zor, unpublished) were prepared as described elsewhere (Tachi, C., 1988). The peritoneal lavage was obtained by injecting i.p. Earl's minimum essential medium (MEM) containing heparin (30 U/ml) to the mice under ether anaesthesia; it was layered onto a Ficoll–Hypaque gradient (d = 1·090 ± 0·001) and centrifuged at about 1200 *g*. The white cells collected at the interface between the lavage and the Ficoll–Hypaque were aspirated and immediately suspended in MEM fortified with fetal calf serum at a concentration of 20% (MEM-FCS/20). Aliquants of the suspension were plated onto Falcon dishes. Relatively high concentrations of the serum were used in the initial phase of the culture to limit the non-specific adherence of B-lymphocytes to the dish (Pennline, 1981). The cells were incubated for 1·0 h at 37°C under an atmosphere of 5% CO_2 and 95% air.

At the end of the incubation, the medium was decanted, the non-adherent cells were removed, and fresh MEM-FCS/20 was added to the cells. After further incubation for 1 h, the detached cells were removed as before, and the medium was replaced with fresh MEM containing FCS at a concentration of 10% (MEM-FCS/10); the incubation was then continued for 16 h. Then the medium was changed with fresh MEM-FCS/10 and the cells were incubated for another 24 h under an atmosphere of 2–3% CO_2 and 98–97% air. The slightly alkaline condition of the medium (pH 7·4–7·6) was optimal, under the conditions we used, for the assay of leukotriene C_4 production, particularly under the influence of a calcium ionophore (C. Tachi, unpublished). The cells remaining firmly adhered to the bottom surfaces of the dishes at the end of the incubation represented a highly purified population of macrophages. Immediately before the start of the experiments when the rates of leukotriene C_4 production into the medium was assayed, fresh MEM containing L-cysteine (4 mM) but no FCS was added to the purified macrophages. They were incubated for 1·5–2·0 h, with or without the test substances, i.e. calcium ionophore, colchicine and cytochalasin B. The amount of leukotriene C_4 released into the medium was measured by radioimmunoassay using the monoclonal antibodies which were a generous gift from Dr F. Kohen (Hormone Research Department, the Weizmann Institute of Science, Rehovot, Israel).

The calcium ionophore, A23187, which has been known as a potent stimulant of leukotriene C_4 production in peritoneal (Bach & Brashler, 1978; Bach *et al.*, 1979) and alveolar (Rankin *et al.*, 1982) macrophages of the rat, induced in our system ~100-fold increase in the rate of leukotriene C_4 synthesis. Concomitantly, the ionophore induced strong elongation of the macrophages (Tachi, C. & Zor, 1986; C. Tachi & U. Zor, unpublished) (Table 1; Fig. 2). However, cytochalasin B (Fig. 2) and colchicine caused strong rounding of the macrophages, and had no effect on leukotriene C_4 production (Tachi, C. & Zor, 1986).

It was tentatively concluded that the rounded macrophages found in the co-culture might be inactive, as far as the production of leukotriene C_4 is concerned, while the elongaged ones are likely to be synthesizing leukotriene C_4 at enhanced rates. However, the possibility remains that the morphological changes which are induced under the influence of the drugs might not be representative of those taking place under natural physiological conditions. The relevance of the findings described herein to the actual processes of implantation which take place *in vivo* are currently being investigated.

We thank Dr F. Kohen and Dr M. Moshonov for the supply of monoclonal antibodies against leukotriene C_4. The work was supported in part by a grant from Ministry of Education, Japan, to C.T. (No. 62109006).

References

Bach, M.K. & Brashler, J.R. (1978) Ionophore A 23187-induced production of slow reacting substance of anaphylaxis (SRS-A) by rat peritoneal cells *in vitro*: evidence for production by mononuclear cells. *J. Immunol.* **120**, 998–1005.

Bach, M.K., Brashler, J.R., Brooks, C.D. & Neerken, A.J. (1979) Slow reacting substances: comparison of some properties of human lung SRS-A and two distinct fractions from ionophore-induced rat mononuclear cell SRS. *J. Immunol.* **122**, 160–165.

Beer, A.E., Billingham, R.E. & Hoerr, R.A. (1971) Elicitation and expression of transplantation immunity in the uterus. *Transplant. Proc.* **3**, 609–611.

Cappell, D.F. (1929) Intravital and supravital staining: II. Blood and organs. *J. Pathol. Bacteriol.* **32**, 629–707.

Glass, R.H., Spindle, A.I., Maglio, M. & Pedersen, R.A. (1980) The free surface of mouse trophoblast in culture is non-adhesive for other cells. *J. Reprod. Fert.* **59**, 403–407.

Hunt, J.S., Manning, L.S. & Wood, G.W. (1984) Macrophages in murine uterus are immunosuppressive. *Cell Immunol.* **85**, 499–510.

Hunt, J.S., Manning, L.S., Mitchel, D., Selanders, J.R. & Wood, G.W. (1985) Localization and characterization of macrophages in murine uterus. *J. Leuk. Biol.* **38**, 255–265.

Kearns, M. & Lala, P.K. (1982) Bone-marrow origin of decidual-cell precursors in the pseudopregnant-mouse uterus. *J. exp. Med.* **155**, 1537–1554.

Lala, P.K., Chatterjee-Hasrouni, S., Kearns, M., Montgomery, B. & Colavincenzo, V. (1983) Immunobiology of the feto-maternal interface. *Immunol. Rev.* **75**, 87–116.

Lala, P.K., Kearns, M., Parhar, R.S., Scodras, J. & Johnson, S. (1986) Immunological role of the cellular constituents of the decidua in the maintenance of semi-allogeneic pregnancy. *Ann. N.Y. Acad. Sci.* **476**, 183–205.

Nicol, T. (1935) The female reproductive system in the guinea pig: intravitam staining: fat production: influence of hormones. *Trans. R. Soc. Edinb.* **58**, 449–483.

Parr, M.B. & Parr, E. L. (1985) Immunohistochemical localization of immunoglobulins A, G, and M in the mouse female genital tract. *J. Reprod. Fert.* **74**, 361–370.

Pennline, K. J. (1981) Adherence to plastic or glass surfaces. In *Manual of Macrophage Methodology*, pp. 63–68. Eds H. B. Herscowitz, H. T. Holden, J. A. Bellanti & A. Ghaffer. Marcel Dekker Inc., New York.

Rachman, F., Casimiri, V. & Bernard, O. (1984) Maternal immunoglobulins G, A, and M in mouse uterus and embryo during the postimplantation period. *J. Reprod. Immunol.* **6**, 39–47.

Rankin, J.A., Hitchcock, M., Merrill, W., Bach, M.K., Brashler, J.R. & Askenase, P.W. (1982) IgE-dependent release of leukotriene C_4 from alveolar macrophages. *Nature, Lond.* **297**, 329–331.

Slapsys, R.M. & Clark, D.A. (1982) Active suppression of the host-vs-graft reaction in pregnant mice. IV. Local suppressor cells in decidual and uterine blood. *J. Reprod. Immunol.* **4**, 355–364.

Tachi, C. (1983) Analysis of local immune responses during implantation in the mouse. *Zool. Mag.* **92**, 505, Abstr. (In Japanese.)

Tachi, C. (1985) Mechanisms underlying regulation of local immune responses in the uterus during early gestation of eutherian mammals. I. Distribution of immuno-competent cells which bind anti-IgG antibodies in the post-nidatory uterus of the mouse. *Zool. Sci.* **2**, 341–348.

Tachi, C. (1988) Cellular mechanisms of the interactions between blastocysts and macrophages co-cultured *in vitro. Proc. 2nd A. Meeting Japan Assoc. Basic Reprod. Immunol.* pp. 71–75.

Tachi, C. & Tachi, S. (1986) Macrophages and implantation. *Ann. New York Acad. Sci.* **476**, 158–182.

Tachi, C. & Zor, U. (1986) Possible correlation between the production of leukotriene C_4 and cytoskeletal organization in mouse peritoneal macrophages cultured *in vitro. Zool. Sci.* **3**, 1011, Abstr.

Tachi, C., Tachi, S., Knyszynskki, A. & Lindner, H.R. (1981) Possible involvement of macrophages in embryo-maternal relationships during ovum implantation in the rat. *J. exp. Zool.* **217**, 81–92.

Tachi, S. & Tachi, C. (1981) Interactions between blastocysts and macrophages *in vitro. Acta anat. Nippon* **56**, 241–242, Abstr.

Tachi, S., Knyszynski, A. & Tachi, C. (1985) Mechanisms underlying regulation of local immune responses in the uterus during early gestation of eutherian mammals. II. Electron microscopic studies in the interactions between blastocysts and macrophages cultured together *in vitro. Zool. Sci.* **2**, 671–680.

Tawfik, O.W., Hunt, J.S. & Wood, G.W. (1986) Partial characterization of uterine cells responsible for suppression of murine maternal anti-fetal immune responses. *J. Reprod. Immunol.* **9**, 213–224.

J. Reprod. Fert., Suppl. **37** (1989), 69–78

Maternal immunological recognition of pregnancy in equids

D. F. Antczak and W. R. Allen*

*James A. Baker Institute for Animal Health, New York State College of Veterinary Medicine, Cornell University, Ithaca, New York, USA; and *Thoroughbred Breeders' Association Equine Fertility Unit, Animal Research Station, Cambridge CB3 OJQ, UK*

Summary. There is little evidence for maternal immunological recognition of pregnancy in most species with the striking exception of the members of the genus *Equus*. Almost all mares make strong cytotoxic antibody responses to paternally inherited fetal antigens by Day 60 of gestation. Most of these responses are directed against antigens of the Major Histocompatibility Complex (MHC), which constitutes the primary immunogenetic barrier to successful organ transplantation.

The source of fetal MHC antigens in the pregnant mare appears to be the specialized trophoblast cells of the chorionic girdle region of the developing placenta. These cells invade the endometrium between Days 36 and 38 after ovulation to form the endometrial cups. The progenitor girdle cells express high levels of paternal MHC antigens, while the non-invasive trophoblast cells of the allantochorion and the differentiated trophoblast cells in the mature endometrial cups do not. This expression of MHC antigens by the chorionic girdle cells is unusual for a trophoblast tissue, and differs from most forms of trophoblast studied in other species. The maternal anti-fetal antibody responses of equine pregnancy do not adversely affect fetal development, nor are they required for successful pregnancy. However, it is possible that fetal loss of an immunological nature could occur in rare cases when the immunoregulatory mechanisms of pregnancy break down.

Keywords: pregnancy; immunology; histocompatibility; equids

Introduction

During pregnancy in mammals the maternal immune system must accommodate an antigenically foreign fetus developing in intimate apposition to maternal tissues. In species with long gestations, such as the domestic farm animals and man, this accommodation lasts for extended periods during which the pregnant female must also maintain an adequate immunological defence system. How is this accomplished?

Several hypotheses have been advanced to explain the immunological paradox of mammalian pregnancy. On the one hand there is evidence for local, non-specific, immunological suppression in the uterus, mediated by hormones, other soluble factors and non-lymphoid cells, which protects the conceptus from maternal immunological recognition and attack (Chaouat *et al.*, 1983; Stites & Siiteri, 1983; Hansen *et al.*, 1989). An opposing view holds that certain types of immune responses to the conceptus are necessary for (Faulk *et al.*, 1987), or are at least beneficial to (Athanassakis *et al.*, 1987), mammalian pregnancy. These two hypotheses are mutually contradictory. Much of the evidence in favour of the former view has been generated using in-vitro systems which are fraught with artefacts, while the latter argument is contradicted by the success of pregnancy in many inbred strains of rodents in which immune responses to conventional histocompatibility antigens cannot occur.

A third hypothesis, based primarily upon the immunological neutrality of the trophoblast, is supported by three lines of investigation. First, expression of Major Histocompatibility Complex (MHC) antigens, which are the principal immunogenetic barriers to the success of clinical organ transplantation (Klein, 1986), is regulated such that most trophoblast tissue in contact with maternal circulation does not express either class I or class II MHC molecules (Redman *et al.*, 1984; Ellis *et al.*, 1986). Second, the trophoblast appears to express few antigens which are not shared by other adult tissues (Bulmer & Johnson, 1985; Anderson *et al.*, 1987), thereby rendering the mother tolerant to most trophoblast molecules. Third, there is evidence for an unusual type of suppressor cell in the uterus which may be activated by the interaction between that cell and the developing trophoblast (Clark *et al.*, 1983).

This paper considers the evidence for maternal immunological recognition of pregnancy in the mare in the light of the hypothesis of immunological neutrality of the trophoblast.

Anti-fetal immune responses in equine pregnancy

In pregnant equids there is evidence for both serological and cellular maternal immune responses against paternally inherited fetal antigens. Antibodies cytotoxic for paternal lymphocytes are found in the serum of almost all foaling mares whereas no such antibodies are found in the serum of stallions, geldings or maiden mares (Antczak *et al.*, 1984).

Evidence for cell-mediated maternal responses to fetal antigens is found in the endometrial cup reaction, the culmination of a series of unusual morphological differentiation changes that occur during early placentation and which is unique to equids. Between Days 25 and 36 after ovulation, a discrete, annulate portion of the chorion, known as the chorionic girdle, is thrown into increasingly elongated and complex folds (Figs 1 and 2). The trophoblast cells at the tips of these villi multiply very rapidly and then actively invade the maternal endometrium between Days 36 and 38 (Figs 1 and 3; Allen *et al.*, 1973). Once in the endometrium the cells round up, enlarge greatly and begin secreting gonadotrophic hormone (horse chorionic gonadotrophin; CG) into the maternal circulation. They retain no further physical contact with the fetal membranes and they become aggregated together in the endometrium to form the so-called endometrial cups. These are seen as a circle of ulcer-like endometrial protuberances around the conceptus in the gravid horn between Days 40 and 120 of gestation (Fig. 1; Allen, 1975).

Shortly after their formation at Day 40 the endometrial cups evoke a striking maternal cell-mediated response. This takes the form of an increasing accumulation of lymphocytes, plasma cells, eosinophils and other leucocytes in the endometrial stroma around each cup (Figs 1 and 3). The invading cells form a dense band which tends to wall off the fetal cup cells from the adjacent maternal tissues and they appear to hasten the degeneration and death of the cup cells between Days 80 and 120. Eventually, during Days 100–120 the necrotic cups are sloughed from the surface of the endometrium to lie free within the uterine lumen (Clegg *et al.*, 1954).

The short life-span and apparent cellular destruction of the fetal endometrial cups has many features of allograft rejection. This is supported by the finding that the cellular response to the cups is greatly increased in both mares and female donkeys when they are carrying interspecific hybrid conceptuses, the mule and hinny, respectively (Allen, 1975). No such accumulations of maternal lymphoid cells occur at the feto-maternal border of the non-invasive trophoblast of the allanto-chorion at any stage of gestation in intra- or interspecific pregnancies (Fig. 1; Allen, 1975). The leucocyte response to the endometrial cups is perhaps the most striking example of a cell-mediated immune response to the feto-placental unit described in any species.

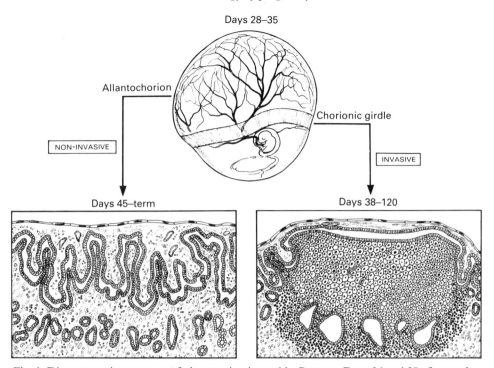

Fig. 1. Diagrammatic summary of placentation in equids. Between Days 36 and 38 after ovulation the specialized trophoblast cells of the annulate chorionic girdle invade the maternal endometrium to form the gonadotrophin (CG)-secreting endometrial cups. Maternal leucocytes surround the cups which degenerate and are sloughed from the endometrium between Days 100 and 120. From Day 45 onwards the non-invasive trophoblast of the allantochorion forms an increasingly complex inter-digitation with the endometrial epithelium over the entire surface of the uterus. However, there is no accumulation of maternal leucocytes in the sub-epithelial endometrial stroma.

First occurrence of maternal immunological recognition of pregnancy

Assay of daily blood samples from pregnant mares for cytotoxic antibodies against paternal lymphocytes first shows the presence of antibody between Days 45 and 70 after ovulation, shortly after invasion of the endometrium by the chorionic girdle cells to form the endometrial cups (Allen, 1979; Antczak *et al.*, 1984). The cellular response to the endometrial cups develops at the same time and, as early as Day 40, small numbers of maternal lymphocytes can be seen at the leading edge of the invading girdle tissue (Fig. 3). The simultaneous appearance of the serological and cellular maternal responses to the conceptus suggests a common antigenic target for these responses.

Type and source of feto-placental antigens

Most of the cytotoxic anti-paternal lymphocyte antibodies produced by mares as a result of allogeneic stimulation during pregnancy are directed against antigens of the Major Histocompatibility Complex, the so-called Equine Lymphocyte Antigen (ELA) system. This has been demonstrated in a number of ways. First, sera from pregnant mares have been the primary source of antisera used to identify the ELA antigens (Antczak *et al.*, 1986). Second, absorption of first pregnancy antisera with lymphocytes from unrelated horses which carry the same MHC types as the mating stallion

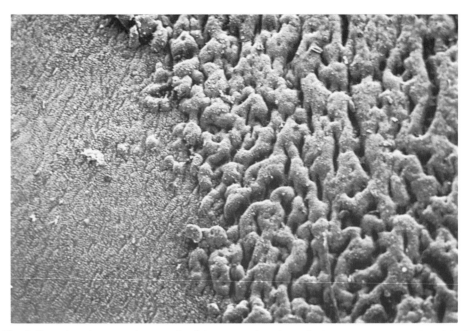

Fig. 2. Scanning electron micrograph of the external surface of a horse conceptus at Day 34 of gestation showing the sharp demarcation between the single cell layer of non-invasive trophoblast of the allantochorion and the villous projections of rapidly multiplying invasive trophoblast cells of the chorionic girdle. × 70.

removes all cytotoxic antibody activity from those sera (Antczak *et al.*, 1982). Third, in experimental matings in which the mare and stallion share the same class I MHC antigens, cytotoxic antibody responses to paternal lymphocyte antigens are usually not detected (Allen *et al.*, 1984).

The MHC codes for two principal types of molecules, the so-called class I and class II histocompatibility antigens. Both are highly polymorphic cell surface glycoproteins (Klein, 1986) and evidence from two types of experiments has shown that anti-MHC antibodies produced in early equine pregnancy are directed almost exclusively against the class I antigens. First, absorption of pregnancy antisera with platelets, which carry class I, but not class II, MHC antigens removes all cytotoxic activity from the sera (Lazary *et al.*, 1980; Antczak, 1984). Second, when using high-titred antisera generated as a result of pregnancy to immunoprecipitate cell-surface molecules from radio-labelled lymphocytes, bands were produced only in the range of M_r 44 000 and 12 000 proteins characteristic of class I antigens, and not in the range (M_r 28 000–34 000) characteristic of class II molecules (Donaldson *et al.*, 1988). There is evidence for the production of maternal anti-fetal antibody responses to non-MHC antigens during equine pregnancy, although such responses occur infrequently (Antczak, 1984).

In an attempt to explain the timing of the maternal antibody responses and the differential cellular responses to the endometrial cups and the allantochorion, the hypothesis was raised that endometrial cup cells, but not the non-invasive trophoblast of the allantochorion, express paternal class I MHC antigens. This was tested in several experiments which revealed unexpected findings.

Effects of maternal immune responses on fetal development

If the endometrial cup reaction is a destructive cellular response to antigens of the feto-placental unit, it should be possible to alter experimentally the intensity of the reaction. This was attempted

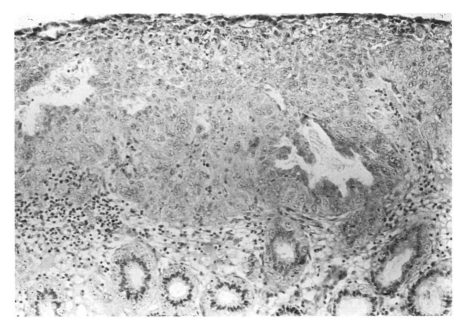

Fig. 3. Low power photomicrograph of a very early endometrial cup at Day 38 of gestation. The invading fetal chorionic girdle cells are seen disrupting the luminal endometrial epithelium and passing down the endometrial glands between the epithelium and the basement membrane. Maternal lymphocytes are already beginning to accumulate in the endometrial stroma. × 120.

through (a) the establishment of pregnancies matched or unmatched for MHC antigens, and (b) by mating mares in 2 consecutive years to a stallion homozygous for an MHC type not carried by the mares. The latter experiment was based on the prediction that secondary immune responses in the repeated pregnancies might produce an accelerated destruction of the endometrial cups relative to that in MHC-incompatible pregnancies established in maiden mares.

The pregnancies were removed surgically at Day 60 to permit sampling of endometrial cups for histological examination. Surprisingly, the leucocyte responses to the cups in MHC-compatible pregnancies appeared as vigorous as those in MHC-incompatible pregnancies, although no cyto-toxic antibody to paternal MHC antigens was detected in the serum of the former mares (Allen *et al.*, 1984). Peak serum concentrations of horse CG and the duration of gonadotrophin secretion were also similar in the two groups. In repeated MHC-incompatible pregnancies strong secondary antibody responses to paternal MHC antigens were generated, thereby demonstrating immunological memory (Antczak *et al.*, 1984). However, there was no histological evidence for any form of anamnestic cellular responses to the endometrial cups in these second pregnancies (unpublished observations). These findings appeared to dissociate the maternal serological responses to paternal MHC antigens from the leucocyte response to the endometrial cups and they suggested that the endometrial cups might not express MHC antigens. A further series of experiments was undertaken to clarify the situation.

Absorption of alloantisera to paternal MHC antigens with fresh endometrial cup tissue from selected pregnancies failed to remove antibody activity consistently from the sera (Crump *et al.*, 1987). Specific absorption was achieved in some experiments but only after repeated absorption of small volumes of antisera with very large volumes of endometrial cup slurry (Allen *et al.*, 1984). Anti-paternal lymphocyte antibody activity was detected in eluates of endometrial cup tissue obtained on Day 60 of gestation although control eluates from non-invasive trophoblast of the allantochorion were not compared in the experiment (Crump *et al.*, 1987). Finally, immunization of horses with isolated endometrial cup tissue failed to produce either primary or secondary antibody responses to paternal MHC antigens (Crump *et al.*, 1987). Taken together, these findings indicated that mature endometrial cup cells either fail to express paternal MHC antigens, or that they do so at very low levels.

Immunohistochemical staining of frozen sections of equine placental tissues obtained between Days 32 and 36 after ovulation revealed that chorionic girdle cells express high levels of paternal MHC antigens, while the adjacent non-invasive trophoblast of the allantochorion is not stained by the same antisera (Crump *et al.*, 1987). The high-titred alloantisera used in the study also precipitated class I, but not class II, MHC antigens from radiolabelled equine lymphocytes (Donaldson *et al.*, 1988). These observations therefore suggested that chorionic girdle cells are the source of paternal MHC antigen which stimulates maternal antibody responses in early equine pregnancy. However, this selective expression of MHC class I antigens is apparently down regulated during transformation of the girdle cells into mature endometrial cup cells.

The presence of strong maternal leucocyte accumulations around the endometrial cups in MHC-compatible pregnancies demonstrates that the target antigens on the cup cells cannot only be MHC antigens. Two other main types of antigens must be considered as candidates: first, the so-called minor histocompatibility antigens which may consist of short fragments of partly digested molecules presented to T-cells by MHC antigens (Loveland & Simpson, 1986; Simpson, 1987); second, molecules expressed only by trophoblast tissue, the so-called trophoblast-specific antigens, to which the mother would not be immunologically tolerant. Minor histocompatibility antigens are detected only by cellular assays and equine minor histocompatibility antigens have not yet been identified.

Monoclonal antibody technology was used to identify trophoblast molecules of the horse. Rats were immunized with isolated horse endometrial cup tissue before fusion of their spleen cells with mouse myeloma cells. Supernatants from over 500 hybrid cell lines secreting antibodies were screened for reactivity with endometrial cups, using an indirect immunoperoxidase assay on cryostat tissue sections. Most antibodies reactive with trophoblast cells also showed broad cross-reactivity with several maternal tissues. Seven of the antibodies showed reactivity that was restricted primarily to horse trophoblast (Antczak *et al.*, 1987a), but only one of these (F67.1) was completely trophoblast specific. This antibody reacts with CG, the principal glycoprotein hormone produced by the endometrial cup cells (Antczak *et al.*, 1987b). Thus, no structural cell surface molecules unique to the horse trophoblast have been identified (Fig. 4).

Discussion

The question arises as to whether the observations on maternal immunological recognition of pregnancy in equids provide a means for choosing between the three hypotheses presented earlier in this paper. Maternal sensitization to paternal MHC antigens in most species, as measured by the production of cytotoxic antibodies reactive with paternal lymphocytes, is a rare event in mammalian pregnancy. For example, it occurs in only about 30% of multiparous women, and in an even lower percentage of primiparous women (see Antczak & Allen, 1984). It could be argued that this relative sparsity of antibody production is evidence for local immunosuppression in the uterus. However, the strong cytotoxic antibody responses of early equine pregnancy demonstrate that the uterus of the mare is a good environment for the induction of both primary and secondary immune responses. It is unlikely, therefore, that local, non-specific immunosuppression in the endometrium plays an important role in the maintenance of pregnancy.

The expression of high levels of paternal MHC antigens by the chorionic girdle cells provides a source of foreign histocompatibility antigens at the appropriate time of pregnancy to account for the temporal correlation between the appearance of antibody and the development of the endometrial cups. Pregnancies develop normally to term in mares that show very high titres of antibodies to

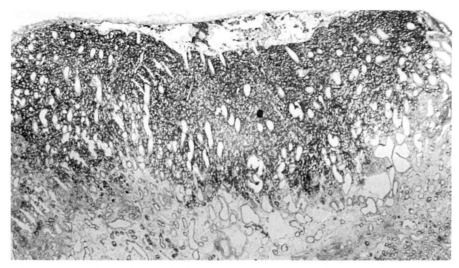

Fig. 4. Low power photomicrograph of an endometrial cup at Day 60 of gestation. The external surface of the fetal endometrial cup cells, but not the overlying non-invasive trophoblast of the allantochorion or the other maternal tissues, is stained specifically with mAb 71.8 (Antczak *et al.*, 1987a) in an indirect immunoperoxidase staining system. × 30.

paternal MHC antigens. The probable reason that such antibodies are ineffective in harming the conceptus is that the trophoblast, with the exception of the specialized cells of the chorionic girdle, fails to express MHC antigens.

The loss of polar trophoblast that occurs between Days 9 and 12 on the equine blastocyst exposes epiblast cells of the embryo to the surface (Enders *et al.*, 1988). However, between Days 6 and 20 the equine conceptus is enveloped by an acellular capsule (Bousquet *et al.*, 1987) which would mask any histocompatibility antigens expressed by the early embryo. It is therefore unlikely that maternal anti-fetal immune responses would be generated during the first 3 weeks of gestation, and none has been observed. Furthermore, maternal antibodies generated in previous pregnancies would probably be unable to reach target cells of the blastocyst while they are protected by the capsule.

The success of MHC-compatible pregnancies in mares demonstrates that immune responses to currently identified equine MHC antigens are not necessary for fetal development. This is consistent with the fertility of many inbred strains of rodents and suggests that histocompatibility differences between mother and fetus may not be required for successful pregnancy. The validity of the second hypothesis is therefore in doubt.

The maternal anti-fetal immune responses measurable in equine pregnancy support the third hypothesis of the immunological neutrality of at least the non-invasive trophoblast. The maturation-related loss of expression of MHC antigens by endometrial cup cells can explain our failure to alter the intensity of the maternal leucocyte response to the cups by increasing or decreasing the feto-maternal differences at the class I MHC barrier. Furthermore, the strong leucocyte accumulations around the endometrial cups observed in mares carrying MHC-compatible pregnancies suggests one of two possibilities; namely, the target of the mononuclear cells is not MHC antigen, or the leucocyte accumulations do not represent a destructive immune response. One consequence of the lack of expression of MHC antigens by trophoblast cells is that immune responses to antigens which can be recognized only in conjunction with MHC antigens will be unlikely to occur; MHC-restricted T cell responses to minor histocompatibility antigens fall into this category. The paucity of trophoblast-specific molecules in the horse, and in other species (Anderson *et al.*, 1987), further limits the range of the antigenic targets on trophoblast and, consequently, the potential for maternal anti-fetal immune responses.

In women there is evidence that the trophoblast cells in contact with maternal blood do not express either class II or the classical polymorphic class I MHC antigens. However, a class I-like molecule with a slightly lower molecular weight than that of the HLA-A, -B antigens has been detected using monoclonal antibody W6/32 (Ellis *et al.*, 1986). Comparable investigations have not been reported for the domestic farm animals, with the exception of the horse.

The third and final part of the hypothesis of immunological neutrality of the trophoblast concerns the evidence for an unusual type of immunoregulatory cell in the uterus (Clark *et al.*, 1983). It is possible that the maternal leucocytes which surround the endometrial cups comprise a diversity of cell types, one of which might have immunosuppressive properties. Our failure to demonstrate traditional immunological attributes to the leucocytes around the cups supports this possibility.

An unusual and particularly interesting feature of the genus *Equus* is the ready ability of its member species to (a) conceive and give birth to a full range of interspecific hybrid offspring (Gray, 1954; Short, 1975) and (b) accept and carry to term a wide range of true, extraspecific conceptuses resulting from between-species embryo transfer (Allen, 1982; Davies *et al.*, 1985; Allen *et al.*, 1987). An important feature of placentation in these inter- and extraspecific equine pregnancies is the marked increase which occurs in the intensity of the maternal leucocyte response to the fetal endometrial cups. For example, in mares carrying interspecific mule conceptuses (male horse × female donkey), very large numbers of lymphocytes begin to accumulate around the cups within a few days of their formation at Day 36–38. Instead of remaining clustered together in a band at the periphery of the cup tissues as described previously for normal intraspecific pregnancies, the lymphocytes begin to invade the cup tissue immediately, thereby hastening the death and degeneration of the cups and the disappearance of horse CG from maternal blood by as early as Day 60–70 of gestation (Allen, 1975). The marked increase in the leucocyte accumulation around the cups in inter- and extraspecific pregnancies strongly suggests that the fetal cup cells express paternally derived antigens which can be recognized by the maternal immune system, and, in addition, that the endometrial cup reaction has a strong immunological component.

One type of extraspecific equine pregnancy which appears to differ markedly from all others is that which results from the transfer of donkey embryos to recipient horse mares. In this case the conceptus seems to develop normally to Day 60–70, but in the absence of any endometrial cup development and CG secretion due to the complete failure of the donkey chorionic girdle to invade the endometrium of the surrogate mare at Day 36. Some 30% of donkey-in-horse pregnancies are able to achieve a sufficient degree of implantation to enable the fetus to continue developing (Allen *et al.*, 1987). In the remaining 70% of pregnancies, however, the non-invasive trophoblast of the enlarging donkey allantochorion lies closely apposed to, but fails to initiate interdigitation with, the horse endometrium. Increasing numbers of lymphocytes and other leucocytes accumulate in the sub-epithelial endometrial stroma throughout the area of endometrium that is in contact with the donkey placenta. The fetus itself becomes progressively more cachexic and wasted in appearance and the amniotic fluid assumes a claret colour due to haemolysis of fetal red blood cells. The accumulated leucocytes begin to pass through the endometrial epithelium, apparently to attack the xenogeneic trophoblast and eventually, between Days 80 and 90 in most cases, the degenerating fetus and pale autolysing placenta are aborted in conjunction with a decline in maternal peripheral plasma progesterone concentrations to baseline values and the consequent relaxation of the cervix (Allen, 1982).

The fact that a domestic mare (*Equus caballus*, 2n = 64) will carry to term a Grant's zebra (*Equus burchelli*, 2n = 46) extraspecific foal (Bennett & Foster, 1985; Kydd *et al.*, 1985) which differs so markedly in genotype and phenotype from itself, and yet will abort the much more genetically similar donkey (*Equus assinus*, 2n = 62) extraspecific foal in association with what appears to be an intense cell-mediated maternal immune rejection response, demands an explanation. The endometrial cup reaction would appear to be the key. It occurs to various degrees in all the successful inter- and extraspecific pregnancy types examined to date, yet is completely absent in the much less successful donkey-in-horse model.

It seems reasonable to suspect that the leucocytes attracted to the fetal endometrial cup cells constitute a much more complex and necessary maternal immune reaction than the rather simple and straight-forward cytotoxic T cell response it has been assumed to be in the past (Allen, 1975). It could well be that specialized uterine lymphocytes with suppressor functions, similar to the non-T-lineage uterine suppressor cells identified in the decidua of pregnant mice (Clark *et al.*, 1983), make up a significant proportion of the leucocytes around the endometrial cups. A vital function of endometrial cup development in normal equine pregnancy may be to present paternally inherited fetal antigens expressed on trophoblast to the mother in such a manner as to stimulate a suppressor cell-mediated immunoprotective type of response within the uterus, rather than the alternative immunodestructive reaction involving cytotoxic T-cells. Investigations of the composition and function of endometrial leucocytes in the mare are hampered by the lack of markers for horse leucocyte subpopulations. However, recent progress in this area (Wyatt *et al.*, 1988; Crump *et al.*, 1988) provides hope for the resolution of questions concerning this unique aspect of equine pregnancy. The evidence already in hand concerning maternal immunological recognition of pregnancy in horses makes this a fascinating and valuable model system.

Research described in this paper was supported by grants from the NIH, USDA, the Zweig Memorial Fund, the Dorothy Russell Havemeyer Foundation, Inc., the Thoroughbred Breeders' Association of Great Britain, and the British Horserace Betting Levy Board.

We thank Dr Elizabeth Lawson for assistance with the preparation of the scanning electron micrograph.

References

Allen, W.R. (1975) Immunological aspects of equine endometrial cup reaction. In *Immunobiology of the Trophoblast*, pp. 217–253. Eds R. G. Edwards, C. Howe & M. H. Johnson. Cambridge University Press, Cambridge.

Allen, W.R. (1979) Maternal recognition of pregnancy and immunological implications of trophoblast-endometrium interactions in equids. In *Maternal Recognition of Pregnancy* (Ciba Fdn Colloq. No. 64), pp. 323–352. Excerpta Medica, London.

Allen, W.R. (1982) Immunological aspects of the endometrial cup reaction and the effect of xenogeneic pregnancy in horses and donkeys. *J. Reprod. Fert., Suppl.* **31**, 57–94.

Allen, W.R., Hamilton, D.W. & Moor, R.M. (1973) The origin of equine endometrial cups. II. Invasion of the endometrium by trophoblast. *Anat. Rec.* **177**, 485–501.

Allen, W.R., Kydd, J., Miller, J. & Antczak, D.F. (1984) Immunological studies on feto-maternal relationships in equine pregnancy. In *Immunological Aspects of Reproduction in Mammals*, pp. 183–193. Ed. D. B. Crighton. Butterworths, London.

Allen, W.R., Kydd, J., Boyle, M.S. & Antczak, D.F. (1987). Extraspecific donkey-in-horse pregnancy as a model of early fetal death. *J. Reprod. Fert., Suppl.* **35**, 197–209.

Anderson, D.J., Johnson, P.M., Alexander, N.J., Jones, W.R. & Griffin, P.D. (1987) Monoclonal antibodies to human trophoblast and sperm antigens: report of two WHO-sponsored Workshops, June 30, 1986-

Toronto. Canada. *J. Reprod. Immunol.* **10**, 231–257.

Antczak, D.F. (1984) Lymphocyte alloantigens of the horse III. ELY-2.1: a lymphocyte alloantigen not coded by the MHC. *Anim. Bld Grps. and Biochem. Genetics* **15**, 103–115.

Antczak, D.F. & Allen, W.R. (1984) Invasive trophoblast in the genus Equus. *Annls Immunol.,—Inst. Pasteur* **135D**, 325–331, 341–342.

Antczak, D.F., Bright, S.M., Remick, L.H. & Bauman, B.E. (1982) Lymphocyte alloantigens of the horse. 1. Serologic and genetic studies. *Tissue Antigens* **20**, 172–187.

Antczak, D.F., Miller, J.M. & Remick, L.H. (1984) Lymphocyte alloantigens of the horse II. Antibodies to ELA antigens produced during equine pregnancy. *J. Reprod. Immunol.* **6**, 283–297.

Antczak, D.F., Bailey, E., Barger, B., Bernoco, D., Bull, R.W., Byrns, G., Guerin, G., Lazary, S., McClure, J., Mottironi, V.D., Symons, R., Templeton, J. & Varewyck, H. (1986) Joint Report of the Third International Workshop on Lymphocyte Alloantigens of the Horse, held 25–27 April 1984, Kennett Square, PA. *Animal Genetics* **17**, 363–373.

Antczak, D.F., Poleman, J.C., Stenzler, L.M., Volsen, S.G. & Allen, W.R. (1987a) Monoclonal antibodies to equine trophoblast. *Trophoblast Research* **2**, 199–214.

Antczak, D.F., Oriol, J.G., Donaldson, W.L., Poleman, J.C., Stenzler, L., Volsen, S.G. & Allen W.R. (1987b) Differentiation molecules of the equine trophoblast. *J. Reprod. Fert., Suppl.* **35**, 371–378.

Athanassakis, I., Bleackley, R.C., Paetkau, V., Guilbert, L., Barr, P.J. & Wegmann, T.G. (1987) The immunostimulatory effect of T cells and T cell lymphokines on murine fetally derived placental cells. *J. Immunol.* **138**, 37–44.

Bennett, S.D. & Foster, W.R. (1985) Successful transfer of a zebra embryo to a domestic horse. *Equine vet. J., Suppl.* **3**, 78–79.

Bousquet, D., Guillomot, M. & Betteridge, K.J. (1987) Equine zona pellucida and capsule: some physiochemical and antigenic properties. *Gamete Res.* **16**, 121–132.

Bulmer, J.M. & Johnson, P.M. (1985) Antigen expression by trophoblast populations in the human placenta and their possible immunobiological relevance. *Placenta* **6**, 127–140.

Chaouat, G., Kolb, J.P. & Wegmann, T.G. (1983) The murine placenta as an immunological barrier between the mother and the fetus. *Immunological Reviews* **75**, 31–60.

Clark, D.A., Slapsys, R.M., Croy, B.A. & Rossant, J. (1983) Suppressor cell activity in the uterine decidua correlates with success or failure of murine pregnancies. *J. Immunol.* **131**, 540–542.

Clegg, M.T., Boda, J.M. & Cole, H.H. (1954) The endometrial cups and allantochorionic pouches in the mare with emphasis on the source of equine gonadotropin. *Endocrinology* **54**, 448–463.

Crump, A., Davidson, W.L., Miller, J., Kydd, J., Allen, W.R. & Antczak, D.F. (1987) Expression of Major Histocompatibility Complex (MHC) antigens on equine trophoblast. *J. Reprod. Fert., Suppl.* **35**, 379–388.

Crump, A.L., Davis, W. & Antczak, D.F. (1988) A monoclonal antibody identifying a T-cell marker in the horse. *Animal Genetics* (in press).

Davies, C.J., Antczak, D.F. & Allen, W.R. (1985). Reproduction in mules: embryo transfer using sterile recipients. *Eq. vet. J., Suppl.* **3**, 63–67.

Donaldson, W.L., Crump, A.L., Zhang, C., Kornbluth, J., Kamoun, M., Davis, W. & Antczak, D.F. (1988) At least two loci encode polymorphic class I MHC antigens in the horse. *Animal Genetics* **19**, 349–357.

Ellis, S.A., Sargent, I.L., Redman, C.W.G. & McMichael, A.J. (1986) Evidence for a novel HLA antigen on human extravillous trophoblast and a choriocarcinoma cell line. *Immunology* **59**, 595–601.

Enders, A.C., Lantz, K.C., Liu, I.K.M. & Schlafke, S. (1988) Loss of polar trophoblast during differentiation of the blastocyst of the horse. *J. Reprod. Fert.* **83**, 447–460.

Faulk, W.P., McIntyre, J.A., Kajino, T. & Torry, D. (1987) TA1 and TLX antigens in human pregnancy. *Colloque INSERM* **154**, 51–62.

Gray, A.P. (1954) *Mammalian Hybrids*, pp. 45–59. Commonwealth Agricultural Bureaux, Farnham Royal, Bucks.

Hansen, P.J., Stephenson, D.C., Low, B.G. & Newton, G.R. (1989) Modifications of immune function during pregnancy by products of the sheep uterus and conceptus. *J. Reprod. Fert., Suppl.* **37**, 55–61.

Klein, J. (1986) *Natural History of the Major Histocompatibility Complex*. John Wiley, New York.

Kydd, J., Boyle, M.S., Allen, W.R., Shephard, A. & Summers, P.M. (1985) Transfer of exotic equine embryos to domestic horses and donkeys. *Equine vet. J., Suppl.* **3**, 80–83.

Lazary, S., de Weck, A.L., Bullen, S., Straub, R. & Gerber, H. (1980) Equine leucocyte antigen system. I. Serological studies. *Transplantation* **30**, 203–209.

Loveland, B. & Simpson, E. (1986) The non-MHC transplantation antigens: neither weak nor minor. *Immunology Today* **7**, 223–229.

Redman, C.W.G., McMichael, A.J., Stirrat, G.M., Sunderland, C.A. & Ting, A. (1984) Class I major histocompatibility complex antigens on human extravillous trophoblast. *Immunology* **52**, 457–468.

Short, R.V. (1975) The evolution of the horse. *J. Reprod. Fert., Suppl.* **23**, 1–6.

Simpson, E. (1987) Non-H-2 histocompatibility antigens: can they be retroviral products? *Immunology Today* **8**, 176–177.

Stites, D.P. & Siiteri, P.K. (1983) Steroids as immunosuppressants. *Immunological Reviews* **75**, 117–138.

Wyatt, C.R., Davis, W.C., McGuire, T.C. & Perryman, L.E. (1988) T lymphocyte development in horses I. Characterization of monoclonal antibodies identifying three stages of T lymphocyte differentiation. *Vet. Immun. Immunopath.* **18**, 3–18.

J. Reprod. Fert., Suppl. **37** (1989), 79–84

Immunopotentiation and pregnancy loss

V. Toder, D. Strassburger, H. Carp, Y. Irlin*, S. Lurie*, M. Pecht* and N. Trainin*

Department of Embryology & Teratology, Tel-Aviv University Medical School, Tel-Aviv 69978, Israel; and *Weizmann Institute of Sciences, Rehovot, Israel

Summary. To test the hypothesis that immunopotentiation of the maternal immune system is beneficial for the developing embryo, we examined (1) the effect of specific preimmunization with paternal leucocytes in women and BALB/c splenocytes in CBA/J × DBA/2J mice (which show increased % fetal resorption) and (2) the influence of non-specific potentiators such as complete Freund's adjuvant and thymus humoral factor on the abortion rate in CBA/J mothers. Subsequent pregnancy was successful in 76% of habitually aborting women after immunization with paternal leucocytes. Immunization of CBA/J mice with complete Freund's adjuvant (2 foot-pad injections) decreased the resorption rate (11·3% vs 34·9% without treatment). The effect was followed by a slight decrease of the L_3H_4-positive lymphocyte subpopulation in the spleen but not in the draining lymph nodes, as measured by flow cytometry analysis. The amount of Lyt-2 positive lymphocytes was not changed as a result of treatment. Thymus humoral factor did not influence the abortion rate in CBA/J females mated with DBA/2J male mice. Our results show that non-specific stimulation of the maternal immune system by complete Freund's adjuvant can improve reproductive success in allogeneic mice with increased pregnancy loss. The exact mechanism of this improvement is still unclear but it seems that systemic cellular mechanisms are not responsible for the effect.

Keywords: pregnancy wastage; animal models; immunopotentiation; maternal recognition; T cell phenotypes

Introduction

Numerous observations of the past decade indicate that maternal recognition of fetal and allo-antigens is of great importance. Active maternal immune responses following early events during pregnancy may play an essential role in conferring selective benefits upon the feto-placental unit from the time of implantation to parturition. The immunological processes responsible for the immunoprotection of the developing embryo are deviant in women with repeated pregnancy loss (Beer, 1985). Several authors have observed that such patients can have their pregnancies successfully brought to term by immunization with paternal or donor leucocytes (Beer *et al.*, 1981; Taylor & Faulk, 1981; Mowbray *et al.*, 1983).

There is a murine allogeneic pregnancy model of habitual abortion in which CBA/J females (H-2^k) are mated with DBA/2J males (H-2^d). These females show a high incidence of fetal resorptions (Clark *et al.*, 1980). Preimmunization of CBA/J females with BALB/c splenocytes compatible with the paternal strain at the Major Histocompatibility Complex (MHC) was able to reverse the tendency to resorb the pregnancy (Chaouat *et al.*, 1983; Clark *et al.*, 1987). Using preimmunization with the spleen cells from various congenic H-2^d strains it was suggested that paternal H-2^d haplotypes must be presented in synergy with some non-MHC-encoded antigens (Kiger *et al.*, 1985).

In women and these mice, reduction of fetal wastage was achieved by the stimulation of the maternal immune system with an additional specific trigger. In addition to data showing the success of specific preimmunization (paternal leucocytes in women and BALB/c splenocytes in the CBA/J × DBA/2J mouse mating combination), we suggest here an alternative approach to potentiate the maternal immune system.

Materials and Methods

Patients. More than 300 women with 3 or more spontaneous abortions were evaluated at the Habitual Abortion Clinic of the Sheba Medical Center. Patients who have no genetic, morphological, endocrinological or other cause for their pregnancy losses are offered treatment by immunization with paternal leucocytes. (The protocol has been approved by the Ethical Committee for experimentation on man of the Israel Ministry of Health.)

Maternal anti-paternal cytotoxic antibody was tested using the standard NIH long-cross math technique (Mittal *et al.*, 1968). The immunization of patients was performed twice with an interval of 4 weeks using intradermal and subcutaneous injection of 60–80 × 10^6 paternal leucocytes (Carp *et al.*, 1988).

Mice. CBA/J (H-2^k), DB2/2J (H-2^d) and BALB/cJ (H-2^d) mice were purchased from Jackson Laboratory (Bar Harbor, Maine, USA).

CBA/J females were checked for oestrus, caged overnight with DBA/2J males and examined for a vaginal plug next morning. The day of finding the plug was considered as Day 1 of pregnancy.

Treatment. To achieve a specific immunopotentiation, CBA/J female mice were immunized i.p. with 3 × 10^7 spleen cells 7 days before mating. BALB/cJ or CBA/J males were used as a source of spleen. Complete Freund's adjuvant (Difco) was injected into the foot pads on Days 1 and 8 of pregnancy in a dose of 0·1 ml.

Thymus humoral factor, obtained from calf thymus as described by Kook *et al.* (1975), was given by 10 daily i.p. injections starting from Day 4 of pregnancy in a dose of 10 mg/kg in 0·1 ml saline.

Control groups of CBA/J females received 10 i.p. injections of saline (9 g NaCl/l) or 2 foot pad injections of Incomplete Freund's Adjuvant (Difco).

Fetal resorption. CBA/J females were checked for resorption of their fetuses on Day 13 of pregnancy by scoring the number of resorbing and viable fetuses. The resorbing fetuses were notably smaller and usually haemorrhagic when compared with the viable fetuses. Statistical analyses were performed by means of χ^2 tests.

Preparation of cells and media. Lymph nodes draining the uterus and spleen were aseptically removed and dispersed into RPMI-1640 medium (Biolab, Jerusalem, Israel) by pressing through a stainless-steel mesh as described elsewhere (Toder *et al.*, 1982). The cells were washed and resuspended in RPMI-1640 medium supplemented with 5 × 10^{-5} M-2-mercaptoethanol, 25 mM-Hepes buffer (Biolab), 100 µg streptomycin/ml and 100 units penicillin/ml (Teva, Jerusalem, Israel).

Flow cytometric analysis. The resulting spleen and lymph node cells were freed from red cells by distilled water lysis for 15 sec followed by restoration to isotonicity with PBS. The lymphocytes were incubated with Anti-L_3H_4 or Anti-Lyt-2 monoclonal antibody (Becton-Dickinson, CA, USA) for 30 min at room temperature. After two washes the cells were exposed to FITC-labelled secondary antibody (Bio-Makor, Jerusalem, Israel) for another 30 min at 4°C in the dark. The cells were washed and fixed in 0·5% paraformaldehyde for 18 h at 4°C in the dark. The expression of surface markers was evaluated using a Fluorescein Activated Cell Sorter (FACS 440, Becton-Dickinson).

Results

Specific stimulation of maternal immune system

Two basic models were chosen to demonstrate the effect of specific immune triggers on maternal recognition of fetal histocompatibility antigens.

Human model. The presence of anti-paternal cytotoxic antibody is generally accepted as an indication of maternal immune recognition and response towards paternal histocompatibility antigens. These antibodies are found in 30–70% of healthy women (Gazit *et al.*, 1977; Beard *et al.*, 1983). Table 1 shows the incidence of antibody-positive patients in our population of habitually aborting women. Antibodies were detected in only 11 of 79 women of this group. To date about 90% antibody-negative women with repeated pregnancy loss converted to antibody-positive after the immunization with paternal leucocytes. More than 76% such women succeeded in their subsequent pregnancies (Table 2). Of 14 women who were antibody-positive without immunization, 11 subsequently delivered a normal child. In the group of patients who did not develop anti-paternal cytotoxic antibody, 54% women aborted again (Table 2).

Table 1. Anti-paternal cytotoxic antibody in habitually aborting women

	Non-immunized	Immunized
Total no. of patients	82	44
Antibody-negative	68 (83%)	13 (29%)
Antibody-positive	14 (17%)	31 (71%)

Table 2. Anti-paternal antibody and pregnancy success in women

	Antibodies present	No. of pregnant women	% of successful pregnancies†
Non-immunized	+	14	78*
	−	21	38
Immunized	+	54	76*
	−	13	46

†As a proportion of total number of patients.
*$P < 0.005$ (χ^2 test).

Murine model. CBA/J females (H-2^k) showing a high rate of spontaneous resorptions after mating with DBA/2J males (H-2^d) were preimmunized with BALB/c (H-2^d) splenocytes compatible with MHC antigens of paternal strain. When injected 2–4 weeks before mating, these splenocytes were able to prevent further pregnancy loss (9·5% vs 34·7%). The immunization did not influence the number of implantations in CBA/J mothers (Table 3). CBA/J (H-2^k) splenocytes could not decrease the resorption rate (26·9% vs 34·7%).

Table 3. Effect of immunostimulation on pregnancy loss in CBA/J × DBA/2J mice

Treatment	No. of mice	No. of implantations per mouse	% of fetal resorptions‡
None	37	8·1 ± 0·8	34·7
Thymic humoral factor	18	8·1 ± 0·9	28·5
Complete Freund's adjuvant	22	8·2 ± 1·3	11·3*
BALB/cJ splenocytes	11	8·3 ± 0·8	9·5*
CBA/J splenocytes	10	8·0 ± 0·7	26·9

†Values are mean ± s.e.
‡Calculated as a proportion of total (R/R + F) × 100 where R = resorptions and F = undamaged fetuses.
*$P < 0.005$ (χ^2 test).

Non-specific stimulation of maternal immune system

Two non-specific immunopotentiators, complete Freund's adjuvant and thymic humoral factor were injected to CBA/J mothers mated with DBA/2J males. Table 3 shows that 2 foot pad injections of complete Freund's adjuvant could reverse the tendency to fetal loss in CBA/J mothers (11·3% *vs* 34·7%). Ten subsequent injections of thymic humoral factor did not decrease significantly the number of fetal resorptions (28·5% *vs* 34·7%). Neither regimen influenced the number of implantation sites (Table 3).

An attempt was made to evaluate possible phenotypic changes in the T-cell population in treated CBA/J mothers. Cell suspensions from the spleen and draining lymph nodes were characterized by indirect immunofluorescence using anti-L_3H_4 and anti-Lyt-2 monoclonal antibodies after FACS analysis. It can be seen from Table 4 that there is a slight decrease of L_3H_4 but not of Lyt-2-positive splenocytes in adjuvant-treated CBA/J mothers as compared to the splenocytes of control mice. Thymic humoral factor did not affect the spleen-derived T-cell population. Neither L_3H_4 nor Lyt-2-positive lymphocyte populations in the draining lymph nodes were affected after treatment by immunopotentiators (Table 4).

Table 4. Incidence of L_3H_4 and Lyt-2-positive lymphocytes in lymphoid organs of CBA/J mice*

Origin of lymphocytes	Treatment	No. of experiments	% of L_3H_4-positive cells	% of Lyt-2-positive cells
Spleen	—	7	18·0 ± 3·0	10·9 ± 2·2
	CFA	6	9·8 ± 1·6	7·5 ± 0·6
	THF	5	12·1 ± 4·1	9·4 ± 2·4
	BALB/c splenocytes	3	15·8 ± 3·6	8·1 ± 1·4
Paraaortic lymph nodes	—	7	40·5 ± 3·8	25·8 ± 5·0
	CFA	5	37·1 ± 3·1	24·6 ± 0·1
	THF	5	41·1 ± 2·4	23·1 ± 3·4
	BALB/c splenocytes	3	40·8 ± 3·5	23·7 ± 2·9

Values are mean ± s.e.
*CBA/J females were mated with DBA/2J males. Lymphoid organs were taken on Day 13–14 of pregnancy.

Discussion

According to our working hypothesis maternal recognition of fetal and/or alloantigens at the feto-maternal interface following maternal immune responses creates various selective immune benefits for the developing embryo. These benefits include specialization of immune responses, e.g. the switching to non-complement fixing IgG_1 in pregnancy serum (Bell & Billington, 1983), accumulation of suppressor cells at the implantation site in human and mouse uterine decidua (Clark *et al.*, 1984, 1985), and non-specific suppressor activity of placental products (Chaouat *et al.*, 1983, 1985). In parallel, maternal T lymphocytes may produce various growth factors such as IL-3 and CSF-GM which may in turn stimulate trophoblast growth (Wegmann, 1984; Athanassakis *et al.*, 1987; Toder, 1988). Also, some non-T cell factors such as epidermal growth factor and placental cells-derived colony-stimulating factors may play roles in trophoblast development (Tsutsumi & Oka, 1987; Toder, 1988). It seems that maternal recognition is impaired in females with repeated pregnancy loss. Our results show a significant decrease of anti-paternal cytotoxic antibodies in the sera of habitually aborting women. An even lower incidence of these antibodies has been found in habitual aborters by Beard *et al.* (1983). The importance of maternal recognition is evident among the antibody-positive patients. After leucocyte immunization about 76% succeeded in their subsequent pregnancies. This is significantly higher than in the group of antibody-negative women with a history of pregnancy loss. The results concur with those of other groups (Mowbray, 1986; Beer *et al.*, 1986). Splenocyte vaccination of CBA/J females mated with DBA/2J males and showing a high rate of spontaneous resorptions also significantly reduces the incidence of abortion. This effect goes along with an increase of local non-specific suppressor activity (Chaouat *et al.*, 1985; Clark *et al.*, 1987).

We have shown here that the high resorption rate in CBA/J mice females can be reversed by the injection of complete Freund's adjuvant. The mechanism by which the abortion rate decreases after immunization with this adjuvant remains obscure although fractions of tubercle bacilli were shown to act as potentiators of cell-mediated immune reactivity and especially of antibody responsiveness (Halperin *et al.*, 1985). Our first attempts to clarify the possible mechanisms of action of complete Freund's adjuvant show that, besides a slight decrease of L_3H_4-positive splenocytes, neither L_3H_4 nor Lyt-2-positive lymphocytes populations in draining lymph nodes are impaired.

Although work on the further characterization of adjuvant-induced reduction of pregnancy loss in CBA/J mothers is still in progress, it seems that systemic cellular mechanisms are not responsible for the effect.

This work was supported by the Israel Academy of Sciences and Humanities, Basic Research Foundation from Tel-Aviv University and M. & F. Eskenazy Institute for Cancer Research.

References

Athanassakis, R., Bleackley, R.C., Paetkau, V., Guilbert, L., Barr, P. & Wegmann, T.G. (1987) The immunostimulatory effect of T cells and T cell lymphokines on murine fetally derived placental cells. *J. Immunol.* **138**, 37–44.

Beard, R.W., Braude, P., Mowbray, J.F. & Underwood, J.L. (1983) Protective antibodies and spontaneous abortion. *Lancet* ii, 1090–1093.

Beer, A.E. (1985) Survival and rejection of the fetal allograft. In *Immunology and Immunopathology of Reproduction*, pp. 114–130. Eds V. Toder & A. E. Beer. Karger, Basel.

Beer, A.E., Guebbeman, J.F., Ayers, J.W.T. & Haines, R.F. (1981) Major Histocompatibility Complex Antigens, maternal and paternal immune responses and chronic habitual abortion. *Am. J. Obstet. Gynecol.* **141**, 987–993.

Beer, A.E., Guebbeman, J.F. & Zhi, X. (1986) Nonpaternal leukocyte immunotherapy to a model of pregnancy failure in equids. In *Reproductive Immunology 1986*, pp. 253–260. Eds D. A. Clark & B. A. Croy. Elsevier, Amsterdam.

Bell, S.C. & Billington, W.D. (1983) Antifetal alloantibody in the pregnant female. *Immunol. Rev.* **75**, 5–30.

Carp, H.J.A., Toder, V., Gazit, E., Mashiach, S., Serr, D.M. & Nebel, L. (1988) Immunization by paternal leucocytes for prevention of habitual abortion. *Acta obstet. gynaec. scand.* (in press).

Chaouat, G., Kiger, N. & Wegmann, T.G. (1983) Vaccination against spontaneous abortion in mice. *J. Reprod. Immunol.* **5**, 389–392.

Chaouat, G., Kolb, J.P., Kiger, N., Stanislawski, M. & Wegmann, T.G. (1985) Immunologic consequences of vaccination against abortion in mice. *J. Immunol.* **134**, 1594–1598.

Clark, D.A., McDermott, M. & Sczwzuk, M.R. (1980) Impairment of the host-vs-graft reaction in pregnant mice. *J. Immunol.* **127**, 1267–1272.

Clark, D.A., Slapsys, R.M., Croy, B.A. & Rossant, J. (1984) Immunoregulation of host versus graft responses in the uterus. *Immunol. Today* **5**, 111–114.

Clark, D.A., Chaput, A., Walker, C. & Rosenthal, K.L. (1985) Active suppression of host-vs-graft reaction in pregnant mice. V. Soluble suppressor activity obtained from decidua of allopregnant mice blocks the response to IL-2. *J. Immunol.* **134**, 1659–1664.

Clark, D.A., Croy, B.A., Wegmann, T.G. & Chaouat, G. (1987) Immunological and para immunological mechanisms in spontaneous abortion: recent insights and future directions. *J. Reprod. Immunol.* **12**, 1–12.

Gazit, E., Elter, T., Mizrachi, Y., Mashiach, I., Mashiach, S. & Serr, D.M. (1977) Acquisition of typing sera from post partum blood clots. *Tissue Antigens* **9**, 66–77.

Halperin, D., Reuben, C., Ben-Efraim, S., Grover, H. & Weiss, D.W. (1985) Effects of the methanol extraction residue (MFR) tubercle bacillus fraction on the production of antibodies in vitro. *Cell Immunol.* **92**, 404–413.

Kiger, N., Chaouat, G., Kolb, J.P., Wegmann, T.G. & Guenet, J.L. (1985) Immunological studies of spontaneous abortion in mice. I. Preimmunization of females with allogeneic cells. *J. Immunol.* **134**, 2966–2970.

Kook, A.I., Yakir, Y. & Trainin, N. (1975) Isolation and partial chemical characterization of THF, a thymus hormone involved in immune maturation of lymphoid cells. *Cell Immunol.* **19**, 151–157.

Mittal, K.K., Mickey, J.R., Singall, D.P. & Terasaki, P.I. (1968) Serotyping for transplantation XVIII.

Refinement of microdroplet cytotoxicity test. *Transplantation* **6**, 913–927.

Mowbray, J.F. (1986) Effect of immunization with paternal cells on recurrent spontaneous abortion. In *Reproductive Immunology*, pp. 269–276. Eds D. A. Clark & B. A. Croy. Elsevier, Amsterdam.

Mowbray, J.F., Gibbins, C.R., Sidgwick, A.S., Ruskiewicz, M. & Beard, R.W. (1983) Effects of transfusion in women with recurrent spontaneous abortion. *Transpl. Proc.* **10**, 896–899.

Taylor, C. & Faulk, W.P. (1981) Prevention of recurrent abortion with leucocyte transfusion. *Lancet* **ii**, 68–71.

Toder, V. (1988) Lymphokines and other growth factors at the feto-maternal interface. In *Perspective in Immunoreproduction: Conception and Contraception*, pp. 368–383. Eds S. Mattur & C. M. Fredericks. Hemisphere, New York.

Toder, V., Blank, M., Drizlikh, G. & Nebel, L. (1982) Placental and embryo cells can induce the generation of cytotoxic lymphocytes in vitro. *Transplantation* **33**, 196–198.

Tsutsumi, O. & Oka, T. (1987) Epidermal growth factor deficiency during pregnancy causes abortion in mice. *Am. J. Obstet. Gynecol.* **156**, 241–244.

Wegmann, T.G. (1984) Foetal protection against abortion. *Annls Immunol.* (Paris) **1350**, 309–315.

LUTEAL AND PLACENTAL CELLS

Chairmen

B. A. Cooke
B. J. Weir
T. A. Bramley
G. E. Lamming

J. Reprod. Fert., Suppl. **37** (1989), 85–89

Comparative aspects of maternal recognition of pregnancy between sheep and pigs

F. W. Bazer, J. L. Vallet, J. P. Harney, T. S. Gross* and W. W. Thatcher*

*Departments of Animal Science and *Dairy Science, Institute of Food and Agricultural Sciences, University of Florida, Gainesville, Florida 32611-0701, U.S.A.*

Summary. Sheep conceptuses secrete a protein, oTP-1, between Days 10 and 21 of gestation which is responsible for establishment of pregnancy. oTP-1 inhibits uterine production of luteolytic amounts of PGF-2α (PGF) produced in response to oestradiol and oxytocin. oTP-1 does not compete with oxytocin for binding to oxytocin receptors, but may interfere with oxytocin stimulation of the inositol phospholipid system. Pig conceptuses secrete oestrogens between Days 10 and 15 of pregnancy which are essential for establishment of pregnancy. Oestrogens, directly or indirectly, alter secretion of PGF from an endocrine direction (towards uterine vasculature) to an exocrine direction (towards the uterine lumen). PGF sequestered in the uterine lumen is unavailable to exert a luteolytic effect on the CL. Pig conceptus secretory proteins stimulate uterine production of PGF and PGE.

Conceptus secretory proteins of sheep and pigs include proteins which have antiviral activity and may be considered interferons. In sheep, oTP-1 has both antiluteolytic and antiviral properties. The specific pig conceptus secretory protein(s) possessing antiviral activity has not been established. Unlike oTP-1, however, it does not appear to possess antiluteolytic activity.

Keywords: conceptus; sheep; pigs; secretions; pregnancy; prostaglandins; protein; endometrium

Introduction

Conceptuses of sheep and pigs produce proteins, steroids and prostaglandins during early pregnancy which may be involved in protecting the CL from the luteolytic effects of prostaglandin (PG) F-2α produced by the uterine endometrium. These secretory products may have a luteotrophic effect on the CL or an antiluteolytic effect by acting directly, in a paracrine manner, on the endometrium, or, in an endocrine manner, on the CL. Available evidence suggests that secretions produced by conceptuses of sheep and pigs are antiluteolytic (Bazer *et al.*, 1986). Conceptus secretory products do not appear to inhibit uterine production of PGF; they either suppress release of episodes of PGF necessary for luteolysis in sheep or redirect secretion of PGF into the uterine lumen where it can be sequestered and/or metabolized in pigs.

Trophoblast protein-1 is the antiluteolytic protein secreted by sheep conceptuses

Sheep conceptuses secrete ovine trophoblast protein-1 (oTP-1) between Days 10 and 21 of pregnancy (Bazer *et al.*, 1986). This protein: (1) has a molecular weight of about 17 000 and isoelectric variants with pI values ranging from 5·3 to 5·7; (2) contains no carbohydrate moiety; (3) is secreted by trophectoderm and taken up by endometrial surface epithelium and superficial glandular epithelium; (4) does not stimulate progesterone secretion by luteal tissue; (5) does not stimulate cAMP, cGMP or inositol phospholipid turnover in endometrial tissue; (6) strongly amplifies endometrial secretion of at least 5 proteins for which functions have not been determined; and (6) has high amino acid sequence homology with interferons of the alpha-2 class (Imakawa *et al.*, 1987; Stewart *et al.*, 1987). oTP-1 appears to be an antiluteolytic paracrine hormone secreted by the sheep conceptus which modifies endometrial secretion of PGF to allow maternal recognition of pregnancy.

The endometrium of cyclic ewes releases PGF in a pulsatile manner on Days 15 and 17 and about 5 episodes of PGF release in 24 h are required for luteolysis (Zarco *et al.*, 1984). McCracken *et al.* (1984) proposed that oestradiol from ovarian follicles induces endometrial oxytocin receptors and that oxytocin stimulates uterine secretion of luteolytic amounts of PGF. Oxytocin from the posterior pituitary and CL appear to control pulsatile secretion of PGF by uterine endometrium (Flint & Sheldrick, 1986; Hooper *et al.*, 1986). Fincher *et al.* (1986) found that pregnant ewes have higher basal concentrations of 15-keto-13,14-dihydro-PGF (PGFM) than do cyclic ewes on Day 15 (193 ± 30 *versus* 67 ± 8 pg/ml), and Lacroix & Kann (1983) demonstrated higher production of PGF from endometrium of pregnant ewes *in vitro*. Therefore, oTP-1 is assumed to exert its antiluteolytic effect on the endometrium by inhibiting the oxytocin-induced pulsatile secretion of PGF necessary for luteolysis in ewes. Hooper *et al.* (1986) reported that the pattern of release of oxytocin was not different between cyclic and pregnant ewes; however, oxytocin receptor numbers are significantly reduced in pregnant ewes (McCracken *et al.*, 1984).

We developed a protocol to test for antiluteolytic activity of total conceptus secretory proteins (oCSP) and purified oTP-1 from Day-16 sheep conceptus culture medium. Fincher *et al.* (1986) infused oCSP or serum proteins into each uterine horn of cyclic ewes between Days 12 and 14 at 08:00 and 17:00 h and injected 0·5 mg oestradiol i.v. at 07:30 h on Day 14 followed by 10 i.u. oxytocin at 08:05 h on Day 15 to determine effects of oCSP on uterine production of PGF. oCSP inhibited uterine production of PGF in response to both oestradiol and oxytocin. Pregnant ewes also failed to respond to the luteolytic effects associated with oestradiol (Kittok & Britt, 1977; Fincher *et al.*, 1986) and oxytocin (Fairclough *et al.*, 1984) treatment. Using this same protocol, Vallet *et al.* (1987) compared effects of intrauterine infusion of purified oTP-1, oCSP, oCSP minus oTP-1 and serum proteins on uterine production of PGF. Purified oTP-1 alone had an antiluteolytic effect equal to that of oCSP. oCSP minus oTP-1 and serum proteins did not inhibit uterine production of PGF in response to oestradiol and oxytocin and did not extend the interoestrous interval. Results from that experiment suggest that oTP-1 alone is the antiluteolytic protein secreted by sheep conceptuses. oTP-1 does not compete with oxytocin for its receptor since tritiated oxytocin can be completely displaced with 100 ng radioinert oxytocin in an endometrial membrane receptor assay, but there was no significant displacement of radiolabelled oxytocin with up to 10 000 ng oTP-1 (A. P. F. Flint, J. L. Vallet & F. W. Bazer, unpublished data). An experiment was then conducted to examine effects of oxytocin and oTP-1 on the phosphatidylinositol cycle which is stimulated by oxytocin (Flint *et al.*, 1986). The results summarized in Table 1 indicate that the overall effect of oTP-1 is to inhibit the phosphatidylinositol cycle; however, failure of oTP-1 to inhibit long-term (180 min) effects of oxytocin are not clear. The mechanism whereby oTP-1 interferes with uterine production of PGF requires further study.

Oestrogens, not conceptus secretory proteins, are responsible for maternal recognition of pregnancy in pigs

The theory of maternal recognition of pregnancy in pigs has been reviewed extensively (Bazer *et al.*, 1986). The theory is based on the assumptions that the uterine endometrium secretes the luteolysin, PGF, and that conceptuses secrete oestrogens which are antiluteolytic. The theory is that PGF is secreted in an endocrine direction, toward the uterine vasculature, in cyclic gilts and transported to the CL to exert its luteolytic effect. However, in pregnant pigs, the direction of secretion of PGF

Table 1. Effects of oxytocin and oTP-1 on inositol phosphate turnover in Day-15 cyclic sheep endometrium

Treatments*†		Turnover (d.p.m.)			
160 min	160–180 min	Inositol	Inositol monophosphate	Inositol bisphosphate	Inositol trisphosphate
None	None	2120	6990	190	1810
None	oTP-1	1645	5070	0	0
None	Oxytocin	1968	12 940	4190	3750
None	oTP-1 + oxytocin	1660	5600	1170	785
oTP-1	oTP-1	2037	5940	0	0
oTP-1	oTP-1 + oxytocin	1690	12 250	3020	2620
Oxytocin	Oxytocin	1592	17 080	5274	6260
Oxytocin	Oxytocin + oTP-1	1940	25 520	8296	13 065

*Treatments were 5 µg oTP-1 and/or 10^{-7} M-oxytocin with 5 replicates per treatment.
†Overall effects of oxytocin were significant ($P < 0.05$), but effects of oTP-1, oTP-1 + oxytocin and control treatments between 160 and 180 min were not different.

is exocrine, into the uterine lumen, where it is sequestered to exert is biological effects and/or metabolized to prevent luteolysis. Secretion of other components of histotroph, e.g., uteroferrin is also in an exocrine direction in pregnant, but not cyclic, pigs after about Day 14 (Chen *et al.*, 1975).

Mean concentrations, peak frequency and peak amplitude of PGF in utero-ovarian vein plasma are lower in pregnant and pseudopregnant than cyclic gilts (Bazer *et al.*, 1982). Shille *et al.* (1979) reported similar results when blood samples from the radial vein of pregnant and cyclic pigs were assayed for PGFM. On the other hand, uterine flushings of pseudopregnant and pregnant gilts have significantly higher amounts of PGF than do those from cyclic gilts (Bazer *et al.*, 1982). These results indicate that PGF is released primarily into the uterine venous drainage (endocrine) in cyclic gilts, but into the uterine lumen (exocrine) in pregnant and pseudopregnant pigs and that secretion of PGF is not inhibited during pregnancy or pseudopregnancy. Lacroix & Kann (1983) developed a perifusion device which allows one to discriminate between release of PGF from the luminal and myometrial sides of the endometrium. Using the perifusion device, Gross *et al.* (1988) confirmed that endometrium from cyclic pigs secretes PGF primarily from the myometrial side (endocrine) and that pregnant gilts secrete PGF primarily from the luminal side (exocrine). The transition from endocrine to exocrine secretion occurs between Days 10 and 12 of pregnancy which is temporally associated with initiation of oestrogen secretion by conceptuses. Oestrogens, secreted by the blastocyst or injected, induce a transient release of calcium into the uterine lumen within 12 h. Re-uptake of that calcium by endometrial and/or conceptus tissues occurs about 12 h after concentrations of calcium in uterine secretions reach maximum values. The switch in direction of secretion of PGF from an endocrine to an exocrine orientation is closely associated with this period of release and re-uptake of calcium by the endometrium in pregnant and pseudopregnant gilts. When endometrium from Day-14 cyclic gilts was treated in the perifusion device with verapamil (calcium channel blocker), 3,4,5-trimethoxybenzoic acid 8-(diethylamino) octyl ester (an inhibitor of intracellular calcium mobilization and calcium–calmodulin interactions) or the calcium ionophore A23187 (an inducer of calcium cycling by epithelium), the calcium ionophore switched secretion of PGF from an endocrine to an exocrine mode during the treatment period. The other two compounds were without effect. These results suggest that induction of calcium cycling across endometrial epithelium redirects secretion of PGF toward the uterine lumen (T. S. Gross & F. W. Bazer, unpublished data).

Recent evidence suggests that an interaction between oestrogen and prolactin enhances uterine secretory activity previously associated with the oestrogen-induced calcium cycling (K. H. Young & F. W. Bazer, unpublished data). Therefore, endometrium from Day-14 cyclic gilts was placed into the perifusion device to determine effects of prolactin on direction of secretion of PGF by endometrium taken before and at 6 or 12 h after injection of 5 mg oestradiol. Prolactin had no effect on direction of secretion of PGF if endometrium was taken before oestradiol treatment. However, endometrium taken at 6 or 12 h after oestradiol treatment responded to prolactin by switching secretion of PGF from an endocrine to an exocrine direction within about 30 min after addition of prolactin to the perifusion buffer. We speculate that oestradiol induces endometrial receptors for prolactin which then allow prolactin to act on the endometrium to induce calcium cycling across the epithelium (T. S. Gross, M. A. Mirando, K. H. Young & F. W. Bazer, unpublished data).

Pig conceptuses secrete two major classes of proteins with molecular weights of 20 000 to 25 000 (pI values ranging from 5·6 to 6·2) and 35 000 to 50 000 (pI values of 8·2–9·0) between Days 10·5 and 18 of gestation (Godkin *et al.*, 1982). Pig conceptus secretory proteins (pCSP) recovered from culture medium of Day-15 conceptuses include a protein(s) with antiviral activity (C. Pontzer, B. Torres, H. M. Johnson & F. W. Bazer, unpublished data). We have conducted an experiment in which 4 mg pCSP plus 4 mg serum proteins or 8 mg serum proteins only were introduced into the lumen of each uterine horn twice daily between Days 12 and 15 after i.m. administration of 1 mg oestradiol on Day 11. Blood samples were collected from the inferior vena cava proximal to entry of the utero-ovarian vein every 15 min between 08:00 h and 11:00 h on Days 12 to 17 and plasma assayed for PGFM, PGE and progesterone. The pCSP had no effect on interoestrous interval or concentrations of progesterone. Peak values for PGFM occurred earlier (Day 13) and coincidentally with initiation of pCSP treatment. Also, pCSP-treated gilts had higher concentrations of PGE (272 ± 35 *versus* 154 ± 35 pg/ml) than did serum protein-treated gilts. These results do not indicate an antiluteolytic role for pCSP (J. P. Harney & F. W. Bazer, unpublished data). Available data support the theory that oestrogens of blastocyst origin are essential for maternal recognition of pregnancy in pigs and that pCSP may play other roles in early pregnancy in this species.

Research reported in this paper has been supported by National Institutes of Health Grant HD 10436 and U.S. Department of Agriculture Grant 86-CRCR-1-2106 and is published as University of Florida Agricultural Experiment Station Journal Series No. 8878.

References

Bazer, F.W., Geisert, R.D., Thatcher, W.W. & Roberts, R.M. (1982) Endocrine vs exocrine secretion of $PGF_{2\alpha}$ in the control of pregnancy in swine. In *Prostaglandins in Animal Reproduction II*, pp. 115–132. Eds L. E. Edqvist & H. Kindahl. Elsevier Science Publishers, Amsterdam.

Bazer, F.W. Vallet, J.L. Roberts, R.M., Sharp, D.C. & Thatcher, W.W. (1986) Role of conceptus secretory products in establishment of pregnancy. *J. Reprod. Fert.* **76**, 841–850.

Chen, T.T., Bazer, F.W. Gebhardt, B & Roberts, R.M. (1975) Uterine secretion in mammals; Synthesis and placental transport of a purple acid phosphatase in pigs. *Biol. Reprod.* **13**, 304–313.

Fairclough, R.J. Moore, L.G. Peterson, A.J. & Watkins, W.B. (1984) Effect of oxytocin on plasma concentrations of 13,14-dihydro-15-keto prostaglandin F and the oxytocin associated neurophysin during the estrous cycle and early pregnancy in the ewe. *Biol. Reprod.* **31**, 36–43.

Fincher, K.B, Bazer, F.W., Hansen, P.J., Thatcher, W.W. & Roberts, R.M. (1986) Proteins secreted by the sheep conceptus suppress induction of uterine prostaglandin F-2α release by oestradiol and oxytocin. *J. Reprod. Fert.* **76**, 425–433.

Flint, A.P.F. & Sheldrick, E.L. (1986) Ovarian oxytocin and maternal recognition of pregnancy. *J. Reprod. Fert.* **76**, 831–839.

Flint, A.P.F., Leat, W.M.F., Sheldrick, E.L. & Stewart, H.J. (1986) Stimulation of phosphoinositide hydrolysis by oxytocin and the mechanism by which oxytocin controls prostaglandin synthesis in the ovine endometrium. *Biochem. J.* **237**, 797–805.

Godkin, J.D., Bazer, F.W., Lewis, G.S., Geisert, R.D. & Roberts, R.M. (1982) Synthesis and release of polypeptides by pig conceptuses during the period of blastocyst elongation and attachment. *Biol. Reprod.* **27**, 977–987.

Gross, T.S., Lacroix, M.C., Bazer, F.W., Thatcher, W.W. & Harney, J.P. (1988) Prostaglandin secretion by perifused porcine endometrium: further evidence for an endocrine versus exocrine secretion of prostaglandins. *Prostaglandins* **35**, 327–341.

Hooper, S.B., Watkins, W.B. & Thorburn, G.D. (1986) Oxytocin, oxytocin-associated neurophysin, and prostaglandin $F_{2\alpha}$ concentrations in the utero-ovarian vein of pregnant and nonpregnant sheep. *Endocrinology* **119**, 2590–2597.

Imakawa, K., Anthony, R.V., Kazemi, M., Mariotti, K.R.,

Polites, H.G. & Roberts, R.M. (1987) Interferon-like sequence of ovine trophoblast protein secreted by embryonic trophectoderm. *Nature, Lond.* **330,** 377–379.

Kittok, R.J. & Britt, J.H. (1977) Corpus luteum function in ewes given estradiol during the estrous cycle or early pregnancy. *J. Anim. Sci.* **45,** 336–341.

Lacroix, M.C. & Kann, G. (1983) Discriminating analysis of in vitro prostaglandin release by myometrial and luminal sides of the ewe endometrium. *Prostaglandins* **25,** 853–869.

McCracken, J.A., Schramm, W. & Okulicz, W.C. (1984) Hormone receptor control of pulsatile secretion of PGF$_{2\alpha}$ from the ovine uterus during luteolysis and its abrogation in early pregnancy. In *Prostaglandins in Animal Reproduction II,* pp. 31–56. Eds L. E. Edqvist & H. Kindahl. Elsevier, Amsterdam.

Shille, V.M., Karlbom, I., Einarsson, S., Larsson, K., Kindahl, H. & Edqvist, L.E. (1979) Concentrations of progesterone and 15-keto-13,14-dihydroprostaglandin F$_{2\alpha}$ in peripheral plasma during the estrous cycle and early pregnancy in gilts. *Zentbl. VetMed. A* **26,** 169–181.

Stewart, H.J., McCann, S.H.E., Barker, P.J., Lee, K.E., Lamming, G.E. & Flint, A.P.F. (1987) Interferon sequence homology and receptor binding activity of ovine trophoblast antiluteolytic protein. *J. Endocr.* **115,** R13–R15.

Vallet, J.L., Bazer, F.W. & Fliss, M.F.V. (1987) Effects of ovine conceptus secretory protein and ovine trophoblast protein-one on uterine production of prostaglandins. *Biol. Reprod.* **36,** Suppl. 1, 155, Abstr.

Zarco, L., Stabenfeldt, G.H., Kindahl, H. Bradford, G.E. & Basu, S. (1984) A detailed study of prostaglandin F$_{2\alpha}$ release during luteolysis and establishment of pregnancy in the ewe. *Biol. Reprod.* **30,** (Suppl. 1), 153, Abstr.

J. Reprod. Fert., Suppl. **37** (1989), 91–99

Antiluteolytic effects of bovine trophoblast protein-1

W. W. Thatcher*, P. J. Hansen*, T. S. Gross*, S. D. Helmer*, C. Plante*
and F. W. Bazer†

*Departments of *Dairy and †Animal Sciences, Institute of Food and Agricultural Sciences,
University of Florida, Gainesville, Florida 32611-0701, U.S.A.*

Summary. Bovine conceptuses exert an antiluteolytic (anti-PGF-2α) effect on the uterus by decreasing the secretion of PGF that results in maintenance of the CL. Basal and oxytocin-stimulated secretion rates of PGF from perifused endometrium are lower at Day 17 of pregnancy than at Day 17 of the oestrous cycle, probably because of increased amounts of an intracellular, endometrial PG-synthesis inhibitor which is present in the 100 000 *g* cytosolic supernatant, is proteinaceous, and acts in a non-competitive manner with respect to arachidonic acid. The antiluteolytic signal in bovine conceptus secretory proteins (bCSP) is bovine trophoblast protein-1 (bTP-1), a group of 7 isomers of N-linked glycoproteins in two size classes (22 000 high-mannose and 24 000 complex types) that are related immunologically to ovine trophoblast protein-1 (oTP-1). Incubation of endometrial explants of Day-17 cyclic cows with bCSP and bTP-1 induced PG-synthesis inhibitor activity and reduced PGF secretion. Intrauterine infusion of bTP-1 from Days 15·5 to 21 extended the interoestrous interval from 19·5 to 26·0 days. Intrauterine infusion of interferon-$\alpha_1$1 through the cervix from Day 15·5 to 21 extended the interoestrous interval from 22·8 to 26·8 days. Platelet-activating factor (PAF) and interferon-$\alpha_1$1 alter PG secretion of endometrial explants (PAF decreases PGF and increases PGE-2; interferon-$\alpha_1$1 does not alter PGF and increases PGE-2 secretion) but neither induces activity of the endometrial PG-synthesis inhibitor. In conclusion, bovine conceptuses exert a paracrine effect through the secretion of bTP-1 to induce an endometrial intracellular inhibitor of PGF synthesis. This antiluteolytic effect is essential to maintenance of the CL and establishment of pregnancy.

Keywords: antiluteolysin; conceptus; prostaglandins; corpus luteum; cow

Introduction

Series of biological signals are elicited from both the conceptus and maternal system to permit establishment of pregnancy and continued development of the conceptus in cattle. One important role for a conceptus signal is to provide for persistence of the CL for an extended period in order to maintain circulating concentrations of progesterone sufficient for maintenance of pregnancy. Associated with regression of the CL during the oestrous cycle is a luteolytic mode of pulsatile prostaglandin (PG) F secretion which is attenuated if the uterus contains a conceptus. This antiluteolytic effect, in which the dynamics of PGF secretion are altered, is referred to as an antiPGF action. Evidence to support this concept has been reviewed extensively (Thatcher *et al.*, 1986). The challenge is to understand the physiological and biochemical events set in motion by the conceptus that result in alteration of endometrial PGF secretion and CL maintenance.

The antiluteolytic–antiPGF system is imprinted in the pregnant endometrium

A perifusion device has been utilized to compare the secretion rates of PGF and PGE-2 from the luminal and stromal surfaces of the endometrium from cyclic and pregnant cows at Day 17 after oestrus (Gross *et al.*, 1988a). Secretion rates of PGF were lower for endometrium of pregnant than cyclic cows, whereas PGE-2 secretion was not affected by pregnancy status. Furthermore, PGF and PGE-2 secretion by endometrium of pregnant cows was not stimulated by oxytocin, although copious amounts of PGF and PGE were secreted by endometrium of cyclic cows (Fig. 1). Recent evidence (Basu & Kindahl, 1987; Gross *et al.*, 1988b) indicates that reduced secretion of prostaglandins in endometrial tissue of early pregnancy is due to the presence of an intracellular, endometrial PG-synthesis inhibitor. The microsomal fraction of parturient bovine cotyledons was utilized as a source of enzymes for PG synthesis (Gross *et al.*, 1988b). Endometrial tissues collected at Day 17 of the oestrous cycle ($n = 12$) and pregnancy ($n = 12$) were homogenized and subjected to differential centrifugation for preparation of microsomes and a high-speed (100 000 g) cytosolic supernatant. Cytosolic supernatant from cyclic cows decreased PGF synthesis by cotyledonary microsomes to a slight extent (21% reduction), whereas preparations from pregnant cows decreased PGF synthesis by 63%. The mechanism of inhibition by endometrial supernatant from pregnant cows appears to be non-competitive with respect to arachidonic acid. The inhibitor appears to be proteinacous and can be precipitated by 20% saturated ammonium sulphate. When resolved by h.p.l.c. gel filtration, activity of the PG synthesis inhibitor occurred in two molecular weight regions (65–70×10^3 and 20–25×10^3) and co-eluted with peroxidase activity that was also higher in pregnant endometrium (Gross *et al.*, 1988c). Additional comparisons between the oestrous cycle, throughout pregnancy and immediately *post partum* (Table 1) indicate that the relative amount of activity of the endometrial PG synthesis inhibitor increases during pregnancy between Days 14 and 17, and is sustained until 250–275 days (T. S. Gross, W. W. Thatcher & P. J. Hansen, unpublished observations). The factors regulating increased PG synthesis inhibitor activity in early pregnant endometrial tissue are likely to be critical for the maintenance of CL function.

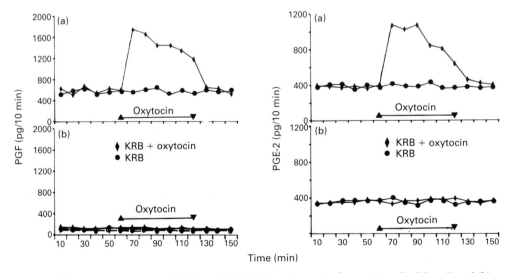

Fig. 1. Mean secretion rates of PGF and PGE-2 for endometria from: (a) cyclic (N = 4) and (b) pregnant (N = 5) cows at Day 17 after oestrus. Tissue was perifused with Kreb's–Ringer–bicarbonate (KRB) (3 ml/10 min) and fractions were collected every 10 min. Oxytocin (1 i.u./ml) was perifused during fractions 7–12.

Table 1. Activity of the intracellular, endometrial PG synthesis inhibitor in cattle during the oestrous cycle, pregnancy and *post partum*

Reproductive stage (days)†	Secretion of PGF* in the presence of cytosol from 0·25 g endometrium	
	ng/h‡	% Reduction
Cycle		
7 (2), 14 (3), 17 (4)	3·6 ± 0·2^a	10
Pregnancy		
7 (3)	3·8 ± 0·2^a	0
14 (4)	3·5 ± 0·2^a	14
17 (5)	2·6 ± 0·2^b	35
21 (4)	2·3 ± 0·2^b	41
30 (3)	2·7 ± 0·2^b	33
60 (2)	2·8 ± 0·1^b	30
120 (2)	2·2 ± 0·3^b	44
250 (2)	3·0 ± 0·3^b	21
275 (2)	3·6 ± 0·2^a	12
Post partum		
0 (3)	3·9 ± 0·2^a	0

*4·1 ng PGF/h secreted by generating system of cotyledonary microsomes from parturient cattle.
†Numbers in parentheses are no. of cows sampled.
‡Means with different superscripts differ ($P < 0.05$; analysis of variance and Student–Newman–Keuls multiple range test of means).

Bovine trophoblastic protein-1 is an antiluteolytic–antiPGF agent

Infusion of bovine conceptus secretory proteins (bCSP; array of proteins secreted by Day 16–18 cow conceptuses during a 24-h incubation; Bartol *et al.*, 1985) from Day 15·5 to Day 21 extended the interoestrous interval (Knickerbocker *et al.*, 1986a), and attenuated uterine PGF production in response to an injection of oestradiol on Day 18 after oestrus (Knickerbocker *et al.*, 1986b). There are two lines of evidence that the antiluteolytic proteins of sheep and cattle conceptuses may be biologically similar. Maintenance of CL occurred in some recipient cows and ewes after interspecies reciprocal transfer of trophoblastic vesicles which secrete antiluteolytic proteinaceous factors (Heyman *et al.*, 1984). Furthermore, antiserum to ovine trophoblastic protein-1 (oTP-1) cross-reacts immunologically with some of the low molecular weight, acidic proteins of bCSP that are defined as the bovine trophoblast protein-1 complex (bTP-1; Helmer *et al.*, 1987). Chemical characterizations of the immunoprecipitated complex indicate that bTP-1 is comprised of 7 isomers of N-linked glycoproteins in two size classes (M_r 22 000 high-mannose and 24 000 complex types; Anthony *et al.*, 1988; Helmer *et al.*, 1988a). The fact that bTP-1 is glycosylated and oTP-1 is not is a striking difference in chemical characteristics between the two classes of molecules. The following procedure was developed for chemical purification of bTP-1 (Helmer *et al.*, 1988b). A pool of bCSP was obtained by culture of Day 17–18 conceptuses for 72 h with minimum essential medium being replaced every 24 h. Medium from the first ($n = 28$), second ($n = 26$), and third ($n = 19$) 24-h periods of culture were pooled. An equal volume of saturated ammonium sulphate was added and incubated for 2 h at 4°C. Supernatants were dialysed and loaded onto a CM-Sepharose column at pH 8·2. Proteins not binding were loaded onto a DEAE column at the same pH, and bound material was eluted with 0·2 M-NaPO$_4$, pH 7·9. Eluted proteins were separated by h.p.l.c. gel filtration on a Zorbax GF-250 column. Protein fractions from the M_r 20–29 000 range were retained for infusion and purity was confirmed by gel electrophoresis. In developing the procedures for the chemical isolation of bTP-1, several points were documented that influence yields of bTP-1. There is an appreciable amount of protease activity within bCSP such that constant attention to inhibiting protease activity (e.g. maintenance of conditions at 4°C and use of protease inhibitors in all buffers) throughout the isolation steps is essential. Secondly, bTP-1 tends to aggregate to form higher molecular weight complexes.

Having purified bTP-1, our objectives were to determine whether it exerts an antiluteolytic–antiPGF effect. Two approaches were taken: (1) to determine whether bTP-1 would cause in-vitro effects that were similar to an antiPGF action and (2) to test whether intrauterine administration would extend the interoestrous interval.

Thatcher *et al.* (1985) proposed that bovine conceptus secretory proteins will selectively stimulate an endometrial protein that inhibits synthesis of PGF. Obviously, bTP-1 would be a likely candidate as a conceptus regulatory protein to induce PG synthesis inhibitor, decrease PGF secretion and therefore maintain the CL. To test these hypotheses, endometrial explants (0·5 g) from cyclic cows at Day 17 after oestrus were incubated for 24 h in 15 ml minimum essential medium with BSA (0, 4·8, 24 or 120 µg/ml gave same responses), 1 µg bTP-1/ml or 12·7 µg bCSP/ml (Table 2; Helmer *et al.*, 1988c). Treatments with bCSP and bTP-1 decreased secretion of PGF. However, PGE-2 secretion was greater for bTP-1 than for bCSP-treated explants. PG synthesis inhibitor was measured as the ability of cytosolic supernatants from the treated endometrial explants to decrease PGF secretion from the cotyledonary generating system (Table 2). Synthesis of PGF by the generating system was slightly decreased by cytosol from BSA-treated explants, whereas cytosol from bCSP- and bTP-1-treated explants markedly decreased PGF synthesis. Both bCSP- and bTP-1 induced synthesis of the inhibitor and reduced PGF secretion; these responses would indicate that bTP-1 has actions on endometrium that *in vivo* would alter PGF secretion in a manner to prevent luteolysis.

To test the in-vivo antiluteolytic effect of bTP-1, cows (3 per group) received twice-daily infusions (Days 15·5–21·0), via a catheter placed in the uterine horn ipsilateral to the CL, with bovine serum albumin (BSA), bCSP or bTP-1 (1·5 mg BSA, 750 µg bCSP + 750 µg BSA or 35 µg bTP-1 + 1·465 mg BSA per infusion; Helmer *et al.*, 1988b). Comparisons of BSA *versus* bCSP + bTP-1 were significant for interoestrous interval (19·5 *versus* 21·5 and 26·0 ± 1·3 days), and the interval for bTP-1 was greater than that for bCSP. Interoestrous intervals after the experiment were 20·2, 17·8 and 21·7 days for BSA, bCSP and bTP-1 groups, respectively. Regression analyses of plasma progesterone concentrations were used to assess CL function. The bCSP and bTP-1 treatments extended luteal phases compared to BSA group, and the difference was due to a longer luteal phase of the bTP-1 group (Fig. 2). Lack of a bCSP effect may be due to low amounts of bTP-1 in conceptus-conditioned medium from cultures carried out for > 24 h. This is in contrast to the extension of interoestrous intervals observed by Knickerbocker *et al.* (1986a) in which only bCSP from the first 24 h of culture was utilized. Some bTP-1 activity was present in the bCSP of the present experiment since it did induce activity of the PG synthesis inhibitor *in vitro* (Table 2). It is clear from the in-vivo and in-vitro experiments that purified bTP-1 was effective in extending CL function via its antiluteolytic–antiPGF effect.

Alpha interferon and platelet-activating factor

Purification of bTP-1 from bCSP is a time consuming and expensive procedure because of the number of conceptuses required for culture. The primary amino acid sequence of oTP-1 has now been elucidated (Imakawa *et al.*, 1987; Stewart *et al.*, 1987) and oTP-1 is probably an α-interferon-like molecule since it displays a 70·3% homology with bovine interferon-α_{II} (Imakawa *et al.*, 1987). The inferred primary structure of bTP-1 also indicated that it could be an interferon. In addition, binding of radiolabelled human α-interferon to membrane receptors from uteri of cyclic ewes could be inhibited by purified oTP-1 (Stewart *et al.*, 1987). These results led us (Plante *et al.*, 1988) to test the possible antiluteolytic effect of recombinant bovine interferon class I, Type 1 (interferon-α_{I}1) that was produced in *Escherischia coli* by recombinant DNA techniques and purified to homogeneity (Capon *et al.*,

Table 2. Effect of potential antiluteolytic antiPGF agents on endometrial prostaglandin secretion and induction of intracellular activity of endometrial PG synthesis inhibitor

	Experiment I				Experiment II			
	BSA (4·8 µg/ml)	bCSP (12·7 µg/ml)	bTP-1 (1 µg/ml)	PAF (5 µg/ml)	Recombinant bovine interferon-α class I (µg/ml)			
					0	4·8	24	120
Explant secretion* (ng/24 h)								
PGF	475[a] ± 13	394[b] ± 9	409[b] ± 20	437[b] ± 16	481[a] ± 21	500[a] ± 15	495[a] ± 18	505[a] ± 15
PGE-2	206[a] ± 5	180[b] ± 5	259[c] ± 8	265[c] ± 5	208[a] ± 9	265[b] ± 22	250[b] ± 8	263[b] ± 13
PG synthesis inhibitor								
Activity† (PGF, ng/h)	3·48[a] ± 0·08 (3·90 ± 0·11)‡	2·25[b] ± 0·12	2·53[b] ± 0·17	3·5[a] ± 0·10	3·6[a] ± 0·2 (4·1 ± 0·2)‡	3·9[a] ± 0·2	4·2[a] ± 0·2	3·8[a] ± 0·2

*Amount of PG secreted by endometrial explants from Day 17 cyclic cows (N = 4, Exp. I; N = 3, Exp. II) treated with appropriate test substances.
†Amount of PGF produced in 1 h by cotyledonary microsomes from parturient cattle when incubated with cytosol from 0·4 g of endometrial explants that were previously incubated with test substances for 24 h.
‡Amount of PGF produced in 1 h by cotyledonary microsomes alone.
Within a row, means with different superscripts within an experiment differ ($P < 0.05$ or $P < 0.01$; analysis of variance and Student–Newman–Keuls multiple range test of means).

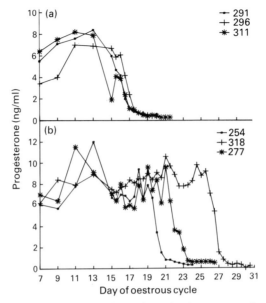

Fig. 2. Effect of intrauterine administration of (a) bovine serum albumin and (b) bovine trophoblast protein-1 from Day 15·5 to 21 after oestrus on concentrations of progesterone in plasma. Individual profiles from each cow in the experiment are plotted.

1985). The interferon-$\alpha_1$1 was kindly provided by CIBA-GEIGY, Basle, Switzerland; such a synthetic source of material permitted design of an experiment with 5 cows per treatment group and an infusion dose of 520 μg interferon-$\alpha_1$1. Twice-daily intrauterine infusion of interferon-$\alpha_1$1, via the transcervical route, from Day 15·5 to 21 extended the interoestrus interval from 22·8 to 26·8 days in cyclic cows and extended CL lifespan accordingly (Fig. 3). In-vitro examination of the antiluteolytic effect indicates that interferon-$\alpha_1$1 did not alter the secretion of PGF by endometrial explants of Day 17 cyclic cows and did not induce intracellular PG synthesis inhibitor activity in the explants after a 24-h culture period (Table 2; C. Plante, T. S. Gross, P. J. Hansen & W. W. Thatcher, unpublished observations). However, interferon-$\alpha_1$1 did increase the endometrial secretion of PGE-2 at each of the doses tested. Collectively, results of these experiments indicate that recombinant interferon-$\alpha_1$1 exerts an antiluteolytic effect, but its mode of action may be different from that of bTP-1. Several explanations may account for this difference. Interferon-$\alpha_1$1 probably does not have 100% homology with bTP-1 (Imakawa *et al.*, 1987). Unlike bTP-1, it is not glycosylated and its action to stimulate endometrial secretion of PGE-2 may permit it to act as an antiluteolytic–luteoprotective agent (Thatcher *et al.*, 1986). In this regard, bTP-1 induced intracellular activity of the PG synthesis inhibitor and selectively decreased PGF secretion, but bTP-1 also stimulated PGE-2 secretion as did interferon-$\alpha_1$1. This is a shared functional link between the two molecules that may contribute to their common net effect of CL maintenance as demonstrated.

There is likely to be an array of molecules produced either by the conceptus or endometrium that have different but complementary effects (antiluteolytic antiPGF or luteoprotective and luteotrophic) to maintain the CL and therefore ensure continued development of the conceptus. Hickey & Hansel (1987) reported that a lipid-like luteotrophic substance is produced by Day 13–18 bovine conceptuses. This material may be analogous to the biologically active phospholipid, embryo-derived platelet-activating factor (PAF) described by O'Neill (1987). When PAF (5 μg PAF + 5 μg BSA/ml) was incubated with Day-17 cyclic endometrial tissues, it caused a decrease in PGF secretion and an increase in PGE-2. However, PAF had no effect on the PG synthesis inhibitor activity of the explants following a 24-h incubation (Table 2; Gross & Thatcher, 1988). If PAF is produced by bovine conceptuses, it may

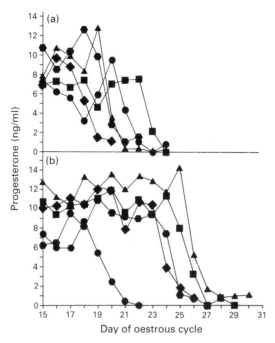

Fig. 3. Effect of intrauterine administration of (a) bovine serum albumin and (b) interferon from Day 15·5 to 21 after oestrus on concentrations of progesterone in serum. Individual profiles from each cow in the experiment are plotted.

contribute to preventing a decrease in endometrial secretion of PGE-2 in early pregnancy (Fig. 1). An increase in the PGE/PGF ratio may serve possible antiluteolytic–luteoprotective and luteotrophic roles that reinforce the predominant antiluteolytic–antiPGF system controlled by bTP-1. One class of antiluteolytic molecules, bTP-1, seems to attenuate PGF secretion via induction of the intracellular PG synthesis inhibitor (antiPGF effect) and also stimulates secretion of PGE-2 (luteoprotective). Additional research is needed to determine whether there are differential regulatory effects of the two molecular weight classes and the various isoelectric variants of bTP-1 (Helmer *et al.*, 1987). It is also essential to determine whether bTP-1 is secreted beyond the period of early pregnancy at the time the CL is maintained. Since bTP-1 is responsible for induction of PG synthesis inhibitor activity, which is elevated throughout pregnancy (Table 1), it would appear that bTP-1 is secreted for extended periods during gestation. Bartol *et al.* (1985) reported that low molecular weight acidic proteins that appear to be similar to bTP-1 were synthesized by Day 69 chorionic tissues of cows.

Physiological importance of bovine trophoblastic protein-1

Based on recent experimentation, a model for blocking luteolysis during early pregnancy involves synthesis of bTP-1 by the conceptus to, in turn, induce synthesis of endometrial PG inhibitor that blocks the actions of endogenous agents which stimulate endometrial PGF secretion leading to luteolysis (e.g. oestradiol, oxytocin receptors and oxytocin). Since the PG-synthesis inhibitor is compartmentalized within the endometrial tissue, it may permit the continued active biosynthesis of prostaglandins by the conceptus and their local associated effects necessary for development. The importance of bTP-1 for embryo survival is indicated by the fact that certain physiological states are associated with higher rates of embryonic death. For example, heat stress reduces both the rate of early embryo development (Putney *et al.*, 1986) and conceptus weights by Day 16 of pregnancy (Biggers *et al.*, 1987). If conceptuses are retarded in their development, they are likely to secrete less bTP-1 and have a smaller probability of exerting an antiluteolytic–antiPGF effect. In fact, Putney *et al.* (1987) demonstrated that hyperthermic temperatures during incubation of Day-17 conceptuses *in vitro* reduced secretion of bTP-1 by 72%. It is likely that embryos that are small for their age may be deficient in bTP-1 secretion. The potential administration of compounds such as bTP-1 for recombinant produced molecules to improve embryo survival in cattle is a rational approach to improve reproductive efficiency.

Research in this paper has been supported by USDA Grants 84-CRSR-22419 and 85-CRSR-1-1871 and is published as University of Florida Agricultural Experiment Station Journal Series No. 9184.

References

Anthony, R.V., Helmer, S.D., Sharif, S.F., Roberts, R.M., Hansen, P.J., Thatcher, W.W. & Bazer, F.W. (1988) Synthesis and processing of ovine trophoblast protein-1 and bovine trophoblast protein-1, conceptus secretory proteins involved in the maternal recognition of pregnancy. *Endocrinology* **123**, 1274–1280.

Bartol, F.F., Roberts, R.M., Bazer, F.W., Lewis, G.S., Godkin, J.D. & Thatcher, W.W. (1985) Characterization of proteins produced in vitro by periattachment bovine conceptuses. *Biol. Reprod.* **32**, 681–693.

Basu, S. & Kindahl, H. (1987) Prostaglandin biosynthesis and its regulation in the bovine endometrium: a comparison between nonpregnant and pregnant status. *Theriogenology* **28**, 175–193.

Biggers, B.G., Geisert, R.D., Wettemann, R.P. & Buchanan, D.S. (1987) Effect of heat stress on early embryonic development in the beef cow. *J. Anim. Sci.* **64**, 1512–1518.

Capon, D.J., Shepard, H.M. & Goeddel, D.V. (1985) Two distinct families of human and bovine interferon-genes are coordinately expressed and encode functional polypeptides. *Molec. cell. Biol.* **5**, 768–779.

Gross, T.S., Thatcher, W.W., Hansen, P.J. & Lacroix, M.C. (1988a) Prostaglandin secretion by perifused bovine endometrium: secretion towards the myometrial and luminal sides at day 17 post-estrus as altered by pregnancy. *Prostaglandins* **35**, 343–358.

Gross, T.S., Thatcher, W.W., Hansen, P.J., Johnson J.W. & Helmer, S.D. (1988b) Presence of an intracellular endometrial inhibitor of prostaglandin synthesis during early pregnancy in the cow. *Prostaglandins* **35**, 359–378.

Gross, T.S., Hansen, P.J., Thatcher, W.W., Helmer, S.D., Plante, C. & Johnson, J.W. (1988c) Peroxidase activity and intracellular inhibitors of prostaglandin synthesis in endometrium during early pregnancy in cattle. *Proc. 11th Int. Congr. Anim. Reprod. & A.I., Dublin* Vol. 2, 91, Abstr.

Gross, T.S. & Thatcher, W.W. (1988) Effect of platelet-activating factor on dynamics of prostaglandin and protein secretion by endometrial explants from pregnant and cyclic cows. *J. Anim. Sci.* **66** (Suppl. 1), 406, Abstr.

Helmer, S.D., Hansen, P.J., Anthony, R.V., Thatcher, W.W., Bazer, F.W. & Roberts, R.M. (1987) Identification of bovine trophoblast protein-1, a secretory protein immunologically related to ovine trophoblast protein-1. *J. Reprod. Fert.* **79**, 83–91.

Helmer, S.D., Hansen, P.J. & Thatcher, W.W. (1988a) Differential glycosylation of the components of the bovine trophoblast protein-1 complex. *Molec. cell. Endocr.* **58**, 103–107.

Helmer, S.D., Hansen, P.J., Thatcher, W.W., Johnson, J.W. & Bazer, F.W. (1988b) Intrauterine infusion of purified bovine trophoblast protein-1 (bTP-1) extends corpus luteum (CL) lifespan in cyclic cattle. *J. Anim. Sci.* **66** (suppl. 1), 415, Abstr.

Helmer, S.D., Gross, T.S., Hansen, P.J. & Thatcher, W.W. (1988c) Bovine conceptus secretory proteins (bCSP) and bovine trophoblast protein-1 (bTP-1), a component of bCSP, alter endometrial prostaglandin (PG) secretion and induce an intracellular inhibitor of PG synthesis in vitro. *Biol. Reprod.* **38**, (Suppl. 1), 153, Abstr.

Heyman, Y., Camous, S., Fevere, J., Meziou, W. & Martal, J. (1984) Maintenance of corpus luteum after uterine transfer of trophoblastic vesicles to cyclic cows and ewes. *J. Reprod. Fert.* **70**, 533–540.

Hickey, G.J. & Hansel, W. (1987) In-vitro synthesis of a low molecular weight lipid-soluble luteotrophic factor by conceptuses of cows at Days 13–18 of pregnancy. *J. Reprod. Fert.* **80**, 569–576.

Imakawa, K., Anthony, R.V., Kazemi, M., Marotti, K.R., Polites, H.G. & Roberts, R.M. (1987) Interferon-like sequence of ovine trophoblast protein secreted by embryonic trophectoderm. *Nature, Lond.* **330**, 377–379.

Knickerbocker, J.J., Thatcher, W.W., Bazer, F.W., Drost, M., Barron, D.H., Fincher, K.B. & Roberts, R.M. (1986a) Proteins secreted by Day-16 to -18 bovine conceptuses extend corpus luteum function in cows. *J. Reprod. Fert.* **77**, 381–391.

Knickerbocker, J.J., Thatcher, W.W., Bazer, F.W., Barron, D.H. & Roberts R.M. (1986b) Inhibition of uterine prostaglandin-F_2 production by bovine conceptus secretory proteins. *Prostaglandins* **31**, 777–793.

O'Neill, C. (1987) Embryo-derived platelet activating factor: a preimplantation embryo mediator of maternal recognition of pregnancy. *Dom. Anim. Endocr.* **4**, 69–85.

Plante, C., Hansen, P.J. & Thatcher, W.W. (1988)

Prolongation of luteal lifespan in cows by intrauterine infusion of recombinant bovine alpha-interferon. *Endocrinology* **122**, 2342–2344.

Putney, D.J., Drost, M. & Thatcher, W.W. (1986) Embryonic development in dairy cattle exposed to elevated temperature between days 1 to 7 post insemination. *Biol. Reprod.* **34** (Suppl. 1), 102, Abstr.

Putney, D.J., Malayer, J.R., Gross, T.S., Hansen, P.J., Thatcher, W.W. & Drost, M. (1987) Heat shock induced alterations in prostaglandin and protein secretion by bovine conceptuses and uterine endometrium. *Biol. Reprod.* **36** (Suppl. 1.), 314, Abstr.

Stewart, H.J., McCann, S.H.E., Barker, P.J., Lee, K.E., Lamming, G.E. & Flint, A.P.F. (1987) Interferon sequence homology and receptor binding activity of ovine trophoblast antiluteolytic protein. *J. Endocr.* **115**, R13–R15.

Thatcher, W.W., Knickerbocker, J.J., Bartol, F.F., Bazer, F.W., Roberts, R.M. & Drost, M. (1985) Maternal recognition of pregnancy in relation to the survival of transferred embryos: endocrine aspects. *Theriogenology* **23**, 129–143.

Thatcher, W.W., Bazer, F.W., Sharp, D.C. & Roberts, R.M. (1986) Interrelationships between uterus and conceptus to maintain corpus luteum function in early pregnancy: sheep, cattle, pigs and horses. *J. Anim. Sci.* **62** (Suppl. 2), 25–46.

J. Reprod. Fert., Suppl. **37** (1989), 101–107

Printed in Great Britain
© 1989 Journals of Reproduction & Fertility Ltd

The continuum of events leading to maternal recognition of pregnancy in mares

D. C. Sharp, Karen J. McDowell*, Joanne Weithenauer and
W. W. Thatcher†

*Animal Science Department and †Dairy Science Department, University of Florida, Gainesville,
FL 32611, U.S.A.; and *Veterinary Science Department, University of Kentucky, Lexington,
KY 40546, U.S.A.*

Summary. Endometria from pregnant mares are able to produce PGF *in vitro*, but when co-incubated with conceptus membranes the amount and rate of PGF production is considerably reduced. To estimate the molecular weight of conceptus factors that inhibited PGF production, Day-14 conceptus membranes were placed inside bags constructed of dialysis tubing and co-incubated with endometria from Day-14 pregnant mares. PGF production was significantly reduced when membranes were in bags with molecular weight exclusion limits of 12 000, 6000, and 3500, but not of 1000, suggesting that conceptus PGF-inhibitory factor(s) is >1000, but $<6000\ M_r$. PGF production at M_r 3500 was only marginally different from control endometria, suggesting proximity to threshold M_r. Because of the apparent transient nature of conceptus factors the importance of conceptus mobility to PGF inhibition from entire uterus was tested. On Day 4, restricting ligatures were placed around uterine horns at the bifurcation ipsilateral or contralateral to the ovulation site. When conceptus mobility was maximally impaired (ipsilateral ligatures) pregnancy failed in 88% (7/8) of mares, whereas when ligatures were placed contralateral to side of ovulation pregnancy failed in 50% (2/4) of mares. Of 5 mares with ligatures around the cranial tip of the uterine horn contralateral to ovulation, 5 established pregnancy. Overall these results suggest that the inhibitory factor has an M_r of 1000–6000 and its transient action necessitates extensive conceptus mobility to block PGF from the majority of the uterus.

Keywords: pregnancy establishment; mare; conceptus; prostaglandin

Introduction

The process of pregnancy establishment appears to be a particularly fragile process in the mare, with a high incidence of errors associated with the maternal recognition of pregnancy. That is, there is a high incidence of inappropriate maintenance of the corpus luteum (CL) or pseudopregnancy in unmated mares (Ginther, 1979; Neely *et al.*, 1979; Sharp, 1980) and a high incidence of early embryonic loss that occurs around the time of pregnancy recognition in mares (Ginther, 1985; Ball & Woods, 1987). In the former case (false positive) the incidence may approach 15–20% of mares in a given herd (Ginther, 1979), while in the latter case (false negative) embryonic loss around the time of maternal recognition of pregnancy has been reported to be as high as 20–25% (Ginther, 1985). Although the reasons for these inappropriate phenomena are not known, it seems reasonable to assume that much of the error is associated with the mechanisms of maternal pregnancy recognition.

Available evidence strongly supports the notion that prostaglandin (PG) F-2α acts as the luteolysin in mares (Sharp, 1980). This evidence includes induction of premature luteolysis by administration of PGF (Douglas & Ginther, 1976), measurement of PGF in the uterine lumen (Zavy *et al.*, 1984), uterine vein (Douglas & Ginther, 1976), and endometrium and in-vitro production rate (Vernon *et al.*, 1981) as well as measurement of the principal PGF metabolite, 13,14-dihydryo-15 keto-prostaglandin F-2α (PGFM), in the peripheral circulation (Kindahl *et al.*, 1982). In all these reports, the secretion of PGF was temporally associated with regression of the CL.

On the other hand, when a conceptus is present, secretion of PGF (or PGFM) is significantly reduced in the uterine vein (Douglas & Ginther, 1976), uterine lumen (Zavy *et al.*, 1984) and periphery (Kindahl *et al.*, 1982). However, Vernon *et al.* (1981) reported that endometrial explants from pregnant mares were as capable of producing PGF *in vitro* as was explanted tissue from non-pregnant mares. This apparent paradox was resolved by Berglund *et al.* (1982) and Sharp *et al.* (1984) when they reported that PGF production *in vitro* was significantly reduced during co-incubation of conceptus membranes and endometrial explants. The significance of these observations lies in the conclusion that the inhibitory effect of the conceptus on PGF secretion is short-lived or transient, at least early in pregnancy establishment, and the endometrium expresses its PGF secretory ability if removed from conceptus influence. It is likely that the extensive mobility of the equine conceptus during the time of maternal pregnancy recognition is an important factor in the recognition process, since it enables the conceptus to interact with the entire endometrial surface repeatedly, thus achieving PGF blockade. These investigations address the continuum of events leading to maternal recognition of pregnancy in mares.

Materials and Methods

Experiment 1: effect of restricting conceptus migration on CL regression. This experiment tested the hypothesis that conceptus migration throughout the entire uterus is necessary for maternal recognition of pregnancy. Uterine horns of mated mares were ligated in one of three positions; at the bifurcation, ipsilateral to side of ovulation (Group 1; N = 5), at the bifurcation contralateral to the side of ovulation (Group 2; N = 4), and at the cranial tip of the horn contralateral to the side of ovulation (Group 3; N = 4), creating 3 experimental groups with: maximal restriction of conceptus mobility (Group 1), intermediate restriction (Group 2) and minimal restriction (Group 3) (see Fig. 1). Ligatures were placed on Day 4 after ovulation and mares were examined daily for the presence of embryonic vesicles with ultrasound echography beginning on Day 9. Blood samples were collected daily for assessment of progesterone concentrations by radioimmunoassay. Progesterone was quantified in plasma by radioimmunoassay using anti-progesterone-C11–BSA generously provided by Dr Juan Troconiz. Sensitivity of the assay was 15·6 pg and intra- and inter-assay coefficients of variation for 16 assays were 8·5 and 17·9% respectively (Knickerbocker, 1985).

Circulating progesterone concentrations were tested for differences in time trends by regression analysis, and the percentage of mares establishing pregnancy was tested by χ^2 analysis. Successful maternal recognition of pregnancy was defined as maintenance of the embryonic vesicle, as determined by ultrasound, to the time of endometrial cup formation (Day 38–40; determined by detection of chorionic gonadotrophin in peripheral plasma), and maintenance of progesterone concentrations > 1 ng/ml. Chorionic gonadotrophin (CG) was detected in plasma using a particle immunoassay system (MIP test; Diamond Laboratories, Des Moines, Iowa 50304, U.S.A.).

Experiment 2. This experiment tested the hypothesis that conceptus loss in the experiment above reflected absence of progesterone. In 2 groups of mares ligatures were placed at the bifurcation ipsilateral to the side of ovulation as above, and mares in Group 1 (N = 3) were treated with vehicle, whereas those in Group 2 (N = 5) were treated with the synthetic progestagen, allyltrenbolone (Regumate: American Hoechst; Somerville, NJ, U.S.A.) beginning on Day 12.

Experiment 3: partial characterization of the conceptus prostaglandin inhibitory factor. Endometrial explants were cultured for 24 h in minimal essential medium (MEM) in the presence of conceptus membranes contained within small chambers constructed of dialysis tubing. Different molecular exclusion limits were used in the construction of the chambers, so that conceptus factors reaching the endometrium had molecular weights less than: (1) 12 000–14 000; (2) 6000–8000; (3) 3500; or (4) 1000. Endometria were cultured for 24 h and media were analysed for PGF by radioimmunoassay. Aliquants of medium were removed from the cultures at 4-h intervals to evaluate the time trends of PGF production and effects of conceptus secretory products over 24 h. Antisera against PGF were generously donated by Dr T. G. Kennedy (London, Ontario, Canada) and the assay was validated for use in MEM in our laboratory. Sensitivity of the assay was between 25 and 100 pg. Inter- and intra-assay coefficients of variation were 8·7 and 17·9%, respectively. Serial dilutions of sample were shown to be parallel to the standard curve.

Experiment 1

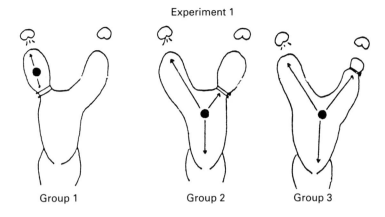

Group 1   Group 2   Group 3

Experiment 2

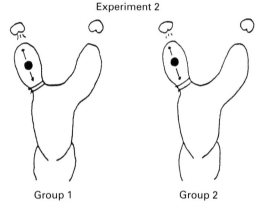

Group 1   Group 2

Fig. 1. Experimental protocol for testing importance of conceptus migration on maternal recognition of pregnancy. Exp. 1—In Group 1, ligatures were placed on Day 4, at the uterine horn–uterine body bifurcation ipsilateral to the side of ovulation, creating maximal restriction of conceptus migration. In Group 2, ligatures were placed at the bifurcation contralateral to the side of ovulation, creating intermediate restriction of conceptus migration. In Group 3, ligatures were placed at the cranial tip of the uterine horn contralateral to the side of ovulation, creating essentially no restriction to conceptus migration, and serving as a surgical control. Exp. 2—In Group 1, ligatures were placed as in Group 1 above. In Group 2, ligatures were placed as in Group 1 above, and synthetic progestagen was administered daily, beginning on Day 12.

Results

Experiment 1

A total of 13 conceptuses was detected in all groups (Group 1 = 5; Group 2 = 4; Group 3 = 4). No conceptuses were lost from Group 3, indicating that the presence of the ligature itself was not detrimental to pregnancy establishment (Table 1). In Group 1, 4 conceptuses were lost by Day 17·0, whereas, in Group 2, 2 conceptuses were lost by Day 15. All mares that failed to recognize pregnancy returned to oestrus at least 1 day before loss of the conceptus. Progesterone concentrations also declined to < 1 ng/ml in all mares before onset of oestrus and loss of the conceptus.

Table 1. Effect of restricted conceptus migration on maternal recognition of pregnancy in mares

Exp.	Group	Conceptuses detected	Conceptuses maintained	Day of return to oestrus	Day of loss
1	1 (ipsilateral)	5	1 (20%)	$16 \cdot 0 \pm 0 \cdot 9$	$17 \cdot 0 \pm 1 \cdot 2$
	2 (contralateral)	4	2 (50%)	$14 \cdot 5 \pm 0 \cdot 7$	$15 \cdot 0 \pm 0 \cdot 7$
	3 (cranial tip)	4	4 (100%)	—	—
2	1 (ipsilateral)	3	0 (0%)	$14 \cdot 5 \pm 3 \cdot 4$	$17 \cdot 3 \pm 4 \cdot 3$
	2 (ipsilateral + progestagen)	5	4 (80%)	$32 \cdot 0$	$16 \cdot 0$

Experiment 2

A total of 8 conceptuses was detected in the two groups (Group 1 = 3; Group 2 = 5). The conceptuses were lost from Group 1 by Day 17, and mares returned to oestrus on Day 14 (Table 1). In Group 2 1 conceptus was lost by Day 16, but this mare did not return to oestrus until after progestagen treatment was discontinued on Day 25.

Experiment 3

PGF production trends over 24 h were significantly affected by co-incubation of endometria with conceptus membranes within dialysis chambers, with a significant interaction of molecular exclusion limit by time (see Fig. 2). PGF production was significantly reduced when endometria were co-incubated with conceptus membranes within dialysis chambers with molecular exclusion limits of 12 000–14 000, 6000–8000, and 3500, but not of 1000. Furthermore, results of PGF production in the 3500 M_r group were less clear. These results suggest that the conceptus secretory product that inhibits PGF production has a molecular weight of > 1000 and < 6000.

Discussion

These results provide evidence for the concept that maternal recognition of pregnancy in mares involves conceptus-secreted factor(s) which inhibit endometrial PGF secretion. Co-incubation of endometria with conceptus membranes contained within dialysis chambers indicated that the conceptus factor(s) which inhibits PGF secretion has a molecular weight of > 1000 and < 6000. Although the chemical characteristics of this factor are not known, the results indicate that it is probably not a steroid, ion, or other prostaglandin. In fact, measurements of PGE in co-incubations of endometrium and conceptus membranes (D. C. Sharp & L. A. Berglund, unpublished observations) suggest that prostaglandins of the E series are also inhibited by conceptus factors. Similarly, administration of PGE to cycling mares did not result in lengthened corpus luteum life-span (D. C. Sharp, unpublished observations). Work is in progress to characterize further the nature of the factor(s).

The demonstration that conceptus migration is necessary for maternal recognition of pregnancy is not surprising. Ginther & First (1971) demonstrated that roughly 50% of hemi-hysterectomized mares underwent luteolysis at the normally expected time, and that the side of ablation relative to side of the CL was not critical. Furthermore, Ginther (1981) reported that the vascular architecture of the equine reproductive tract was not suggestive of a local pathway for PGF transport to the ovary bearing the CL. Therefore, the presence of endometrium, regardless of its location relative to the CL, may cause luteolysis, provided there is a sufficient amount of endometrium present. The report of Ginther & First (1971) suggests that luteolysis can occur with only approximately 50% of the uterus remaining. This information, coupled with the transient nature of the conceptus

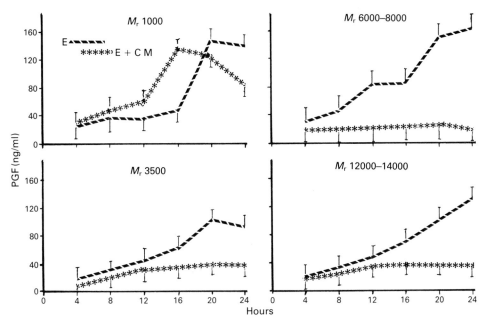

Fig. 2. PGF-2α in endometrial explant cultures (E) and in the presence of conceptus membranes (CM) within dialysis chambers. Similar amounts of endometrium from Day-14 pregnant mares were added to culture plates, and the conceptus membranes were coincubated within dialysis chambers of different molecular exclusion limits as defined in each quadrant. Values are mean ± s.e.m. for 5 observations.

PGF-inhibitory factor, suggests that it is necessary for the conceptus to migrate in order to maintain PGF blockade throughout the entire uterus. It is significant that conceptus mobility ceases about Day 16 or 17 (Ginther, 1983), presumably having accomplished the objective of PGF blockade by the critical deadline. Furthermore, it is likely, although not tested, that conceptus migration offers the opportunity to garner histotrophe throughout the uterus. It may be that the migration of the horse conceptus serves much the same function as elongation of the conceptus in other domestic species (McDowell *et al.*, 1985).

Hershman & Douglas (1979) reported that the life-span of the corpus luteum was not significantly extended in mares from which conceptuses were removed by uterine lavage on Days 10, 12 or 14, but was extended in mares from which conceptuses were removed on Day 16. These authors interpreted their data as indicating the presence of a 'critical period' for maternal recognition of pregnancy. We would suggest, instead, that the conceptus must deal with a 'critical deadline'. That is, we know that corpus luteum regression will occur unless endometrial PGF secretion is abrogated. Furthermore, measurements of PGF secretion in uterine vein (Douglas & Ginther, 1976), uterine lumen (Zavy *et al.*, 1984), endometrium (Vernon *et al.*, 1981), in-vitro production rate (Vernon *et al.*, 1981) and measurements of PGFM in the peripheral circulation (Kindahl *et al.*, 1982) all suggest that PGF secretion begins around Day 14 to 15 after ovulation in mares. Therefore, the 'critical deadline' appears to be at that time. However, we know less of the events which lead to the appropriate endometrial and/or conceptus response by that time. Vernon *et al.* (1981) and Zavy *et al.* (1984) reported that PGF secretion by endometrium in ovariectomized mares required exposure to progesterone, and that acute exposure to oestrogen *in vitro* resulted in greater production of PGF (Vernon *et al.*, 1981). This is in agreement with the results of Poyser (1984) and McCracken *et al.* (1984) that oestradiol is involved in the final stimulus for PGF secretion in a progesterone-primed uterus. Although the mechanisms by which progesterone priming prepares the equine endometrium for PGF secretion are unknown, there is evidence that the process requires some time. Pretreatment of ovariectomized mares with oestradiol for 7 days, followed by 14 days of progesterone treatment did not result in uterine luminal PGF concentrations as high as in mares treated with only progesterone for 21 days (Zavy *et al.*, 1984). Likewise, Betteridge *et al.* (1985) reported that the PGFM response to oxytocin administration was essentially non-existent in a single ovariectomized mare treated with oestradiol and progesterone for 7 days, but that the response was similar to that of intact mares after 14 days of progesterone administration. Therefore, these results indicate that the ability of the endometrium to secrete PGF is acquired over time of progesterone exposure, with between 7 and 14 days required for PGF secretion similar to that of intact mares. The importance of these observations is that we do not know when the conceptus begins to suppress PGF secretion by the endometrium, or whether it is important to begin in advance of the ability of the uterus to secrete PGF maximally. Uterine luminal PGF concentrations in pregnant mares, however, were already considerably lower than in non-pregnant mares on Day 12 (Zavy *et al.*, 1984), suggesting that conceptus factors may already be inhibiting endometrial PGF secretion. It seems reasonable to suggest that conceptuses that are delayed, or retarded to some extent, may not accomplish the blockade of PGF in time to prevent luteolysis, although firm evidence for this idea is not available at present.

These results provide further support for the idea that maternal recognition of pregnancy in the mare involves suppression of endometrial prostaglandin secretion by conceptus factors, and that conceptus migration is an important mechanism by which the PGF inhibitory factor(s) are delivered throughout the entire uterus.

We thank Lynn Peck, Steve Davis, Michael Seroussi, and Peter Sheerin for help in these projects. The authors also acknowledge support from the Morris Animal Foundation, and the Grayson Foundation. Florida Agricultural Experiment Station Journal Series No. 9238.

References

Ball, B.A. & Woods, G.L. (1987) Embryonic loss and early pregnancy loss in the mare. *Compendium for Cont. Ed. Pract. Vet.* **9**, 459–469.

Berglund, L.A., Sharp, D.C., Vernon, M.W. & Thatcher, W.W. (1982) Effect of pregnancy and collection technique on prostaglandin F in the uterine lumen of pony mares. *J. Reprod. Fert., Suppl.* **32**, 335–341.

Betteridge, K.J., Renard, A. & Goff, A.K. (1985) Uterine prostaglandin release relative to embryo collection, transfer procedures and maintenance of the corpus luteum. *Eq. vet. J., Suppl.* **3**, 25–34.

Douglas, R.H. & Ginther, O.J. (1976) Concentration of prostaglandins F in uterine venous plasma of anesthetized mares during the estrous cycle and early pregnancy. *Prostaglandins* **11**, 251–260.

Ginther, O.J. (1979) *Reproductive Biology of the Mare. Basic and Applied Aspects.* Equiservices, Inc. Cross Plains.

Ginther, O.J. (1981) Local versus systemic utero ovarian relationships in farm animals. *Acta vet. scand., Suppl.* **77**, 103–115.

Ginther, O.J. (1983) Mobility of the early equine conceptus. *Theriogenology* **19**, 603–661.

Ginther, O.J. (1985) Dynamic physical interactions between the equine embryo and uterus. *Equine vet. J., Suppl.* **3**, 41–48.

Ginther, O.J. & First, N.L. (1971) Maintenance of the corpus luteum in hysterectomized mares. *Am. J. vet. Res.* **32**, 1687–1691.

Hershman, L. & Douglas, R.H. (1979) The critical period for the maternal recognition of pregnancy in pony mares. *J. Reprod. Fert., Suppl.* **27**, 395–401.

Kindahl, H., Knudsen, O., Madej, A. & Edqvist, L.E. (1982) Progesterone, prostaglandin F-2α, PMSG and oestrone sulphate during early pregnancy in the mare. *J. Reprod. Fert., Suppl.* **32**, 353–359.

Knickerbocker, J.J. (1985) *Pregnancy recognition in cattle: effects of conceptus products on uterine prostaglandin production.* Ph.D. Dissertation, University of Florida, Gainesville, FL.

McCracken, J.A., Schramm, W. & Okulicz, W.C. (1984) Hormone control of pulsatile secretion of PGF$_{2\alpha}$ from the ovine uterus during luteolysis and its abrogation in early pregnancy. *Anim. Reprod. Sci.* **7**, 31–57.

McDowell, K.J., Sharp, D.C., Peck, L.S. & Cheves, L.L. (1985) Effect of restricted conceptus mobility on maternal recognition of pregnancy in mares. *Equine vet. J., Suppl.* **3**, 23–24.

Neely, D.P., Kindahl, H., Stabenfeldt, G.H., Edqvist, L.E. & Hughes, J.P. (1979) Prostaglandin release patterns in the mare: physiological, pathophysiological and therapeutic responses. *J. Reprod. Fert., Suppl* **27**, 181–189.

Poyser, N.L. (1984) Prostaglandin production by the

uterus of the non-pregnant and early pregnant guinea pig. *Anim. Reprod. Sci.* **7**, 1–30.

Sharp, D.C. (1980) Factors associated with the maternal recognition of pregnancy in mares. *Vet. Clinics of North America: Large Animal Practice* **2**, 277–290.

Sharp, D.C., Zavy, M.T., Vernon, M.W., Bazer, F.W., Thatcher, W.W. & Berglund, L.A. (1984) The role of prostaglandin in the maternal recognition of pregnancy in mares. *Anim. Reprod. Sci.* **7**, 269–282.

Vernon, M.W., Zavy, M.T., Asquith, R.L. & Sharp, D.C. (1981) Prostaglandin $F_{2\alpha}$ in the equine endometrium: steroid modulation and production capacities during the estrous cycle and early pregnancy. *Biol. Reprod.* **25**, 581–589.

Zavy, M.T., Vernon, M.W., Asquith, R.L., Bazer, F.W. & Sharp, D.C. (1984) Effect of exogenous gonadal steroids and pregnancy on uterine luminal prostaglandin F in mares. *Prostaglandins* **27**, 311–320.

J. Reprod. Fert., Suppl. **37** (1989), 109–113

Characteristics of pregnancy-specific protein B in cattle

R. G. Sasser, J. Crock and C. A. Ruder-Montgomery

Department of Animal Science, University of Idaho, Moscow, Idaho 83843, U.S.A.

Summary. Pregnancy-specific protein B (PSPB) has been isolated from placental tissue of cows. Antisera were developed against PSPB and by immunohistochemical techniques the protein was localized to the binucleated cells of the trophoblastic ectoderm. A radioimmunoassay (RIA) was also developed and used to detect PSPB in sera of pregnant animals. The RIA has been used successfully in pregnancy testing in cattle and other ruminants. The assay can also be used to detect time of embryonic death. Chemical characterization of PSPB showed that it was an acidic glycoprotein with an apparent molecular weight of 78 000. It has several isoelectric variants with pIs of 4·0–4·4.

Keywords: pregnancy; protein; pregnancy-specific protein B; embryo; cattle

Introduction

Proteins produced by the placenta have been reported for many years in several species. For example Aschheim & Zondek (1928) reported that a protein named human chorionic gonadotrophin (hCG) was present in urine of pregnant women. This can be measured in urine or blood at about 10 days after conception (Marshall *et al.*, 1968). Several other pregnancy proteins have been found in the human but not all reach the maternal blood or urine (Bohn, 1985).

Several pregnancy proteins are reported in domestic animals. Pregnant mare serum gonadotrophin was found in serum of mares (Cole & Hart, 1930) and used as a pregnancy marker (Cole & Hart, 1942). Rowson & Moor (1967) showed that a heat-labile substance in the 13-day-old sheep embryo, when infused into the uterus of the cyclic sheep, would extend the life-span of the corpus luteum. Later, Godkin *et al.* (1982) studied proteins produced by the conceptus of this species and showed that the major secretory protein was a low molecular weight acidic protein produced between Days 13 and 21 of pregnancy. This was termed ovine trophoblast protein-1 (oTP-1). This protein is probably the same as trophoblastin, a substance earlier identified by Martal *et al.* (1979). oTP-1 is secreted at a time corresponding to the time of maternal recognition of pregnancy in the ewe and is involved in regulation of protein secretion by the endometrium (Vallet *et al.*, 1987). Chemical characteristics of this protein suggest that it is similar to a human alpha interferon (Imakawa *et al.*, 1987). As in sheep, the early bovine conceptus, when homogenized and infused into the uterus, will extend luteal life-span (Betteridge *et al.*, 1980; Northey & French, 1980; Dalla Porta & Humblot, 1983). The major protein secreted by the bovine embryo between Days 16 and 24–27 has properties similar to those of oTP-1 (Bartol *et al.*, 1984) and is termed bovine trophoblast protein-1. Godkin *et al.* (1988) have identified several proteins of the bovine conceptus near Days 30 to 40 of gestation.

Pregnancy-specific protein B (PSPB) has been found in the serum of pregnant cattle (Sasser *et al.*, 1986) and has been used as a pregnancy marker. This paper will summarize currently understood biological and chemical characteristics of this protein.

Pregnancy-specific protein B

This protein was found after immunizing rabbits with homogenates of whole bovine placenta and adsorbing the antisera with somatic tissues to remove antibodies to proteins not specific to the placenta. Remaining antibodies were against alpha-fetoprotein and PSPB of the placenta (Butler et al., 1982). Adsorbed antisera were used as a marker in immunodiffusion and immunoelectrophoresis methods to isolate a preparation of PSPB (R-37) from bovine placenta (Sasser et al., 1986). A new antiserum (RGS 38-1) was then developed in a rabbit for use in development of a double-antibody radioimmunoassay (RIA) for PSPB (Sasser et al., 1986) and for further characterization of PSPB.

Biological characteristics

Source of PSPB. Immunohistochemical methods were used to find that PSPB was present in the giant binucleated cells of the trophectoderm of the placenta (Eckblad et al., 1985). Also, studies by Reimers et al. (1985) showed that PSPB secretion into media was greater by placental cell fractions enriched in binucleated cells than by those enriched in mononucleated cells.

The presence of PSPB in body fluids other than blood has been investigated. Cross-reacting antigens have not been found in urine, tears, saliva, or vaginal or cervical secretions; however, milk contains PSPB when collected at a time when it is excessively high in plasma of cows, i.e. within the week after parturition (R. G. Sasser, unpublished).

Pregnancy testing with PSPB. Cross-reactions of antigens in sera from the cow, sheep and goat, compared to the PSPB standard for this RIA, are shown in Fig. 1. The sera of pregnant cows paralleled the standard curve while that of pregnant sheep and goats did not. The assay was therefore quantitative for cow but only qualitative for sheep or goat PSPB. However, a qualitative assay is adequate for a test for pregnancy. There were no cross-reacting antigens in sera of non-pregnant animals and so the RIA can be used to detect pregnancy in these ruminants.

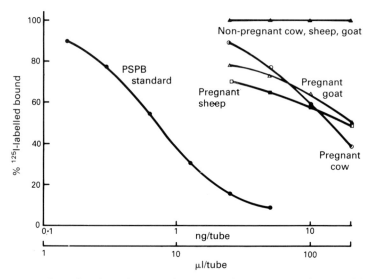

Fig. 1. Cross-reaction of antigens in sera of pregnant sheep, goats and cows with Antiserum RGS 38-1 compared to R-37 PSPB standard. (From Sasser & Ruder, 1987.)

Sasser et al. (1986) have shown that the RIA for cattle was appropriate for pregnancy testing in large numbers of animals. Additionally, they showed that PSPB was present in serum from the 3rd week until the end of pregnancy in most cows and, in some, as early as the 2nd week of gestation.

The time during the 3rd–4th week that the test could first be used and detect a high percentage of pregnancies was evaluated in dairy cattle by Humblot *et al.* (1988a). Cows (N = 76) and heifers (N = 71) were subjected to 177 artificial inseminations (AI) followed by analyses of blood for PSPB by RIA on Days 24, 26 and 30–35 and some on Day 70 after AI. All data were compared for accuracy with rectal examination data at Day 70.

As shown in Table 1, accuracy improved as gestation age increased. The accuracy of the test was acceptable by 30–35 days and was considerably more accurate than the milk progesterone assay administered to these same animals on Days 22 and 24 after insemination: 70, 77 and 79% on Days 22, 24, and Days 22 + 24 combined.

Table 1. Accuracy of pregnancy detection at different days of pregnancy in 177 cows and heifers

Pregnancy status at 70 days	Day of gestation			
	24	26	30–35	70
Pregnant	86 (50/58)	88	90 (83/92)	99 (77/78)
Non-pregnant	72 (86/119)	89 (84/94)	100 (83/83)	100 (36/36)
Overall	77 (136/177)	89 (157/177)	95 (166/175)*	99 (113/114)†

Values are % with the numerator being the total no. of pregnant or non-pregnant animals by PSPB assay and the denominator the no. that returned to oestrus before 70 days or were palpated at 70 days as pregnant or non-pregnant.
*Two animals returned to oestrus and were not included in this calculation.
†Serum was collected and analysed for PSPB on Day 70 in only 114 of the 177 animals initially started on the project.

The sensitivity of the RIA has been modified by changing first antibody dilution and incubation conditions. Estimates of pregnancy with high accuracy before 30–35 days are anticipated (R. G. Sasser, unpublished).

Post-partum PSPB. Ruder & Sasser (1986) showed that PSPB remains in the serum for a considerable time after parturition in cows. The half-life was estimated to be 7·3 days from Days 21 to 53 *post partum* in cows which were hysterectomized on Day 21. This long half-life poses a problem for pregnancy testing in re-mated post-partum cows. Studies are being conducted with the above-mentioned sensitive RIA to determine the time that an acceptable low level of PSPB is reached during the post-partum interval in order that a higher level of PSPB of a new pregnancy at 26–28 days can be determined.

Estimates of embryo death. We have also shown that PSPB can be used in conjunction with the milk progesterone assay for monitoring time of embryonic death (Humblot *et al.*, 1988b). Milk or serum progesterone concentration at 21–24 days is indicative of the presence or absence of an embryo at 16–17 days since this is the time that the embryo signals its presence to the maternal system (Northey & French, 1980). Later embryo death can be determined by the PSPB assay. The time of embryo death can therefore be surveyed from Day 16 until term pregnancy.

Chemical characteristics

Since the success of the RIA for pregnancy detection relies upon the displacement of radio-labelled PSPB (preparation R-37), all chemical isolation and analysis has relied upon displacement of radiolabelled PSPB from Antiserum RGS 38-1. Additionally, polyacrylamide gel electrophoresis (PAGE) has been analysed by Western blotting of immunoreactive proteins on nitrocellulose paper using Antiserum RGS 38-1 (R. G. Sasser & J. Crock, unpublished).

The R-37 preparation of PSPB contained several immunoreactive bands as determined by Western blotting after SDS-PAGE. Most were removed by column chromatography of radio-labelled PSPB during the iodination procedure (Sasser *et al.*, 1986) and before use in the RIA. A band containing the majority of the radioactivity remained and had an apparent molecular weight of 78 000 (SDA-PAGE estimate).

Extraction of PSPB from bovine cotyledons yielded a single major immunoreactive band and 2 minor bands with apparent respective molecular weights of 78 000, 85 000 and 90 000 by SDS-PAGE. Migration of the band of M_r 78 000 was not affected by β-mercaptoethanol, suggesting that PSPB exists as a monomer and that disulphide linkages are not important in maintaining tertiary structure of the molecule.

Cultures of whole cotyledons from bovine placenta of 90 days of age secreted proteins into medium (Hanks' balanced salt solution). Five proteins, when separated on SDS-PAGE were detectable by Antiserum RGS 38-1 on a Western blot. The major band had an estimated molecular weight of 78 000 and 4 minor bands had molecular weights of 48 000, 65 000, 85 000 and 90 000. Antisera were produced against the bands of M_r 78 000, 85 000 and 90 000 which had been cut from PAGE gels and injected, with polyacrylamide, into rabbits. Immune sera against each antigen cross-reacted with the other two in the Western blot. All antisera also bound the radiolabelled R-37 preparation of PSPB.

Radiolabelled R-37 preparation of PSPB and the M_r 78 000 preparation from culture media were subjected to two-dimensional IEF-SDS-PAGE. Both of these proteins of M_r 78 000 contained 7 isoelectric variants with isoelectric points between 4·0 and 4·4. Two variants with pIs of approximately 4·2–4·25 were most abundant. Peptide maps of these isomers were similar, indicating that all variants are charge isomers and not different proteins with similar molecular weights and pIs. The protein of M_r 78 000 contained ~5% hexose sugars and ~3% sialic acid.

Conclusion

PSPB is a glycoprotein produced by the binucleate cells of the placenta of ruminant animals. The biological function of this protein awaits determination. Measurement of it in plasma or serum but probably not in other biological fluids can be used as a pregnancy test. Care must be taken in evaluating sera of animals in the early post-partum period for a new pregnancy. A false positive test may be obtained.

It is anticipated that PSPB can be formatted into a field test kit that can be purchased by producers and applied at their own facilities. Such tests are available for measurement of other chemical substances. Actual assay time is only 3–10 min.

This study was supported by the Idaho Agricultural Experiment Station, U.S.A; the United Dairymen of Idaho, U.S.A.; and UNCEIA Laboratoire d'Hormonologie, Maisons Alfort, France.

References

Aschheim, S. & Zondek, B. (1928) Diagnosis of pregnancy by demonstrating the presence of the hormone of the anterior hypophysis in the urine. *Klin. Wschr.* **7,** 1404–1411.

Bartol, F.F., Roberts, R.M., Bazer, F.W., Lewis, G.S., Godkin, J.D. & Thatcher, W.W. (1984) Characterization of proteins produced *in vitro* by periattachment bovine conceptuses. *Biol. Reprod.* **32,** 681–694.

Betteridge, K.J., Eaglesome, M.D., Randall, G.C.B. & Mitchell, D. (1980) Collection, description and transfer of embryos from cattle 10–16 days after oestrus. *J. Reprod. Fert.* **59,** 205–216.

Bohn, H. (1985) Biochemistry of pregnancy proteins—an overview. In *Early Pregnancy Factors*, pp. 127–139. Eds F. Ellendorff & E. Koch. Perinatology Press, Ithaca.

Butler, J.E., Hamilton, W.C., Sasser, R.G., Ruder, C.A., Hass, G.M. & Williams, R.J. (1982) Detection and partial characterization of two bovine pregnancy-specific proteins. *Biol. Reprod.* **26,** 925–933.

Cole, H.H. & Hart, G.H. (1930) The potency of blood serum of mares in progressive stages of pregnancy in affecting the sexual maturity of the immature rat. *Am. J. Physiol.* **93,** 57–68.

Cole, H.H. & Hart, G.H. (1942) Diagnosis of pregnancy in the mare by hormonal means. *J. Am. vet. med. Ass.* **101,** 124–128.

Dalla Porta, M.A. & Humblot, P. (1983) Effect of embryo removal and embryonic extracts or PGE₂ infusions on luteal function in the bovine. *Theriogenology* **19,** 122–131.

Eckblad, W.P., Sasser, R.G., Ruder, C.A., Panlasigui, P. & Kuczynski, T. (1985) Localization of pregnancy-specific protein B (PSPB) in bovine placental cells using a glucose oxidase-anti-glucose oxidase immunohistochemical stain. *J. Anim. Sci.* **61,** (Suppl.), 149–150, Abstr.

Godkin, J.D., Bazer, F.W., Moffatt, J., Sessions, F. & Roberts, R.M. (1982) Purification and properties of a major, low molecular weight protein released by the trophoblast of sheep at Day 13–21. *J. Reprod. Fert.* **65,** 141–150.

Godkin, J.D., Lifesy, Jr. B.J. & Gillespie, B.E. (1988) Characterization of bovine conceptus proteins produced between the peri- and post attachment periods of early pregnancy. *Biol. Reprod.* **38,** 703–712.

Humblot, P., Camous, S., Martal, J., Charlery, J., Jeanguyot, N., Thibier, M. & Sasser, R.G. (1988a) Diagnosis of pregnancy by radioimmunoassay of a pregnancy-specific protein in plasma of dairy cows. *Theriogenology* **30,** 257–268.

Humblot, P., Camous, S., Martal, J., Charlery, J., Jeanguyot, N., Thibier, M. & Sasser, R.G. (1988b) Pregnancy-specific protein B, progesterone concentrations and embryonic mortality during early pregnancy in dairy cows. *J. Reprod. Fert.* **83,** 215–223.

Imakawa, K., Anthony, R.V., Kazemi, M., Marotti, K.R., Polites, H.G. & Roberts, R.M. (1987) Interferon-like sequence of ovine trophoblast protein secreted by embryonic trophectoderm. *Nature, Lond.* **330,** 337–379.

Marshall, J.R., Hammond, C.B., Ross, G.T., Jacobson, A., Rayford, P. & Odell, W.D. (1968) Plasma and urinary chorionic gonadotrophin during early human pregnancy. *Obstet. Gynec., N.Y.* **32,** 760–764.

Martal, J., Lacroix, M.C., Loudes, C., Saunier, M. & Wintenberger-Torres, S. (1979) Trophoblastin, an antiluteolytic protein present in early pregnancy in sheep. *J. Reprod. Fert.* **56,** 63–67.

Northey, D.L. & French, L.R. (1980) Effect of embryo removal and intrauterine function of embryonic homogenates on the lifespan of the bovine corpus luteum. *J. Anim. Sci.* **50,** 298–302.

Reimers, T.J., Sasser, R.G. & Ruder, C.A. (1985) Production of pregnancy-specific protein by bovine binucleate trophoblastic cells. *Biol. Reprod.* **32,** (Suppl.), 65, Abstr.

Rowson, L.E.A. & Moor, R.M. (1967) The influence of embryonic tissue homogenate infused into the uterus on the life-span of the corpus luteum in sheep. *J. Reprod. Fert.* **13,** 511–516.

Ruder, C.A. & Sasser, R.G. (1986) Source of bovine pregnancy-specific protein B (bPSPB) during the postpartum period and estimation of half-life of bPSPB. *J. Anim. Aci.* **63,** (Suppl.), 335, Abstr.

Sasser, R.G. & Ruder, C.A. (1987) Detection of early pregnancy in domestic ruminants. *J. Reprod. Fert., Suppl.* **34,** 261–271.

Sasser, R.G., Ruder, C.A., Ivani, K.A., Butler, J.E. & Hamilton, W.C. (1986) Detection of pregnancy by radioimmunoassay of a novel pregnancy-specific protein in serum of cows and a profile of serum concentrations during gestation. *Biol. Reprod.* **35,** 936–942.

Vallet, J.L., Bazer, F.W. & Roberts, R.M. (1987) The effect of ovine trophoblast protein-one on endometrial protein secretion and cyclic nucleotides. *Biol. Reprod.* **37,** 1307–1316.

J. Reprod. Fert., Suppl. **37** (1989), 115–119

Measurement and clinical significance of preimplantation blastocyst gonadotrophins

Brij B. Saxena

Division of Reproductive Endocrinology, Department of Obstetrics & Gynecology, Cornell University Medical College, New York, New York 10021, U.S.A.

Keywords: gonadotrophin; blastocyst; corpus luteum

Introduction

Psychoyos (1967) first proposed that the blastocyst and the uterus exchange information before implantation. On theoretical grounds there is no particular reason why the blastocyst should not be able to secrete chorionic gonadotrophin (CG) before implantation. The fact that after fertilization the life-span of the corpus luteum is extended is the most compelling rationale to search for such a preimplantation luteotrophic stimulus.

The mechanism of the rescue of the corpus luteum of pregnancy has not been completely elucidated. The detection of CG-like material on the surface of mouse and rabbit morulae (Wiley, 1974; Asch *et al.*, 1978) was confirmed by the presence of gonadotrophin, namely luteinizing hormone (LH) and CG-like material, in the blastocyst before implantation (Haour & Saxena, 1974; Fujimoto *et al.*, 1975; Channing *et al.*, 1978). These observations have provided one of the most important clues for the sustenance of the functional life of the corpus luteum until the fetal–luteal transfer for the maintenance of the endometrium in early pregnancy has been established. In this paper, I shall consider the biological and clinical significance of the luteotrophin in the blastocyst of various species before implantation.

There is evidence to indicate that maternal recognition of pregnancy exists in different species. For example, the occurrence of luteotrophic or antiluteolytic substances and steroidogenesis in the embryos of mice, rat, rabbit, hamster, pig, sheep, dog, monkey and human before or at the time of implantation has been described (Huff & Eik-Nes, 1966; Perry *et al.*, 1973; Dickman & Dey, 1974; Saxena *et al.*, 1974; Kosasa *et al.*, 1974; Hodgen *et al.*, 1974; Catt *et al.*, 1975; Dickmann, 1976; Batta & Channing, 1979; Moudgal *et al.*, 1978; Pope *et al.*, 1982).

Luteotrophin in the rabbit blastocyst

On the basis of the presence of hCG-like material in the blastocyst before implantation (Haour & Saxena, 1974), and of the significantly greater increase in the secretion of progesterone from Day 4 *post coitum* in pregnant than in pseudopregnant rabbits, Fuchs & Beling (1974) suggested that the maternal ovary recognizes the presence of blastocysts before implantation. Chatterton *et al.* (1975) recognized the secretion of progesterone synthesis-promoting substance by the unimplanted rat blastocyst *in vitro*. It was suggested that the steroidogenesis in the rabbit blastocyst may be activated by a luteotrophic material of blastocyst origin. The maintenance of the corpus luteum of pregnancy in the presence of the blastocyst, implanted under the kidney capsule in the rat, further emphasized the blastocyst as the source of preimplantation luteotrophic stimulus (Zeilmaker & Verhamme, 1978). The secondary rise of CG–LH-like material in the serum of pregnant rabbits on Days 3 and 5 after an ovulatory LH surge is of interest. Our findings (Varma *et al.*, 1979) and those of Singh & Adams (1978) are in agreement with those of Fuchs & Beling (1974) that pregnant rabbits show a greater increase in progesterone during the preimplantation phase than do pseudopregnant rabbits, and that the blastocyst is the source of a preimplantation luteotrophic stimulus. If a CG-like substance is produced in the rabbit blastocyst, its presence in the blood suggests an active transport of material through the uterine wall before implantation and before establishment of vascular connections. Exogenous hCG introduced into the rabbit uterus appeared in the peripheral circulation within 30 min (Saxena *et al.*, 1977).

A logit-log relationship of a standard curve obtained with hCG yielded a slope of -0.70 in the presence of 10, 20, 40, 60 and 80 µl of blastocyst fluid, which was similar to those of hCG and LH. The blastocyst fluid also competed with ^{125}I-labelled hCG for binding to the receptor, prepared from rat ovaries and rat testes. Estimates from 16 independent radioreceptor assays using the bovine corpus luteum receptor yielded 0.83–1.0 ng hCG–LH-like luteotrophin per blastocyst. On Days 5–6 after mating, 6–8 ng hCG-like material/ml plasma were present (Haour & Saxena, 1974). The radioreceptor assay estimate of luteotrophic material ($\sim$87 ng/ml) is higher than the radioimmunoassay estimate of 20 ng/ml blastocyst fluid of Day 6. About 1–1.5 ng hCG in 15 µl fluid per blastocyst was measured.

We have attempted to purify the hCG-like material from rabbit blastocysts. New Zealand White rabbits (36 adult females, 6 normal males and 2 vasectomized males) (3–4 kg) were maintained at room temperature in 12 h of light (06:00–18:00 h). The animals were provided with compressed food and water *ad libitum*. The day of mating was designated as Day 0. Blastocysts were removed by laparotomy performed on Day 6 after mating. The blastocysts were punctured by a needle and centrifuged at 2600 *g* at 4°C for 30 min to recover the blastocyst fluid. A total of 3.3 ml blastocyst fluid was recovered from 196 eggs. Two batches of 4.5 and 5 ml blastocyst fluid were also contributed by Dr Cornelia Channing and Dr Ricardo Asch respectively.

In a typical purification procedure, a 4.5-ml sample of the blastocyst fluid was lyophilized and redissolved in 1 ml 0.01 M-Tris–HCl buffer of pH 7.5 containing 0.1 MNaCl, and centrifuged. The supernatant was applied to a 0.7 × 20 cm column of Concanavalin A–Sepharose 4B, which was previously equilibrated with the same buffer. After the elution of the unadsorbed protein fraction, the column was eluted with 0.1 M-α-methyl mannoside in the same buffer. The fractions were assayed for hCG-like activity in the radioreceptor assay. The adsorbed fraction contained the hCG–LH-like activity. This fraction was lyophilized, dissolved in 0.5 ml 0.1 M-ammonium bicarbonate buffer, and fractionated on a 1 × 115 cm column of Sephadex G-100 equilibrated in the above buffer. The k_{av} of this fraction on Sephadex G-100 was similar to that of hCG. The hCG–LH-like activity (mi.u./µg protein) of the purified blastocyst luteotrophin in the various assays was 20 in the radioreceptor assay, 7.8 in an hCG-β subunit radioimmunoassay, 14 in the rat Leydig cell assay for testosterone production and 25 for progesterone production after 5 days of culture of monkey granulosa cells (Saxena, 1979). Carbohydrate analysis of the purified luteotrophic fraction showed 1.4% fucose, 1.8% mannose, 5.8% galactose, 5.6% *N*-acetylglucosamine, 7.4% *N*-acetylgalactosamine and trace amounts of sialic acid. These observations suggested that the luteotrophic material present in the preimplanted rabbit blastocyst is a glycoprotein and similar to hCG in biological activity. Moudgal *et al.* (1978) found that the serum progesterone concentrations in pregnant monkeys (*Macaca radiata*) were higher than those in the normal cycling animals before the establishment of implantation, thus suggesting the presence of a stimulus to the corpus luteum from the unimplanted blastocyst. The presence of gonadotrophin was also detected in the monkey uterine venous effluent at the time of implantation (Hodgen *et al.*, 1974).

Secretion of luteotrophin by monkey blastocysts

The presence and secretion of hCG-like material of the blastocyst of rhesus monkeys and its ability to stimulate steroidogenesis in cultured granulosa cells obtained from preovulatory monkey follicles were demonstrated by Batta & Channing (1979). Starting at the onset of menstruation until the end of the cycle, 5 ml femoral blood samples were obtained daily from 9 cycling female rhesus monkeys during ketamine anaesthesia. The serum was assayed for oestrogen and progesterone by radioimmunoassay. On the day of the oestrogen surge, each female was left for 48–72 h with a fertile male. After the vaginal plug was observed the female was isolated and for 7 days daily 5 ml femoral blood samples were obtained. Oocytes were also obtained from 3 monkeys during the oestrogen surge. In one monkey, superovulation was induced by the use of PMSG, hCG and prostaglandin E-1: blastocysts and morulae were obtained 7 days after mating. The oocytes, morulae and blastocysts were cultured individually in Falcon microtest plates in a volume of 0·2 ml Medium 199 with 25 mM-Hepes buffer (Grand Island Biological Co., NY), containing 50 µg Gentamicin/ml, 1 µg insulin/ml and 15% (v/v) fasting male monkey serum. The conditioned culture medium was frozen at $-35°C$ and later tested for hCG-like activity, using cultured monkey granulosa cells as an assay system. At the end of the incubation, the cultures were fixed in 10% formalin and stained with oil red O and haematoxylin. Control cultures were incubated in 50% control medium, which previously had been incubated under conditions comparable to the experimental cultures.

Out of a total of 5 untreated mated monkeys, 2 did not have normal post-ovulatory progesterone concentrations and did not yield blastocysts, whereas 3 had normal luteal function as indicated by a post-ovulatory rise of progesterone. Of the 3 normally ovulating monkeys, 2 yielded degenerate oocytes in the uterine lavage 7 days after mating and the 3rd provided a morula of normal appearance. The morula was cultured and grew to become a blastocyst within 3 days of culture. The 3 oocytes obtained during the oestrogen surge matured in culture and expelled a polar body. The medium obtained from the morula exerted a 173–242% stimulation in progesterone secretion whereas medium from the 2 cultured unfertilized oocytes exerted little stimulation of progesterone secretion.

Two blastocysts, 2 morulae and 2 oocytes were recovered from the superovulated treated monkey. Each was cultured individually. The progesterone secretion by the granulosa cell culture was increased in the presence of culture medium from the blastocysts and morulae (Table 1). Addition of medium obtained from the morulae and blastocysts showed an average increase in the progesterone secretion of 110, 112, 196 and 400% on Days 3, 5, 7 and 9 of culture. The stimulation of progesterone secretion in the presence of the morulae and blastocysts varied from 106 to 408% on Day 7 and from 226 to 2826% on Day 9. The medium from the blastocysts also stimulated morphological luteinization of the granulosa cells in culture. Medium from the blastocysts had a greater ability to stimulate progesterone secretion compared to the morulae. Medium from the oocytes increased progesterone stimulation up to 315% only up to Day 7; by Day 9 values were decreased to control levels. These studies show that the monkey morula and blastocyst have the potential to secrete an agent(s) capable of stimulating progesterone secretion by cultured monkey

Table 1. Effect of medium conditioned by rhesus monkey oocyte, blastocyst and morulae on progesterone secretion (pg/cell/day/monkey) by cultured monkey granulosa cells (adapted from Channing *et al.*, 1978)

Source of medium	Days in culture			
	3	5	7	9
Control	0·44	0·57	0·58	0·19
Oocyte	0·53	0·63	1·09	0·37
Morulae and blastocysts	0·48	0·64	1·14	1·72

granulosa cells. It is tempting to speculate that monkey CG is similar to hCG, since hCG has a similar activity in stimulating progesterone secretion by monkey granulosa cells.

Secretion of luteotrophin by human blastocysts

The ability of the blastocyst to produce luteotrophin material on its own is clearly demonstrated by ectopic implantation of the blastocyst at sites other than the endometrium, suggesting that the blastocyst is biochemically equipped to produce CG to support the corpus luteum of gestation. It has long been assumed that the secretion of CG is initiated at the time of implantation. It is now apparent that the human embryo is present in the uterus as early as 3·5 days after ovulation. The human blastocyst is quite large, having as many as 186 cells before implantation. In fact, in recent years there have been several observations which indicate that the blastocyst is able to provide a signal to the corpus luteum even before implantation. Saxena *et al.* (1974) and Kosasa *et al.* (1974) have been able to demonstrate hCG in human serum as early as 6–8 days after ovulation, whereas Catt *et al.* (1975) detected hCG in the plasma only after the initiation of implantation of the blastocyst. It is difficult to ascertain the exact time of implantation in these studies since, according to Hertig *et al.* (1956) implantation could begin as early as 4·5 days and as late as 9 days after ovulation. The disagreement on the presence of hCG in the blastocyst, in the serum and in the urine before implantation appears to be due to the use of non-specific assays at the limit of their sensitivity. The direct evidence to confirm our findings in women is provided by the observations of Fishel *et al.* (1984) who collected human oocytes by laparoscopy (Table 2). When the fertilized embryos were cultured *in vitro*, hCG was detected in the medium surrounding the embryos cultured for more than 7 days after fertilization, presumably secreted by the preimplantation embryos.

Table 2. Production of hCG by human blastocysts (adapted from Fishel *et al.*, 1984)

Culture medium	Hours after insemination	hCG (m i.u/ml)
Control		Not detected
Compacted	110	Not detected
Blastocyst	170	25
Blastocyst	216	43
Trophoblast outgrowth	288	6033

The foregoing clearly demonstrates the role of hCG-like material in the blastocyst in the maternal recognition of pregnancy, before implantation. The clinical significance of the blastocyst luteotrophin and its interrelationship with other endocrine and metabolic factors may be realized in relation to the early diagnosis and management of high risk pregnancy and pregnancy wastage, as well as their usefulness in in-vitro fertilization and fertility regulation.

I thank Dr Ricardo Asch, Dr Cornelia P. Channing and Dr R. G. Edwards for collaboration.

References

Asch, R.H., Fernandez, E.O., Magnasco, L.A. & Pauerstein, C.J. (1978) Demonstration of a chorionic gonadotropin-like substance in rabbit morulae. *Fert. Steril.* **29**, 444–446.

Batta, S.K. & Channing, C.P. (1979) Preimplantation Rhesus Monkey blastocyst: secretion of substance capable of stimulating progesterone secretion by granulosa cell cultures. *Life Sci.* **25**, 2057–2063.

Catt, K.J., Dufau, M.L. & Vaitukaitis, J.L. (1975) Appearance of hCG in pregnancy plasma following the initiation of the implantation of the blastocyst. *J. clin. Endocr. Metab.* **40**, 537–539.

Channing, C.P., Stone, S.L., Sakai, C.L., Haour, F. & Saxena, B.B. (1978) A stimulatory effect of the fluid from preimplantation rabbit blastocysts upon luteinization of monkey granulosa cell cultures. *J. Reprod. Fert.* **54**, 215–220.

Chatterton, R.J., Jr, McDonald, G.J. & Ward, D.A. (1975) Effect of blastocysts on rat ovarian steroidogenesis in early pregnancy. *Biol. Reprod.* **13**, 77–82.

Dickmann, Z. (1976) A new concept. Control of early pregnancy by steroid hormones originating in the preimplantation embryo. *Vitams Horm.* **36**, 215–242.

Dickmann, Z. & Dey, S.K. (1974) Steroidogenesis in the preimplantation rat embryo and its possible influence on morula–blastocyst transformation and implantation. *J. Reprod. Fert.* **37**, 91–93.

Fishel, S.B., Edwards, R.G. & Evans, C.J. (1984) Human chorionic gonadotropin secreted by preimplantation embryos cultured in vitro. *Science, N.Y.* **223**, 816–818.

Fuchs, A.R. & Beling, C. (1974) Evidence for early ovarian recognition of blastocysts in rabbits. *Endocrinology* **95**, 1054–1058.

Fujimoto, S., Euker, J., Riegel, G. & Dukelow, W. (1975) On a substance cross-reacting with luteinizing hormone in the preimplantation blastocyst fluid of the rabbit. *Proc. Japan Acad.* **51**, 123–125.

Haour, F. & Saxena, B.B. (1974) Detection of a gonadotropin in rabbit blastocyst before implantation. *Science, N.Y.* **185**, 444–445.

Hertig, A.T., Rock, J. & Adams, E.C. (1956) A description of 34 human ova within the first 17 days of development. *Am. J. Anat.* **98**, 435–493.

Hodgen, G.D., Tullner, W.W., Vaitukaitis, J.L., Ward, D.N. & Ross, G.T. (1974) Specific Radioimmunossay of chorionic gonadotropin during the implantation in rhesus monkeys. *J. clin. Endocr. Metab.* **39**, 457–464.

Huff, R.L. & Eik-Nes, K.B. (1966) Metabolism *in vitro* of acetate and certain steroids by six-day-old rabbit blastocysts. *J. Reprod. Fert.* **11**, 57–63.

Kosasa, T., Levesque, L., Goldstein, D.P. & Taymor, M.L. (1974) Clinical use of a solid phase radioimmunoassay specific for hCG. *Am. J. Obstet. Gynec.* **119**, 784–791.

Moudgal, R.N., Mukku, V.R., Prahalada, S., Murty, G.S.R.C. & Li, C.H. (1978) Passive immunization with an antibody to the β-subunit of ovine luteinizing hormone as a method of early abortion—a feasibility study in monkeys (Macaca radiata). *Fert. Steril.* **30**, 223–229.

Perry, J.S., Heap, R.B. & Amoroso, E.C. (1973) Steroid hormone production by pig blastocysts. *Nature, Lond.* **245**, 45–47.

Pope, V.Z., Pope, C.E. & Beck, L.R. (1982) Gonadotropin production by baboon embryos in vitro. In *In Vitro Fertilization and Embryo Transfer*, pp. 129–134. Ed. E. S. E. Hafez. MTP Press Ltd, Lancaster.

Psychoyos, A. (1967) The hormonal interplay controlling egg-implantation in the rat. In *Advances in Reproductive Physiology*, vol. 2, pp. 257–277. Ed. A. McLaren. Academic Press, London.

Saxena, B.B. (1979) Current studies of a gonadotropin-like substance in preimplanted rabbit blastocyst. In *Recent Advances in Reproduction and Regulation of Fertility*, pp. 319–332. Ed. G. P. Talwar. Elsevier/North Holland Biomedical Press, Amsterdam.

Saxena, B.B., Hasan, S., Haour, F. & Schmidt-Gollwitzer, M. (1974) Radioreceptor assay of human chorionic gonadotropin detection of early pregnancy. *Science, N.Y.* **184**, 793–795.

Saxena, B.B., Kaali, S. & Landesman, R. (1977) The transport of chorionic gonadotropin through the reproductive tract, *Eur. J. Obstet. Gynec. Reprod. Biol.* **7**, 1–4.

Singh, M.M. & Adams, C.E. (1978) Luteotropic effect of the rabbit blastocyst. *J. Reprod. Fert.* **53**, 331–333.

Varma, S.K., Dawood, M.Y., Haour, F., Channing, C. & Saxena, B.B. (1979) Gonadotropin-like substance in the preimplanted rabbit blastocyst. *Fert. Steril.* **31**, 68–75.

Wiley, L.D. (1974) Presence of a gonadotropin on the surface of preimplanted mouse embryos. *Nature, Lond.* **252**, 715–716.

Zeilmaker, G.H. & Verhamme, C.M.P.M. (1978) Luteotropic activity of ectopically developed rat blastocyst. *Acta endocr., Copenh.* **88**, 589–593.

J. Reprod. Fert., Suppl. **37** (1989), 121–126

Steroid hormone regulation of the earliest endometrial responses to implantation in the rat

P. F. Kraicer, U. Barkai and T. Kidron

Department of Zoology, George S. Wise Faculty of Life Sciences, Tel Aviv University, Ramat Aviv 69978, Israel

Keywords: decidualization; oestrogen; progesterone; receptors; implantation; rat

Introduction

In deciduate mammals, such as rodents, carnivores and primates, the most remarkable progesterone-dependent response is the decidual cell response (DCR). Although usually a response to the blastocyst, production of decidual tissue can be elicited experimentally in the non-pregnant but appropriately sensitized endometrium. In every known respect, this experimentally induced decidual cell response, the deciduoma, mimics the uterine response at the site of embryonic implantation. In both conditions, the growth and differentiation of decidual tissue is referred to by the generic term decidualization.

This study was directed to analysis of hormonal aspects of the induction phase, first using the experimental induction of decidualization in the non-pregnant animal, and subsequently to apply the information derived to analysis of implantation. This approach was critically dependent on the exploitation of a non-traumatic technique for the induction of decidual cell response, namely intraperitoneal injection of pyrathiazine. We have found corroboration for our supposition that pyrathiazine provides a reasonably accurate model for the induction of decidualization. Of all inducers examined, only blastocyst implantation and pyrathiazine required oestrogen pretreatment in addition to progesterone. Not only was systemic oestrogen effective, but also locally applied (parametrial) oestrogen could produce a unilateral response. This was not found to be true for any other induction stimulus.

Experimental work

First of all, it was necessary to define the duration of induction stage of decidualization. This was done by exploiting the well-known increase in ornithine decarboxylase activity appearing with induction of growth and/or differentiation of all kinds. Decidualization was induced by intraperitoneal pyrathiazine and the ornithine decarboxylase activity was determined at intervals after this induction treatment. A sharp increase was seen after $4\frac{1}{2}$ h, signalling the beginning of the production phase (Barkai & Kraicer, 1978). This induction of ornithine decarboxylase activity could be prevented by injection of antiserum to progesterone, ovariectomy or pretreatment with ergocornine, indicating that it was obviously contingent on the continued presence of progesterone. These results clearly implied (1) that the induction events occurred within the first 4 h and (2) were progesterone-dependent.

The nature of the progesterone-dependence, causal or permissive, was not clear. It was reasoned that, if the effect were more than permissive, a change in the uterine uptake of progesterone might be expected during the induction period. At 30-min intervals after induction of decidualization, rats were injected with tracer doses of [³H]progesterone and the uptake into the uterus measured 30 min later. The accumulation of labelled progesterone was not uniform but showed a short sharp peak of uptake at about 90 min after pyrathiazine administration (Table 1). The peak of uptake had been passed by the time that ornithine decarboxylase activity began to increase.

Were the absolute concentration of progesterone in the blood to fall, the contribution of the labelled progesterone to the total would rise. A peak in uptake of radioactivity might therefore reflect a constant rate of uptake of progesterone in the face of an increased specific activity of the blood progesterone. First, the concentration of progesterone in the blood did not fall. Second, the concentration of progesterone in the uterus was measured by extraction and radioimmunoassay, and it showed an augmentation the timing of which precisely paralleled the timing of the increased uptake of [^{3}H]progesterone (Barkai & Kraicer, 1979). Clearly, decidual induction caused a real increase in the uterine uptake of progesterone.

Table 1. Uptake of [^{3}H]progesterone by the uterus during a 30-min pulse

Time after induction (min)	Radioactivity 30 min after injection	
	Uterus (d.p.m./mg)	Serum (d.p.m./μl)
0	101 ± 12·1 (18)	135 ± 8·0 (5)
30	122 ± 13·9 (5)	111 ± 12·3 (5)
60	325 ± 61·3 (6)	133 ± 7·2 (5)
90	425 ± 82·1 (11)	132 ± 7·5 (5)
120	238 ± 62·3 (6)	Not done
180	169 ± 23·7 (5)	Not done
210	Not done	129 ± 2·5 (5)

Values are means ± standard errors for the no. of rats indicated in parentheses.

Table 2. The effect of pyrathiazine injection on uterine uptake (d.p.m./mg tissue) of steroids

Steroid mixture*	Induction of decidual cell response	
	No	Yes
[^{3}H]Progesterone	3·19 ± 0·51	11·58 ± 1·12
[^{14}C]Testosterone	2·39 ± 0·41	9·81 ± 0·74
[^{3}H]Progesterone	3·26 ± 0·66	12·44 ± 3·72
[^{14}C]Pregnenolone	0·93 ± 0·18	3·84 ± 0·77

Values are mean ± s.e. for 5 rats/group, killed 30 min after the steroid injection.
*Injected 60 min after the pyrathiazine or solvent control.

Progesterone, like other steroids, is believed to pass the cell membrane by free diffusion. An increase in steroid uptake would therefore be expected to reflect an increase in its concentration in the blood and extracellular fluid. There was, however, no correlation between concentration of progesterone in blood and its uptake (Table 1). To test whether the heightened uptake reflected a change specific to progesterone, two other irrelevant steroids, pregnenolone or testosterone, were administered concurrently with labelled progesterone. The uptake of the irrelevant steroid was affected to precisely the same degree as that of progesterone (Table 2). In other words, the induction of decidualization is followed by a change in permeability to steroid hormones. We presume that this is the permeability change which permits implantation sites to be located by extravasated dyed albumin (Psychoyos, 1961).

The proportion of the radioactive material present in the uterine tissue which was actually progesterone was approximately 50% for all times of administration (Table 3). That the bulk of the label remained unchanged suggested that much or most of the [³H]progesterone was receptor-bound. Scatchard-type analysis of the extractable receptors (then referred to as cytosolic receptors) revealed their rapid disappearance at a time coincident with the increased uptake of [³H]progesterone (Barkai *et al.*, 1981). Subsequently, it was shown that the [³H]progesterone was compartmentalized in a predictable fashion: the earliest uptake was into the 'cytosolic' fraction. Its concentration in this compartment reached a maximum within 30 min, and then fell. Meanwhile the concentration rose in the 'nuclear' fraction, reaching a plateau after 90 min. Thus, the progesterone was translocated in a way consistent with action on the genome.

Table 3. Thin-layer chromatographic fractionation of radioactive compounds in the uterus 30 min after injection of 15 μCi [³H]progesterone

t.l.c. fraction	No pyrathiazine	Time between pyrathiazine and [³H]progesterone (min)	
		30	60
Progesterone	56 ± 4·0	56 ± 5·0	53 ± 3·1
5-Dihydroprogesterone	2 ± 0·4	3 ± 0·4	3 ± 0·4
17-Hydroxy- and 20-dihydroprogesterone	38 ± 3·8	37 ± 5·2	38 ± 4·2
Others	4 ± 2·3	5 ± 0·2	6 ± 1·8

Values are in % of recovered radioactivity, means ± standard errors.

Table 4. Effect of oestradiol (1·25 μg injected s.c. in 0·1 ml sesame oil) on decidual induction

Time (h)	Group size	DCR weight* (mean ± s.e.m.)
−9·5	5	17·8 ± 5·08
−8	8	4·9 ± 3·78
−6	5	5·6 ± 2·58
−4	5	0
−2	5	0
0	6	8·0 ± 3·88
2	7	16·5 ± 6·64
5	7	17·6 ± 6·77
7	6	37·3 ± 8·29

*Expressed as % of the total uterine weight.

Since decidualization is growth and differentiation of new tissue, activity at the genomic level would be anticipated. In other words, our first assumption was that the surge of progesterone uptake was an integral part of the induction process. Later evidence showed that this is not so. Apparently the change in permeability during induction of decidualization is not contingent on decidual cell response. Increase in the accumulation of [³H]progesterone was seen in the contra-lateral horn after ipsilateral induction of decidualization, for example by unilateral intraluminal vegetable oil. Progesterone uptake was even enhanced in a totally irrelevant tissue, the rectum, after systemic induction of decidualization by pyrathiazine. This raised the possibility that the increased permeability and uptake of progesterone was an irrelevant concomitant to decidual induction.

In a direct test of the necessity for the presence of progesterone at the time of decidual induction, antiserum to progesterone was injected into rats directly before the induction with pyrathiazine. The 'neutralization' of progesterone prevented the induction of decidualization (Barkai & Kraicer, 1979). The surge of uptake must therefore be considered a necessary condition for the decidual cell response but not a requisite part of the induction process itself.

Table 5. Inhibition of decidual induction by clomiphene (0·25 mg, in 0·1 ml dimethyl sulphoxide)

Time (h) after induction	Group size	% DCR weight (mean ± s.e.m.)
−9	8	1·4 ± 1·44
−6	5	8·7 ± 1·63
−4	5	9·0 ± 0·83
−2	5	11·8 ± 4·84
0	4	33·5 ± 2·78
3	6	45·7 ± 2·45
5	5	42·2 ± 2·24
7	5	48·0 ± 0·36

Table 6. Time of blastocyst→epithelium attachment estimated by reduction of numbers of preimplantation embryos in uterine flushings of Day 4 of pregnancy

Clock time (h)*	Age of pregnancy (h)†	No. of free blastocysts (mean ± s.e.m.)	Group size	Zona-free blastocysts (%)
06:00–08:00	103	7·0 ± 1·51	6	0/42 (0)
10:00–12:00	107	8·1 ± 0·69	8	0/65 (0)
12:00–14:00	109	6·3 ± 0·73	11	6/69 (9)
14:00–16:00	111	1·0 ± 0·68	6	3/12 (25)
16:00–18:00	113	1·0 ± 0·45	10	4/9 (44)
18:00–20:00	115	0·1 ± 0·14	7	

*On Day 4.
†Hours after 24:00 h of Day 0.

What is the relevance of these experimental findings on deciduoma to implantation? In collaboration with Dr D. Eichler, we examined the possible role of progesterone at the time of implantation. Unilaterally ovariectomized rats were made pregnant. The uptake of [³H]progesterone during a 30-min pulse was measured in the pregnant and non-pregnant horns. Two findings were clear: (1) there were 2 surges of uptake, one early on Day 4 and the other, a sharp peak, at around 17:00 h; and (2) there was no difference between the pregnant and the non-pregnant horns. We guessed that the second, sharper peak represented the nidational surge. We have now measured the actual hour of blastocyst attachment in our rats, and it is at ∼ 14:00–16:00 h (see Table 6). The peak of progesterone uptake (which should take place at 90 min after induction) at 17:00 h is, therefore, found at the expected time.

In other words, induction of decidualization is followed by a generalized increase in permeability. In the uterus, at least, this causes an accumulation of progesterone. The progesterone is receptor-bound and accumulated in the nucleus. To test the meaning of this finding, we are currently searching for specific genes whose activity is significantly enhanced or suppressed by induction of decidualization. Only if and when such genes are identified shall we be able to test their dependence on progesterone.

In addition to progesterone, the uterus requires oestrogen to sensitize it for implantation (Shelesnyak *et al.*, 1963); in an ovariectomized rat, about 50 ng oestrogen must be given. However, in larger doses oestrogen can upset the progesterone dominance and inhibit decidualization. It is believed that the oestrogen acts in an antagonistic fashion to progesterone. We therefore tested the effect of a relatively large dose of oestradiol, 1·25 µg, on decidual induction (Table 4). A strong inhibition of decidualization was observed when the oestrogen was administered at or about the time of systemic induction of decidualization. Curiously, oestradiol proved inhibitory even at the actual time of decidual induction. This timing of the inhibitory phase was not consistent with an action at the level of the nucleus, which should exhibit a latency of 10–20 h.

Table 7. Preimplantation losses (as % of CL) of embryos after subcutaneous injections of clomiphene or oestradiol at different times on Day 4 of gestation

Time of pregnancy (h)	Clomiphene*	Oestradiol†
105	23 ± 7 (8)	23 ± 6 (5)
107	19 ± 8 (5)	29 ± 9 (5)
109	48 ± 15 (8)	33 ± 6 (5)
111	69 ± 16 (8)	35 ± 12 (5)
113	30 ± 6 (8)	16 ± 5 (5)

Values are mean ± s.e.m. for the no. of animals given in parentheses.
*0·25 mg clomiphene citrate in 0·1 ml DMSO, s.c.
†6·25 µg oestradiol in 0·1 ml oil, s.c.

Oestrogen is known to have non-genomic actions on uterine permeability. However, this could hardly be the explanation since increased permeability should induce, not inhibit, induction of decidualization. We speculated that oestradiol was disrupting some uterine response which the blastocyst elicited.

In continuing this study we sought another substance which would also bind the oestrogen receptor, but not be an oestrogen itself. Clomiphene citrate proved to be such a material (Clark & Markaverich, 1982). Although the precise timing of the clomiphene action was not identical, it was sufficiently close to indicate a similarity of mechanism (Table 5). Furthermore, the two enantiomers of clomiphene, enclomiphene and zuclomiphene, prove equally effective in blocking decidual induction despite the fact that (in the rat) the former is a weak oestrogen and the latter an anti-oestrogen. Taken together, we have found that the induction of the decidual response is equally blocked by a potent oestrogen (oestradiol), a weak oestrogen (zuclomiphene), an oestrogen antagonist (enclomiphene) or the commercial mixture of the two (enclomiphene:zuclomiphen ratio 62:38). The only obvious common denominator of these substances appears to be their affinity for oestrogen binders.

Oestradiol and clomiphene were also tested for their effect on implantation. To compare the actions in pseudopregnancy to those in pregnancy, it was necessary to establish a common time scale. We assumed that the time at which the blastocyst induces decidualization is somewhere between the time that the zona pellucida is shed and the blastocyst is fixed to the uterine epithelium. This time (Table 6) is at approximately 110 h of pregnancy, i.e. at 14:00 h of Day 4. Clomiphene citrate and oestradiol were injected during the periimplantation period, i.e. from 105 ± 1 to

113 ± 1 h. At the dose levels administered to pseudopregnant rats there was a weak inhibitory response to clomiphene and none to oestradiol. When the dose of oestradiol was increased 5-fold, a weak inhibitory response was obtained (Table 7).

Conclusions

Although these results must be considered preliminary, it does appear that (1) both oestradiol and clomiphene can interfere with implantation at times close to the time of induction of the decidual cell response; and (2) their effectiveness in pregnancy is far less than against induction of deciduoma in the pseudopregnant animal. Taken together, these results lead us to speculate that there is a protective action of the blastocyst on induction of decidualization. The work of Dey & Johnson (1986) on the involvement of catecholoestrogens in implantation suggests that (a) the oestradiol may be blocking the effect of catecholoestrogens and (b) the blastocyst is able to secrete protective amounts of catecholoestrogens.

References

Barkai, U. & Kraicer, P.F. (1978) Definition of the period of induction of decidua in the rat using ornithine decarboxylase as a marker of growth onset. *Life Sci.* **23**, 679–682.

Barkai, U. & Kraicer, P.F. (1979) The role of progesterone in induction of decidualization in the uterus of the pseudopregnant rat. *Adv. Biosci.* **25**, 199–207.

Barkai, U., Sherizly, I. & Kraicer, P.F. (1981) A rapid assay for progesterone receptors in rat uterine cytosol: technique, changes at induction of decidualization. *J. Steroid Biochem.* **14**, 713–720.

Clark, J.H. & Markaverich, B.M. (1982) The agonistic-antagonistic properties of clomiphene: a review. *Pharmac. Ther.* **15**, 467–519.

Dey, S.K. & Johnson, D.C. (1986) Embryonic signals in pregnancy. *Annls N. Y. Acad. Sci.* **476**, 49–62.

Psychoyos, A. (1961) Permeabilite capillaire et decidualisation uterine. *C. r. hebd. Séanc. Acad. Sci., Paris D* **252**, 1515–1517.

Shelesnyak, M.C., Kraicer, P.F. & Zeilmaker, G.H. (1963) Studies on the mechanism of decidualization. I. The estrogen surge of pseudopregnancy and progravidity and its role in the process of decidualization. *Acta endocr., Copenh.* **42**, 225–232.

J. Reprod. Fert., Suppl. **37** (1989), 127–138

Antiluteolytic effects of blastocyst-secreted interferon investigated *in vitro* and *in vivo* in the sheep

H. J. Stewart*, A. P. F. Flint†, G. E. Lamming‡, S. H. E. McCann* and T. J. Parkinson‡

AFRC Research Group on Hormones and Farm Animal Reproduction at: *Institute of Animal Physiology and Genetics Research, Babraham, Cambridge, CB2 4AT, U.K.;* †*Institute of Zoology, Regent's Park, London NW1 4RY, U.K.; and* ‡*University of Nottingham, Faculty of Agricultural Science, Sutton Bonington, Loughborough, Leics LE12 5RD, U.K.*

Keywords: blastocyst; interferon; antiluteolysin; trophoblastin; embryo

Introduction

The establishment of pregnancy in domestic ruminants depends upon the continued secretion of progesterone by the corpora lutea. In non-pregnant cycles the corpora lutea regress on Days 12–15 after oestrus; this process must be blocked in early pregnancy in order to ensure continued exposure of the uterus to progesterone. Inhibition of luteolysis results from the secretion by the developing blastocyst of a protein which has been termed trophoblast antiluteolysin, trophoblastin or (in sheep) ovine trophoblast protein-1 (oTP-1) (Rowson & Moor, 1967; Martal *et al.*, 1979; Bazer *et al.*, 1986). To ensure inhibition of the process of luteal regression, this protein must be secreted by the blastocyst between Days 12 and 14 after oestrus in sheep (between Days 16 and 17 in cattle). This important period of early gestation has been termed the time of "the maternal recognition of pregnancy" by Short (1969), and it corresponds to a period in early gestation when pregnancy frequently fails in domestic animals (Sreenan & Diskin, 1986).

The trophoblast antiluteolysin is an acidic protein of molecular weight approximately 18 000, which represents a major secretory product of the blastocyst between Days 13 and 21 of pregnancy (Godkin *et al.*, 1982). The protein has been purified and characterized, and has been shown to delay luteal regression in cyclic ewes after intrauterine administration (Godkin *et al.*, 1984a); endometrial receptors for the antiluteolysin have been demonstrated and characterized by Godkin *et al.* (1984b). The mechanism of action of the antiluteolysin is thought to involve the inhibition or re-direction of endometrial secretion of prostaglandin (PG) F-2α (see Flint & Hillier, 1975, and references therein), although the mechanism by which this effect is exerted is uncertain (Fincher *et al.*, 1986).

We describe here the sequence analysis of the antiluteolysin by amino acid and cDNA sequencing, studies on the binding of the antiluteolysin to endometrial receptors and an investigation of the effects of a related protein produced by genetic engineering on cycle length following administration *in vivo*.

Structure of antiluteolysin

Incubation media from Day-16 sheep blastocysts cultured in the presence of [^{3}H]leucine were fractionated by ion exchange chromatography and gel filtration to purify the antiluteolysin (Fig. 1a, b; Godkin *et al.*, 1982). In order to prepare the protein sufficiently pure for N-terminal amino acid sequencing the resultant material was further purified by high performance liquid chromatography (h.p.l.c., Fig. 1c). On SDS polyacrylamide electrophoresis the purified protein consisted of a single major component after silver staining, and a single ^{3}H-labelled compound was detected by fluorography (Fig. 2). Using these methods an M_r of 18 700 $\pm$ 340 was obtained for the antiluteolysin.

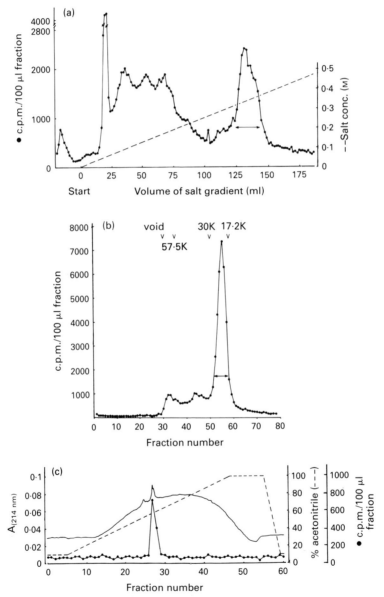

Fig. 1. Purification of oTP-1 from sheep blastocysts flushed from uteri on Day 16 of gestation and incubated for 24 h at 37°C with 50–100 μCi [4,5-^{3}H]leucine in 15–20 ml MEM under O_2: CO_2:N_2 (50:5:45) (Godkin *et al.*, 1982). (a) DEAE-cellulose chromatography; (b) Sephacryl S200 gel filtration; (c) h.p.l.c. using a C_1-silicate reverse phase column (TSK TMS-250, LKB), eluted with a gradient of acetonitrile into water. Both eluate solutions contained 0·1% trifluoroacetic acid. oTP-1 eluted in approximately 57% acetonitrile. Arrows in (a) and (b) indicate material taken for further purification.

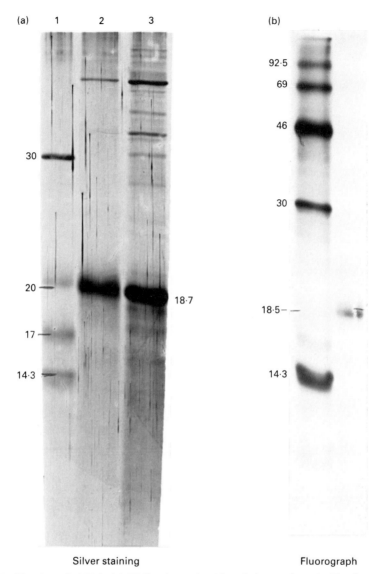

Fig. 2. Purification of oTP-1. (a) SDS polyacrylamide gel electrophoresis. Tracks were loaded with: 1, molecular weight markers ($M_r \times 10^{-3}$ indicated to left); 2, oTP-1 purified by h.p.l.c.; 3, oTP-1 before h.p.l.c. Material after h.p.l.c. was used for amino acid sequence determination. The M_r ($\times 10^{-3}$) of purified oTP-1 is indicated to the right. (b) Fluorograph showing that the oTP-1 preparation is pure with respect to proteins labelled with [³H]leucine. ¹⁴C-molecular weight markers ($M_r \times 10^{-3}$) are on the left.

The eluate from h.p.l.c. containing approximately 5 μg protein was reduced in volume (< 100 μl) and the N-terminal sequence was determined by gas-phase Edman degradation (Applied Biosystems 470A, Warrington, Cheshire, U.K.). The N-terminal amino acid sequence obtained is given in Fig. 3. Computer-aided analysis of this sequence, using the Los Alamos/NBRF DNA and protein sequence analysis software to detect homology with other proteins, revealed that 40% of amino acids in the N-terminal region of the antiluteolysin are identical to those in bovine interferon (IFN) α2 and 37% are identical to those in human IFN-α1 (Stewart *et al.*, 1987). The amino acid sequence derived from the sequence of the antiluteolysin cDNA confirmed an overall 70·3% similarity between oTP-1 and bovine IFN-α2 (Imakawa *et al.*, 1987). No sequence data are available for sheep interferons. Differences were observed between the amino acid sequence obtained by sequencing of the protein and those derived from the cDNA sequences published by Imakawa *et al.* (1987).

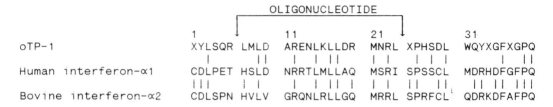

Fig. 3. N-terminal amino acid sequence of oTP-1; homology with human interferon-α1 and bovine interferon-α2. The amino acid residues from which the oligonucleotide was derived are indicated. Amino acids are given by the single letter convention; X = identity uncertain.

To investigate these differences and to confirm the cDNA sequence, cDNA clones were isolated. An oligonucleotide sequence for use as a probe for the antiluteolysin cDNA clones was derived from the amino acid and cDNA sequences (Fig. 3) and synthesized using a Biosearch 8750 four channel DNA synthesizer (Biosearch, San Rafael, CA, U.S.A.) by β-cyanoethyl phosphoamidite chemistry. Isolation and purification were by 7 M-urea denaturing polyacrylamide gel electrophoresis followed by ion exchange column chromatography. Total RNA was prepared from Day-13–23 sheep blastocysts (Chirgwin *et al.*, 1979) and poly(A)$^+$ mRNA was isolated using oligo(dT) chromatography (Aviv & Leder, 1972). In-vitro translation of Day-16 sheep blastocyst RNA synthesized a major protein of M_r 22 000 and demonstrated the integrity of the RNA (Fig. 4). This major translation product is the expected size for the antiluteolysin before removal of the signal peptide by post-translational processing. Northern blotting of total RNA from sheep blastocysts at between Days 13 and 23 of pregnancy demonstrated a single mRNA species of ~900 bases which was present in 13-, 15- and 16-day blastocysts but declined from Day 17 to 23 (Fig. 4). Similar results were obtained using the full length cDNA (see below) as probe. The stages of pregnancy at which oTP-1 mRNA was detected are consistent with those upon which the antiluteolysin is produced (Godkin *et al.*, 1982) and with the stages at which blastocyst extracts contain antiluteolytic principles (Rowson & Moor, 1967; Martal *et al.*, 1979). The oligonucleotide also hybridized to RNA of a similar size in Day-16 cow blastocysts, but not to that from Day-14–19 pig blastocysts. It is known that antibodies against the antiluteolysin will cross-react with bTP-1 (Bazer *et al.*, 1986).

Fig. 4. Synthesis of oTP-1 mRNA by sheep blastocysts and in-vitro translation of Day-16 blastocyst RNA. (a) Northern blotting of sheep blastocyst RNA (20 μg total RNA in each lane) and hybridization to the ^{32}P-labelled oTP-1 oligonucleotide by a method modified from Taylor *et al.* (1984) by the exclusion of formamide from the hybridization buffer and the use of 6% polyethylene glycol instead of dextran sulphate. Hybridization was carried out at 37°C. Size markers are those of eukaryotic ribosomal RNA. (b) In-vitro translation of Day-16 sheep blastocyst total RNA and mRNA using a reticulocyte lysate and labelling with [^{35}S]methionine (Jackson & Hunt, 1983). ^{14}C-molecular weight markers are on the left ($M_r \times 10^{-3}$) and the M_r of the major protein product is indicated as 22 000 (representing the translated protein, including signal peptide, see Fig. 5). TMV = translation products of tobacco mosaic virus mRNA as quality control.

(a)

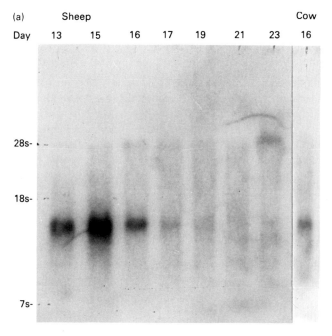

(b)

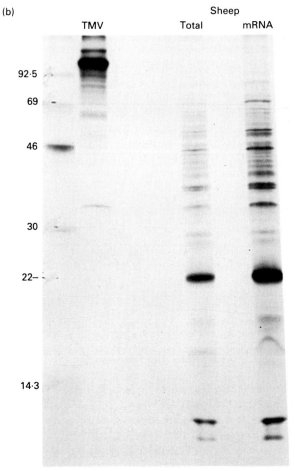

A cDNA library was prepared from Day-16 sheep blastocyst mRNA (see Fig. 4b) in λgt10 (cDNA cloning kit: Amersham International, Aylesbury, Bucks, U.K.). The library consisted of 5×10^5 clones of which $>0.6\%$ were positive on screening with ^{32}P-labelled oTP-1 oligonucleotide. Twelve positive clones were selected all of which contained inserts of 900–1000 bases. Single-strand DNA sequencing (Sanger *et al.*, 1977) of the largest cDNA isolated showed it to have a sequence largely identical to that of the antiluteolysin (Fig. 5; Imakawa *et al.*, 1987). Minor differences noted were base 398 resulting in aspartate instead of glutamate at residue 83 and bases 973–974 in the poly(A) tail. The amino acid sequence at residues 5 and 6 (gln-arg) obtained by analysis of the purified protein (Fig. 3) differs from those of Imakawa *et al.* (1987) and this was confirmed by cDNA sequencing. Sequence heterogeneity is to be expected in view of the presence of several isoforms of antiluteolysin on 2-dimensional gel electrophoresis (Godkin *et al.*, 1982; Imakawa *et al.*, 1987).

Receptor binding studies

In view of the structural similarities demonstrated above between the trophoblast antiluteolysin and the interferon-α family of proteins, a study was undertaken of the ability of interferons to bind to, and to displace labelled antiluteolysin from, endometrial receptors. By this means it was sought to confirm the structural relationship between the proteins, and to compare the functional properties of the interferons with those of the antiluteolysin.

Initial studies were conducted using human interferon (Sigma, Poole, Dorset, U.K.), which was labelled with ^{125}I to a specific activity of 37 mCi/mg using iodogen (see Stewart *et al.*, 1987). This material bound to membrane preparations from sheep endometrium in a displaceable manner; binding was proportional to endometrial protein concentration and the dissociation constant of the binding reaction was approximately 4×10^{-11} M (Figs 6a–d). Binding of ^{125}I-labelled human interferon was displaced by purified antiluteolysin (Fig. 6c).

Subsequent investigations utilized ^{125}I-labelled antiluteolysin and ^{125}I-labelled bovine recombinant interferon-α1 (brIFN; kind gift of Ciba-Geigy, Basle, Switzerland). Labelled antiluteolysin (prepared by iodination of h.p.l.c.-purified material described in Figs 1 and 2) bound to sheep endometrial receptors, as shown previously (Godkin *et al.*, 1984b), and binding was blocked by unlabelled brIFN (Fig. 6d). Binding of labelled brIFN was approximately one-fifth that obtained with hIFN (Fig. 6b).

To confirm that the ^{125}I-labelled human interferon and brIFN were isotopically pure, these preparations were analysed by h.p.l.c. using the elution system and the C_1 column described previously (Figs 1 & 2). Both labels eluted from h.p.l.c. in positions close to the unlabelled material, and both also eluted at acetonitrile concentrations similar to the antiluteolysin. Therefore isotopic impurity was unlikely to account for the lower binding activity of ^{125}I-labelled brIFN. Some of the properties of the interferons (particularly their propensity to bind to plastics or glass, which was not reduced by siliconization) caused technical difficulties, but these were encountered with all three of the labelled preparations used, and were probably not responsible for the low affinity of receptors for brIFN.

Effects of intrauterine infusion of brIFN

Ewes were used during the breeding season (November 1987–February 1988) to study the effects of the intrauterine administration of brIFN. Oestrus was detected by the use of a raddled vasectomized ram, and 6 or 7 days after spontaneous oestrus the ewes were anaesthetized using thiopentone induction, and halothane maintenance. A catheter (1·2 mm o.d., 0·9 mm i.d.) was placed in the lumen of the uterine horn ipsilateral to a corpus luteum bearing ovary. The catheter

```
                              30                                                    80
                              GGTTCCCCCTGACCCCATCTCAGCCAGCCCAGCAGCAGCCGCATCTTCCCC
  81                                                                                140
  ATG GCC TTC GTG CTC TCT CTA CTG ATG GCC CTG GTG CTG GTC AGC TAT GGC CCA GGA GGA
  S1                                                                                S20
  Met Ala Phe Val Leu Ser Leu Leu Met Ala Leu Val Leu Val Ser Tyr Gly Pro Gly Gly
 141                                                                                200
  TCT CTG GGT TGT TAC CTA TCT CAG AGA CTC ATG CTG GAT GCC AGG GAG AAC CTC AAG CTC
  S21           1                                                                    17
  Ser Leu Gly Cys Tyr Leu Ser Gln Arg Leu Met Leu Asp Ala Arg Glu Asn Leu Lys Leu
 201                                                                                260
  CTG GAC CGA ATG AAC AGA CTC TCC CCT CAT TCC TGT CTG CAG GAC AGA AAA GAC TTT GGT
   18                                                                                37
  Leu Asp Arg Met Asn Arg Leu Ser Pro His Ser Cys Leu Gln Asp Arg Lys Asp Phe Gly
 261                                                                                320
  CTT CCC CAG GAG ATG GTG GAG GGC GAC CAG CTC CAG AAG GAC CAG GCC TTC CCT GTG CTC
   38                                                                                57
  Leu Pro Gln Glu Met Val Glu Gly Asp Gln Leu Gln Lys Asp Gln Ala Phe Pro Val Leu
 321                                                                                380
  TAC GAG ATG CTC CAG CAG AGC TTC AAC CTC TTC TAC ACA GAG CAC TCC TCT GCT GCC TGG
   58                                                                                77
  Tyr Glu Met Leu Gln Gln Ser Phe Asn Leu Phe Tyr Thr Glu His Ser Ser Ala Ala Trp
 381                                                                                440
  GAC ACC ACC CTC CTG GAC CAG CTC TGC ACT GGA CTC CAA CAG CAG CTG GAC CAC CTG GAC
   78                                                                                97
  Asp Thr Thr Leu Leu Asp Gln Leu Cys Thr Gly Leu Gln Gln Gln Leu Asp His Leu Asp
 441                                                                                500
  ACC TGC AGG GGT CAA GTG ATG GGA GAG GAA GAC TCT GAA CTG GGT AAC ATG GAC CCC ATT
   98                                                                                117
  Thr Cys Arg Gly Gln Val Met Gly Glu Glu Asp Ser Glu Leu Gly Asn Met Asp Pro Ile
 501                                                                                560
  GTG ACC GTG AAG AAG TAC TTC CAG GGC ATC TAT GAC TAC CTG CAA GAG AAG GGA TAC AGC
  118                                                                                137
  Val Thr Val Lys Lys Tyr Phe Gln Gly Ile Tyr Asp Tyr Leu Gln Glu Lys Gly Tyr Ser
 561                                                                                620
  GAC TGC GCC TGG GAA ATC GTC AGA GTC GAG ATG ATG AGA GCC CTC ACT GTA TCA ACC ACC
  138                                                                                157
  Asp Cys Ala Trp Glu Ile Val Arg Val Glu Met Met Arg Ala Leu Thr Val Ser Thr Thr
 621                                                             666                683
  TTG CAA AAA AGG TTA ACA AAG ATG GGT GGA GAT CTG AAC TCA CCT TGA TGACTCTTGCCGACT
  158                                                             172
  Leu Gln Lys Arg Leu Thr Lys Met Gly Gly Asp Leu Asn Ser Pro
                                                                                    763
  AAGATGCCACATCAGCCTCCTACACCCGCCTGTGTTCATTTCAGAAGACTCTGATTTCTGCTCCAGCCACCAAATTCATT
                                                                                    843
  GAATTACTTTAGCTGATACTTTGTCAGTAGTAAAAAGCAAGTAGATATAAAAGTATTCAGCTGTAGGGGCATGAGTCCTG
                                                                                    923
  AAATGATGCCTTCCCTGATGTTATCTGTTGCTGATTTATTTATACCTTCTAGCATTTAACATACTTAAAATATTAGGAAA
                                                                                    990
  TTTGTTAAGTTACATTTCATCTGTACATCATATTAAAATTTCTAAAACATGAAAAAAAAAAAAAAAAA
```

Oligonucleotide

Fig. 5. cDNA and derived amino acid sequence of cloned trophoblast antiluteolysin mRNA. The sequence of the oligonucleotide used to probe the cDNA library and the polyadenylation site are underlined. Amino acids comprising the signal peptide are prefixed 'S'. Nucleotides numbered after Imakawa *et al.* (1987).

was externalized through a sub-lumbar stab incision. At the same time one jugular vein was also catheterized. From the 8th day after oestrus daily 5-ml blood samples were collected for progesterone determination using sodium heparin as anticoagulant. On the next day ewes were divided into 7 groups and given continuous intrauterine infusions of one of the following treatments: (1) 20 µg meclofenamic acid in 9·6 ml saline (0·154 M-NaCl) per 24 h as a positive control to prolong luteal function (N = 2); (2) 2 mg meclofenamic acid in 9·6 ml saline per 24 h (N = 2); (3) controls for meclofenamate treated groups, given 9·6 ml saline per 24 h (N = 2); (4) 0·2 mg brIFN in 9·6 ml saline per 24 h (N = 4); (5) controls for Group 4 given vehicle in 9·6 ml saline per 24 h (N = 2);

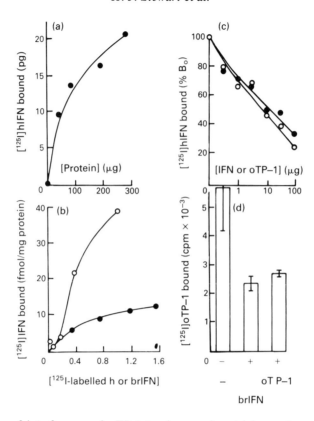

Fig. 6. Binding of interferons and oTP-1 to sheep endometrial receptor preparations. (a) Binding of ^{125}I-labelled human IFN-α with various concentrations of endometrial protein; (b) binding of ^{125}I-labelled human IFN-α (○) and ^{125}I-labelled brIFN (●), with various ligand concentrations (nM); (c) competition for binding of ^{125}I-labelled human IFN with various concentrations of unlabelled hIFN (●) or oTP-1 (○); (d) competition for binding of ^{125}I-labelled oTP-1 with unlabelled brIFN or oTP-1 (both at 500 ng/ml). Incubation conditions were as described by Stewart *et al.* (1987).

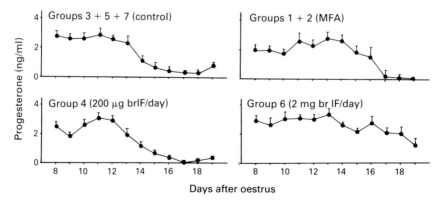

Fig. 7. Daily plasma progesterone concentrations (mean ± s.e.m.) of control (Groups 3, 5 & 7), meclofenamate- (Groups 1 & 2) and brIFN- (Groups 4 & 6) treated ewes.

Table 1. Effects of brIFN treatment in ewes (Groups 5 and 7, controls; Group 4, 0·2 mg brIFN/day; Group 6, 2 mg brIFN/day)

Group	Ewe	Day of progesterone fall*	State of ovary	Corpus luteum weight at autopsy (g)	Oxytocin receptor conc. (fmol/mg protein)
5	6	15	FO	0·1; 0·13	433
5	33	15	CA	0·39	558
7	17	18	FO	0·03; 0·04	99
4	4	15	FO	0·11; 0·14	672
4	5	16	FO	0·12; 0·11	359
4	7	16	FO	0·24	2721
4	46	17	FO	0·07; 0·05	1160
6	60	18	CL	0·39; 0·32	2166
6	13	>19	CL	0·50; 0·53	291
6	35	>19	CL	0·46; 0·42	188
6	45†	19	CA	0·16; 0·17	993

FO = fresh ovulation; CA = corpus albicans; CL = corpus luteum of appearance resembling normal mid-cycle structure.
*Day when progesterone concentration was first observed below 0·3 ng/ml.
†Infusion catheter leaky at autopsy, and so the full dose was probably not received.

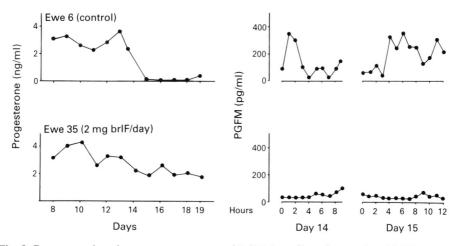

Fig. 8. Representative plasma progesterone and PGFM profiles of control and brIFN-treated ewes.

(6) 2 mg brIFN in 5·5 ml saline per 24 h (N = 4); and (7) control for Group 6, given vehicle in 5·5 ml saline per 24 h (N = 1).

On Day 14, 5-ml blood samples were collected every hour for 9 h and, on Day 15, hourly samples were collected for 12 h for assay of 13,14-dihydro-15-keto-PGF (PGFM). Treatment was continued until slaughter on Days 19 or 20. At slaughter the position and patency of the uterine catheters was confirmed, the corpora lutea present were noted and normality of the uterine tissues was confirmed by gross examination. In one animal partial leakage of infusate had occurred from the uterus as a result of a suture failure. Endometrial tissue was taken for preparation of membrane fractions for oxytocin receptor measurement (by the method of Sheldrick & Flint, 1985).

Results for the 3 control groups (3, 5 and 7) were similar and data from the 5 control animals were therefore pooled. Results from Groups 1 and 2, treated with meclofenamic acid, were also similar and were pooled. Composite daily plasma progesterone profiles are shown in Fig. 7. The day on which progesterone concentrations fell to <0.3 ng/ml was used to indicate luteal regression and these data, together with corpus luteum weights and oxytocin receptor concentrations, are given in Table 1.

The high dose brIFN treatment (Group 6) significantly extended the luteal phase ($P < 0.001$) compared with all control groups. Meclofenamic acid treatment did not significantly extend the cycle when compared to controls, but the effect was significant ($P < 0.05$) when compared to the Group 3 controls alone. The day following that of slaughter (Day 20) was used for statistical purposes for ewes not showing a decline of progesterone concentration by the day of slaughter.

Representative progesterone and PGFM profiles for animals in the 4 pooled treatment groups are shown in Fig. 8. There was a significant decrease in mean PGFM concentrations on Days 14 and 15 in Groups 1, 2 and 6. The mean amplitude of PGFM episodes was not different between groups or days, but there was a trend for ewes in Group 6 to have lower amplitude episodes on both Days 14 and 15, and for ewes in Groups 1 and 2 to have lower amplitude episodes on Day 14 than controls but higher amplitude episodes on Day 15, reflecting the later onset of luteal regression in these animals.

As shown in Table 1, mean ($\pm$ s.e.m.) total corpus luteum weights/animal were raised in Group 6 ewes (2 mg brIFN) (0.74 ± 0.15 g) compared with those in Groups 5 and 7 (vehicle) (0.23 ± 0.09 g) or in Group 4 (0.2 mg brIFN) (0.22 ± 0.05 g).

Measurements of endometrial oxytocin receptor concentrations in ewes receiving interferon showed that brIFN failed to block the rise normally occurring in non-pregnant ewes on Days 13–16 after oestrus (Table 1; Sheldrick & Flint, 1985). Mean ($\pm$ s.e.m.) oxytocin receptor concentrations (fmol/mg protein) on Day 19 were 363 ± 137 in control animals (N = 3, Groups 5 & 7), 1228 ± 524 in Group 4 (N = 4, 0.2 mg brIFN/day) and 909 ± 455 in Group 6 (N = 4, 2 mg brIFN/day). The value determined in control ewes was significantly lower than that observed previously at oestrus (approx. 1000–2000 fmol/mg protein), presumably because the samples were obtained some time after oestrus at a time when receptor concentrations have previously been shown to decline (Sheldrick & Flint, 1985). The range of values in ewes treated with 2 mg brIFN/day was large (188–2166 fmol/mg) and did not correlate with the circulating progesterone concentration on Day 19. Receptor concentrations were, however, low in the 2 animals in which corpus luteum weight was highest, and in which progesterone concentrations were maintained, compared to those in which progesterone fell (Ewe 60) or when the full dose of infusate was not received (Ewe 45).

Conclusions

The in-vitro and in-vivo results presented above provide strong evidence that the blastocyst antiluteolytic protein oTP-1 is an interferon. Not only are the amino acid and cDNA sequences indicative of a strong homology with interferons, but the molecular sizes of oTP-1 and the alpha interferons (both in the range 17 000–18 000), the fact that both are acidic proteins (see Pestka *et al.*, 1987) and their similar elution positions on h.p.l.c. support this conclusion. The result of northern blotting of sheep blastocyst mRNA, using an oligonucleotide probe synthesized on the basis of the amino acid sequence provides further confirmation; the time at which blastocyst levels of oTP-1 mRNA were highest corresponded to the period during which it has been shown that the blastocyst contains the antiluteolytic protein.

The structural relationship between oTP-1 and the interferons was further indicated by the binding studies carried out with these compounds. It was initially considered possible that there may be more than one interferon binding site in endometrial tissues, only one of which controls the antiluteolytic effect and binds oTP-1; however, the ability of oTP-1 to displace ^{125}I-labelled interferon binding and *vice versa* clearly indicates that the same receptor(s) are utilized by both compounds. The concentration of binding sites and their affinity for interferon determined in extracts of endometrium were similar to those described previously for interferon receptors in membrane preparations from bovine lung and placenta (Branca, 1986). The reason for the relatively low binding of bovine recombinant interferon is uncertain; it appears possible that although the homology between the sequences of bovine recombinant interferon and antiluteolysin is high there may be specific amino acid differences between the sequences, resulting in reduced receptor affinity.

The results of structural analysis and receptor binding studies indicate a clear homology between the antiluteolysin and the interferons, and this is confirmed by the observation that infusion of bovine recombinant interferon into the uterine lumen *in vivo* delays the onset of luteolysis and reduces circulating concentrations of PGF-2α metabolites. However, large doses of bovine recombinant interferon were required to exert this effect, possibly reflecting the relatively low binding affinity of bovine recombinant interferon for the endometrial antiluteolysin binding site.

While the data reviewed above indicate that the trophoblast antiluteolytic protein is an interferon, they are not sufficient to allow a conclusion that this protein is the only antiluteolytic compound present. This is indicated by two pieces of evidence. Firstly the infusion of bovine recombinant interferon, using the conditions described here, resulted in the prolongation of luteal function beyond Day 19 in only 2 of the 4 ewes treated. Secondly the treatment failed to reduce endometrial oxytocin receptor concentrations to those characteristic of pregnancy in any of the animals to which it was administered. These observations therefore raise the question of whether blastocyst extracts contain a second unidentified antiluteolytic protein acting at the same time as blastocyst interferon, and perhaps in synergy with it.

Although the mechanism by which blastocyst interferon acts to reduce uterine PGF-2α secretion is not known, it appears from the results presented here that interferon is unlikely to affect oxytocin receptor concentrations directly. An action on post-receptor events controlling prostaglandin synthesis is possible, however, and the report by Chandrabose & Cuatracasas (1981) that interferon-α reduces the concentration of unsaturated fatty acids in membrane phospholipids suggests that a similar effect may be involved in the mechanism of action of the antiluteolytic signal. The production of interferon by the developing conceptus is a relatively widespread phenomenon (man; see Chard *et al.*, 1986; mouse: Fowler *et al.*, 1980). Its principal function may be antiviral (Isaacs & Lindenmann, 1957), although roles in regulation of the maternal immune response or cellular differentiation also appear possible (Taylor-Papadimitriou & Rozengurt, 1985). In evolutionary terms, therefore, the acquisition of an antiluteolytic function by blastocyst interferon in ruminants may represent the use of a pre-existing secretory product in a novel paracrine role.

We thank Miss L. J. Jenner for assistance with the preparation of endometrial extracts; Dr J. C. Pascall for advice on cloning techniques; and Mr A. J. Northrop and Mr P. J. Barker for oligonucleotide synthesis and amino acid sequencing, respectively. The sequence data presented in this paper will appear in the EMBL/GenBank/DDBJ Nucleotide sequence Databases under the accession number X07920.

References

Aviv, H. & Leder, P. (1972) Purification of biologically active globin messenger RNA by chromatography on oligothymidylic acid-cellulose. *Proc. natn. Acad. Sci. U.S.A.* **69**, 1408–1412.

Bazer, F.W., Vallet, J.L., Roberts, R.M., Sharp, D.C. & Thatcher, W.W. (1986) Role of conceptus secretory products in establishment of pregnancy. *J. Reprod. Fert.* **76**, 841–850.

Branca, A.A. (1986) High affinity receptors for human interferon in bovine lung and human placenta. *J. Interferon Res.* **6**, 305–311.

Chandrabose, K. & Cuatrecasas, P. (1981) Changes in

fatty acyl chains of phospholipids induced by interferon in mouse sarcoma S-180 cells. *Biochem. Biophys. Res. Commun.* **98,** 661–668.

Chard, T., Craig, P.H., Menabawey, M. & Lee, C. (1986) Alpha interferon in human pregnancy. *Br. J. Obstet. Gynaec.* **93,** 1145–1149.

Chirgwin, J.M., Przybyla, A.E., MacDonald, R.J. & Rutter, W.J. (1979) Isolation of biologically active ribonucleic acid from sources enriched in ribonuclease. *Biochemistry, N.Y.* **18,** 5294–5299.

Fincher, K.B., Bazer, F.W., Hansen, P.J., Thatcher, W.W. & Roberts, R.M. (1986) Proteins secreted by the sheep conceptus suppress induction of uterine prostaglandin F-2α release by oestradiol and oxytocin. *J. Reprod. Fert.* **76,** 425–433.

Flint, A.P.F. & Hillier, K. (1975) Prostaglandins and reproductive processes in female sheep and goats. In *Prostaglandins and Reproduction,* pp. 271–308. Ed. S. M. M. Karim. MTP Press Ltd, Lancaster.

Fowler, A.K., Reed, C.D. & Giron, D.J. (1980) Identification of an interferon in murine placentas. *Nature, Lond.* **286,** 266–267.

Godkin, J.D., Bazer, F.W., Moffatt, J., Sessions, F. & Roberts, R.M. (1982) Purification and properties of a major, low molecular weight protein released by the trophoblast of sheep blastocysts at Day 13–21. *J. Reprod. Fert.* **65,** 141–150.

Godkin, J.D., Bazer, F.W., Thatcher, W.W. & Roberts, R.M. (1984a) Proteins released by cultured Day 15–16 conceptuses prolong luteal maintenance when introduced into the uterine lumen of cyclic ewes. *J. Reprod. Fert.* **71,** 57–64.

Godkin, J.D., Bazer, F.W. & Roberts, R.M. (1984b) Ovine trophoblast protein 1, an early secreted blastocyst protein, binds specifically to uterine endometrium and affects protein synthesis. *Endocrinology* **114,** 120–130.

Imakawa, K., Anthony, R.V., Kazemi, M., Marotti, K.R., Polites, H.G. & Roberts, R.M. (1987) Interferon-like sequence of ovine trophoblast protein secreted by embryonic trophectoderm. *Nature, Lond.* **330,** 377–379.

Isaacs, A. & Lindenmann, J. (1957) Virus interference. I. The interferon. *Proc. R. Soc. B* **147,** 258–267.

Jackson, R.J. & Hunt, T. (1983) Preparation and use of nuclease-treated rabbit reticulocyte lysate for the translation of eukaryotic messenger RNA. *Methods in Enzymology* **96,** 50–74.

Martal, J., Lacroix, M-C., Loudes, C., Saunier, M. & Wintenberger-Torres, S. (1979) Trophoblastin, an antiluteolytic protein present in early pregnancy in sheep. *J. Reprod. Fert.* **56,** 63–73.

Pestka, A., Langer, J.A., Zoon, K.C. & Samuel, C.E. (1987) Interferons and their actions. *Ann. Rev. Biochem.* **58,** 727–777.

Rowson, L.E.A. & Moor, R.M. (1967) The influence of embryonic tissue homogenate, infused into the uterus, on the life span of the corpus luteum in the sheep. *J. Reprod. Fert.* **13,** 511–516.

Sanger, F., Nicklen, S. & Coulson, A.R. (1977) DNA sequencing with chain-terminating inhibitors. *Proc. natn. Acad. Sci. U.S.A.* **74,** 5463–5467.

Sheldrick, E.L. & Flint, A.P.F. (1985) Endocrine control of uterine oxytocin receptors in the ewe. *J. Endocr.* **106,** 249–258.

Short, R.V. (1969) Implantation and the maternal recognition of pregnancy. In *Foetal Autonomy* (Ciba Fdn Symp.), pp. 2–26. Eds G. Wolstenholme & M. O'Connor. Churchill, London.

Sreenan, J.M. & Diskin, M.G. (1986) The extent and timing of embryonic mortality in the cow. In *Embryonic Mortality in Farm Animals,* pp. 1–11. Eds J. M. Sreenan & M. G. Diskin. Martinus Nijhof, Dordrecht.

Stewart, H.J., McCann, S.H.E., Barker, P.J., Lee, K.E., Lamming, G.E. & Flint, A.P.F. (1987) Interferon sequence homology and receptor binding activity of bovine trophoblast antiluteolytic protein. *J. Endocr.* **115,** R13–R15.

Taylor, J.B., Craig, R.K., Beale, D. & Ketterer, B. (1984) Construction and characterization of a plasmid containing complementary DNA to mRNA encoding the N-terminal amino acid sequence of the rat glutathione transferase Ya subunit. *Biochem. J.* **219,** 223–231.

Taylor-Papadimitriou, J. & Rozengurt, E.A. (1985) Interferons as regulators of cell growth and differentiation. In *Interferons: Their Impact in Biology and Medicine,* pp. 81–98. Ed. J. Taylor-Papadimitriou. Oxford University Press.

STEROIDOGENESIS

Chairmen

Z. Ben Rafael
Z. Kraiem
P. Humblot
A. P. F. Flint

J. Reprod. Fert., Suppl. **37** (1989), 139–145

Printed in Great Britain
© 1989 Journals of Reproduction & Fertility Ltd

Control of multiple transducing systems by LH which results in the modulation of adenylate cyclase, protein kinase C, lipoxygenases and cyclooxygenases

B. A. Cooke, E. A. Platts, R. Abayasekera, L. O. Kurlak, D. Schulster* and M. H. F. Sullivan

*Department of Biochemistry, Royal Free Hospital School of Medicine, Rowland Hill Street, London NW3 2PF, U.K. and *Department of Endocrinology, National Institute for Biological Standards and Control, South Mimms, Herts EN6 3QG, U.K.*

Keywords: LH; Leydig cells; cyclic AMP; leukotrienes

Introduction

It is well established that gonadotrophic hormones such as luteinizing hormone (LH) interact with their plasma membrane receptors to activate the adenylate cyclase system to form cyclic AMP followed by a subsequent increase in steroidogenesis. Repeated administration of the hormone leads to a desensitization of that same hormonal response and eventually to loss of receptors (down regulation). Recent evidence suggests that trophic hormones, including LH, may also directly activate other transducing mechanisms leading to activation of phospholipase C and A_2 and the subsequent formation of inositol 1,4,5-trisphosphate (IP_3), diacylglycerol and arachidonic acid metabolites. This is followed by an increase in intracellular calcium and activation of protein kinase C. Some or all of these intracellular second messengers may be involved in the stimulation and desensitization of the trophic hormone responses (see review by Rommerts & Cooke, 1988). The following is a summary of some of our recent work on LH receptor transducing mechanisms in testis Leydig cells. It addresses the following questions:

(1) What are the mechanisms and factors controlling cyclic AMP production?

(2) Does LH through its receptor directly modulate other transducing systems leading to formation of other second messengers?

Formation of cyclic AMP

Stimulation of Leydig cells with LH results in the stimulation of adenylate cyclase activity. Stimulation occurs within several minutes after addition of the hormone, is dose-dependent and can also be demonstrated in isolated membranes. The stimulatory effects of LH on the adenylate cyclase system have been assumed to be mediated by the putative stimulatory GTP binding protein (G_s). This is because cholera toxin, which specifically activates the G_s protein, increases cyclic AMP production and steroidogenesis in intact Leydig cells. LH and hCG stimulation of adenylate cyclase in plasma membranes from Leydig cells is increased in the presence of GTP and non-hydrolysable GTP analogues again indicating the involvement of a G_s protein (see Rommerts & Cooke (1988) for references).

The presence of an inhibitory GTP binding protein (G_i), which has been demonstrated in many different cell types, has also been inferred from indirect studies to be present in Leydig cells. Evidence for this was obtained from studies with cultured Leydig cells in which it was shown that the inhibitory effects of arginine vasotocin on steroidogenesis could be abolished by pertussis toxin, which inactivates G_i via ADP ribosylation (Adashi *et al.*, 1984). Similar studies with forskolin (Khanum & Dufau, 1986) demonstrated that low concentrations of this compound inhibited hCG-stimulated cyclic AMP production and this inhibition was prevented by pertussis toxin.

We have recently obtained direct evidence for the presence of the G_s and G_i proteins. Highly purified Leydig cells (98%) were homogenized in a hypotonic medium and the plasma membranes were isolated from the homogenate in a dextran–polyethylene glycol 2-phase system (Levi *et al.*, 1982). The membrane protein (50–100 mg) was incubated for 30 min with [^{32}P]NAD, cholera and pertussis toxin in incubation mixtures which provided optimal conditions either for cholera toxin ($+MgCl_2$ + phosphate) or for pertussis toxin ($-MgCl_2$ − phosphate) (Ribeiro-Neto *et al.*, 1985). The membrane proteins were then separated by SDS–polyacrylamide gel electrophoresis and the gels were dried and autoradiographed.

It was found that toxin substrates occurred in both testis and tumour Leydig cell membranes (Fig. 1). Pertussis toxin ADP-ribosylated a protein with an apparent molecular weight of 40 000–41 000. The protein ADP-ribosylated by cholera toxin had molecular weights of 50 000 and 52 000. This agrees with the known molecular weights of the α_s and α_i subunits of the G_s and G_i proteins from other systems, especially from hepatocytes (Gilman, 1984).

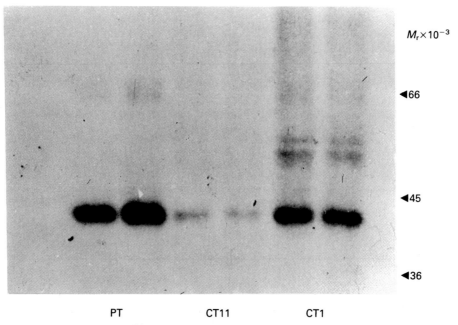

$M_r \times 10^{-3}$

◀66

◀45

◀36

PT   CT11   CT1

Fig. 1. Autoradiograph of ^{32}P-ADP-ribosylated Leydig cell plasma membrane. The membranes were incubated with ^{32}P-NAD as indicated in the text in the presence of pertussis toxin (PT), pertussis toxin, cholera toxin and an excess of unlabelled ADP (CT11), or pertussis toxin and cholera toxin (CT1). The mobility of standard molecular weight markers on the same polyacrylamide electrophoresis gels as the membranes are shown.

Desensitization of adenylate cyclase

In addition to the stimulatory actions of LH and hCG on steroidogenesis in Leydig and ovarian cells, these hormones also cause a refractoriness or desensitization of that same steroidogenic response. This may involve a loss of LH receptors (down regulation), an uncoupling of the LH receptor from the adenylate cyclase, an increase in the metabolism of cyclic AMP due to an increased phosphodiesterase activity and a decrease in the activities in some of the enzymes in the pathways of steroidogenesis (see Rommerts & Cooke (1988) for references). Our work has concentrated mainly on the desensitization of LH-stimulated cyclic AMP production. Evidence from in-vivo experiments after administration of hCG suggested that a lesion develops between the LH receptor and the adenylate cyclase in rat testicular and ovarian cells (see Rommerts & Cooke (1988) for references). Further work carried out *in vitro* with tumour Leydig cells demonstrated that LH produced a decrease in LH stimulation of adenylate cyclase in intact cells. This loss of response persisted in plasma membranes prepared from the desensitized cells (Dix *et al.*, 1982). The response of the intact cells to cholera toxin and of the plasma membranes to fluoride and guanosine 5′-[β,γ-imido]triphosphate (p(NH)ppG) were not decreased. These studies suggested that the lesion occurred between the LH receptor and G_s whereas the coupling between G_s and the adenylate cyclase catalytic unit was intact (see Fig. 2). Such a conclusion is in agreement with that of other workers investigating the catecholamine-induced desensitization of S49 lymphoma cells (Iyengar *et al.*, 1981; Green & Clark, 1981). This lesion may be necessary before internalization of the receptor can occur.

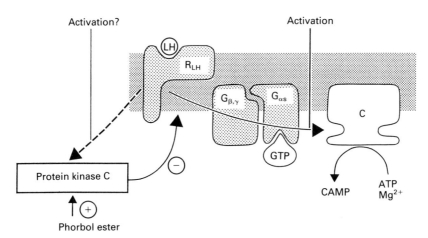

Fig. 2. Scheme showing possible activation and site of action of protein kinase C on the LH receptor–G protein–adenylate cyclase transducing system.

Interactions between different transducing systems i.e. adenylate cyclase and protein kinase C, have been reported in both mouse and rat Leydig cells (Mukhopadhyay & Schumacher, 1985; Themmen *et al.*, 1986; Dix *et al.*, 1987) and in many other cell types (Nishizuka, 1984). Treatment with the phorbol ester 12-0-tetradecanoylphorbol-13-acetate (TPA) can mimic hormone-induced desensitization and has been demonstrated both in tumour Leydig cells (Rebois & Patel, 1985; Dix *et al.*, 1987) and in other cell types, e.g. avian erythrocytes (Sibley *et al.*, 1984). However, differences between hormone- and TPA-induced desensitization have also been noted (see Dix *et al.*, 1987).

In further studies, using testicular Leydig cells, we have now found that, although both LH and TPA induced desensitization of adenylate cyclase, there were marked differences between the effects of these compounds upon adenylate cyclase activity subsequently stimulated by cholera toxin. This effect may have been due to a modification of the G_s protein such that activity is increased or to an inhibitory effect upon the G_i protein. These differential effects of LH and TPA were therefore investigated further, using pertussis toxin (which ADP-ribosylates and hence inactivates G_i), to examine whether this protein is inhibited by TPA (Platts *et al.*, 1988). Cyclic AMP production from cultured Leydig cells of rats was stimulated by both LH and cholera toxin. Pre-treatment with LH for 1 h inhibited, i.e. desensitized, the ability of the cells to respond subsequently to further LH. In agreement with previous results (Habberfield *et al.*, 1987), it was found that in LH-treated cells the 'basal' production of cyclic AMP was increased and the addition of further LH had little effect. When 'basal' levels were subtracted, the response (mean $\pm$ s.d., $n = 3$; pmol cyclic AMP/10^6 cells/h) to cholera toxin by LH-desensitized cells ($66\cdot9 \pm 8\cdot3$) was not significantly different from that found in the control ($76\cdot5 \pm 10\cdot0$), i.e. LH did not desensitize the response to cholera toxin.

Pretreatment of the cells with TPA also caused an inhibition of subsequent LH-stimulated cyclic AMP production from $188\cdot3 \pm 4\cdot8$ to $120\cdot6 \pm 4\cdot1$ pmol/10^6 cells/h. However, TPA-desensitized cells had an enhanced response (pmol cyclic AMP/10^6 cells/h) to cholera toxin ($189\cdot5 \pm 8\cdot8$) compared to control cells ($76\cdot5 \pm 10\cdot0$). These effects were not observed in cells treated with phorbol-12,13-didecanoate, a phorbol ester which does not activate protein kinase C.

To examine whether this effect was due to an interaction of TPA with the G_i protein, cells were incubated in the presence of pertussis toxin before being desensitized. Pertussis toxin potentiated cyclic AMP production in basal and stimulated cells. Pertussis toxin also potentiated LH- and cholera toxin-stimulated cyclic AMP production in LH-desensitized cells, although the effect of LH upon pertussis toxin-treated LH-desensitized cells was still less than the effect of LH upon pertussis-treated non-desensitized cells. Thus inactivation of G_i protein did not reverse LH-induced desensitization. The effects of TPA were not modified by culture with pertussis toxin. The fact that pertussis toxin was not able to potentiate further the enhanced response to cholera toxin implied that TPA and pertussis toxin have a common site of action (see Fig. 3).

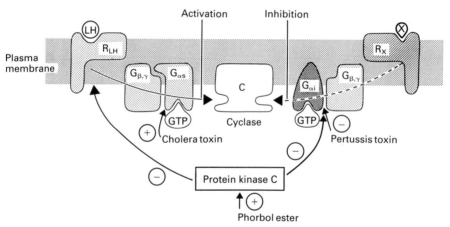

Fig. 3. Scheme showing proposed sites of action of phorbol ester-activated protein kinase C on the LH receptor–G protein–adenylate cyclase transducing system.

It is concluded that the normal Leydig cell differs from the tumour Leydig cell (Dix *et al.*, 1987) in that TPA enhances the normal response to cholera toxin. That this effect is not potentiated further by pertussis toxin demonstrates that the difference between LH- and TPA-induced desensit-ization is probably due to a modification of G_i protein by TPA but not LH. Phosphorylation of G_i and attenuation of G_i activity in platelets and S49 lymphoma cells by TPA has been demonstrated (Katada *et al.*, 1985; Jakobs *et al.*, 1985; Bell & Brunton, 1986). The difference between LH- and TPA-induced desensitization may then be that LH brings about homologous desensitization, whereas TPA desensitizes in a heterologous manner, i.e. it inhibits G protein function generally (Sibley & Lefkowitz, 1985).

Formation and possible roles of leukotrienes in the control of Leydig cells

Arachidonic acid, the precursor of prostaglandins and leukotrienes, is released by the action of phospholipase A_2 on phospholipids. Little is known about the mechanism controlling this enzyme in the ovaries and testes. Recent evidence from other cells indicates that it might be a target for protein kinase C as well as the known modulators Ca^{2+} and lipocortin. It has been established for many years that prostaglandins are formed in the ovaries and testes, but, with the exception of a possible role in follicle rupture, their physiological status remains uncertain. Recently attention has focussed on the alternate pathway of arachidonic acid metabolism via the lipoxygenases leading to the leukotrienes. This is because of the roles of leukotrienes as chemical mediators in allergies and inflammations; they have astonishingly high histamine-like activity in producing contraction of capillaries and permeabilization of capillary vessels (leading to oedema) and they are powerful chemotactic agents (Samuelsson, 1982). Recent evidence also suggests that certain endocrine glands many be regulated by the leukotrienes; these include the pituitary (Snyder *et al.*, 1983), pancreas (Metz *et al.*, 1982), adrenal cortex (Hirai *et al.*, 1985), ovaries (Reich *et al.*, 1983) and testes (Dix *et al.*, 1984).

Our previous studies have shown that inhibitors of lipoxygenase but not cyclo-oxygenase activity inhibited LH, LH-releasing hormone (LHRH) and dibutyryl cyclic AMP-stimulated steroidogenesis in purified normal and tumour Leydig cells (Dix *et al.*, 1984; Sullivan & Cooke, 1985a). The metabolites of [^{14}C]arachidonic acid formed in these cells had similar mobilities on thin-layer chromatograms (t.l.c.) to 5-HETE (5-L-hydroxy-6,8,11,4-eicosatetraenoic acid), 12-HETE (12-L-hydroxy-5,8,10,14-eicosatetraenoic acid) and LTB_4 (leukotriene B_4) (Dix *et al.*, 1984). Further work using a radioimmunoassay (RIA) for LTB_4 showed that this compound was synthesized and secreted by Leydig cells (Sullivan & Cooke, 1985b). Addition of the calcium ionophore A 23187 increased LTB_4 production 6-fold within 10 min but the effects of LH and hCG were variable (Sullivan & Cooke, 1984b). Recently, our attention has focussed on the contribution of other testicular cells that may synthesize LTB_4 and also whether LH increases LTB_4 synthesis. A specific RIA is available for this leukotriene and therefore, because LTB_4 is one of the end products of arachidonic acid metabolism, it can be used to address the question of whether the lipoxygenase pathway is controlled by LH. In our current studies LTB_4 production has been determined in highly purified Leydig cells and compared with impure preparations. The effects of various stimulants on LTB_4 production in Leydig cells *in vitro* with and without treatment *in vivo* with hCG have been determined.

Rat testes were incubated with collagenase to give a crude interstitial cell preparation (Leydig cells 20%). This was purified on a Percoll gradient (Leydig cells 85%) or the cells were separated by elutriation and then on Percoll gradients (Leydig cells 97%). Small increases in LTB_4 production following incubation with LH or hCG were found in the purified cells but not in the crude preparation. When the latter was mixed with either of the other two, the response to LH/hCG was lost. Very high levels of LTB_4 were produced in response to A 23187 in the crude preparation (~ 2500 pg/106 cell/3 h) compared to the purified cells (~ 400 pg/106 cells/3 h). However, there was little difference between the effect of A 23187 on the two purified preparations indicating that the 15% non-Leydig cells in the Percoll purified cells did not contribute to the LTB_4 production. Extensive metabolism of LTB_4 added to the crude preparation took place, indicating that the values obtained are an underestimation of the actual production. In a further series of experiments with purified cells it was found that the response to LH/hCG was inconsistent, although A 23187 always gave an increase. The effect of hCG *in vivo* on the subsequent LTB_4 production *in vitro* was therefore investigated. It was found that the levels of LTB_4 and response to A 23187 *in vitro* in elutriator/Percoll purified cells increased with the time after administration of hCG; they were low after 3 h (158 ± 15 and 194 ± 29 pg/10^6 cells/2 h respectively) but had not reached a maximum after 12 h (424 ± 50 and 1096 ± 168 pg/10^6 cells/2 h respectively; $\pm$s.d., $n = 5$). Little or no additional response to hCG added *in vitro* was obtained. HCG given *in vivo* increased PGF-2α levels *in vitro* and these had declined after 12 h. Neither hCG nor A 23187 had any effect *in vitro* on PGF-2α levels. The testosterone production *in vitro* showed a typical desensitization response after hCG *in vitro*.

We conclude that Leydig cells and other testis cell types form LTB₄. Although the response to LH/hCG *in vitro* is variable (possibly because of the short incubation times used), the Leydig cells isolated from hCG-treated rats contained higher levels of LTB₄ which increased with the time after administration of hCG. No extra effect of hCG added *in vitro* was found but A 23187 further increased LTB₄ levels. PGF-2α concentrations were also increased by hCG *in vivo* but they did not parallel LTB₄ and were not increased by A 23187 or hCG *in vitro*.

These experiments demonstrate that the synthesis of LTB₄ can be stimulated by hCG (LH). However, long periods are required (4–6 h) and so it is possible that this represents a trophic effect of hCG on the lipoxygenase enzymes rather than an acute stimulatory effect on phospholipase A₂. Also, the kinetics of LTB₄ production indicate that this leukotriene is not involved in the control of steroidogenesis. Preliminary data on the results of addition of 5-HPETE indicate that this short half-life derivative directly stimulates steroidogenesis in Leydig cells (unpublished results), and so it is possible that short-lived precursors of LTB₄ may be involved rather than LTB₄.

Conclusions

It is apparent that the control of one of the main second messengers, cyclic AMP, in Leydig cells is a complex process. The formation of cyclic AMP involves the GTP-mediated protein (G_s) activation of adenylate cyclase. It may also be negatively regulated by the inhibitory GTP-binding protein G_i although no direct effect of LH has yet been demonstrated. Phorbol esters do, however, inhibit G_i protein as shown by the potentiation of the cholera toxin effects on cyclic AMP. The LH-induced desensitization of adenylate cyclase is not regulated by cyclic AMP and is only partly restored by inactivation of G_i. The lesion occurs between the coupling of the LH receptor with G_s. Evidence from the similar effects of phorbol esters indicates that protein kinase C activation may be involved. This in turn implies that LH activates an additional transducing system involving polyphospho-inositide metabolism leading to release of diacylglycerol and protein kinase C activation.

Yet another transducing system is that involving phospholipase A₂ activation leading to arachidonic acid release. Inhibition of the lipoxygenase pathway but not the cyclooxygenase pathway leads to rapid inhibition of steroidogenesis. This implies that LH activates arachidonic acid release and metabolism to the leukotrienes. This possible acute effect requires further investigation. A chronic effect of LH (hCG) on the synthesis of the powerful chemotactic compound LTB₄ has, however, been demonstrated; this leukotriene is probably not involved in the control of steroidogenesis but may control interstitial fluid volumes and the chemotactic movement of polymorphonucleocytes into the interstitial fluid.

We thank the MRC, SERC and the AFRC for financial support.

References

Adashi, E.Y., Resnick, C.E., Cronin, M.J. & Hewlett, E.L. (1984) "Antigonadal" activity of the neurohypophysial hormones in cultured rat testicular cells: abolition by pertussis toxin. *Endocrinology* **115**, 839–841.

Bell, J.D. & Brunton, L.L. (1986) Enhancement of adenylate cyclase activity in S49 lymphoma cells by phorbol esters: withdrawal of GTP-dependent inhibition. *J. biol. Chem.* **261**, 12036–12041.

Dix, C.J., Schumacher, M. & Cooke, B.A. (1982) Desensitization of tumour Leydig cells by lutropin: evidence for uncoupling of the lutropin receptor from the guanine nucleotide binding protein. *Biochem. J.* **202**, 739–745.

Dix, C.J., Habberfield, A.D., Sullivan, M.H.F. & Cooke, B.A. (1984) Inhibition of steroid production in Leydig cells by non-steroidal anti-inflammatory and related compounds: evidence for the involvement of lipoxygenase products in steroidogenesis. *Biochem. J.* **219**, 529–537.

Dix, C.J., Habberfield, A.D. & Cooke, B.A. (1987) Similarities and differences in phorbol ester- and luteinizing hormone-induced desensitization of rat tumour Leydig-cell adenylate cyclase. *Biochem. J.* **243**, 373–377.

Gilman, A.G. (1984) G proteins and dual control of adenylate cyclase. *Cell* **36**, 577–579.

Green, D.A. & Clark, R.B. (1981) Adenylate cyclase coupling proteins are not essential for agonist-specific desensitization of lymphoma cells. *J. biol. Chem.* **256**, 2105–2108.

Habberfield, A.D., Dix, C.J. & Cooke, B.A. (1987) Effects of lutropin (LH) receptor internalization and recycling on the apparent numbers of LH receptors in rat testis Leydig cells at different temperatures. *Molec. cell. Endocrinol.* **51**, 153–161.

Hirai, A., Tahara, Y., Saito, H., Terano, T. & Yoshida, S. (1985) Involvement of 5-lipoxygenase metabolites in ACTH-stimulated corticosteroidogenesis in rat adrenal glands. *Prostaglandins* **30**, 749–767.

Iyengar, R., Vhat, M.K., Riser, M.E. & Birnbaumer, L. (1981) Receptor-specific desensitization of the S49 lymphoma cell adenylyl cyclase. Unaltered behaviour of the regulatory component. *J. biol. Chem.* **256**, 4810–4815.

Jakobs, K.H., Bauer, S. & Watanabe, Y. (1985) Modulation of adenylate cyclase of human platelets by phorbol ester. Impairment of the hormone-sensitive inhibitory pathway. *Eur. J. Biochem.* **151**, 425–430.

Katada, T., Gilman, A.G., Watanabe, Y., Bauer, S. & Jakobs, K.H. (1985) Protein kinase C phosphorylates the inhibitory guanine-nucleotide-binding protein regulatory component and apparently suppresses its function in hormonal inhibition of adenylate cyclase. *Eur. J. Biochem.* **151**, 431–437.

Khanum, A. & Dufau, M.L. (1986) Inhibitory action of forskolin on adenylate cyclase activity and cyclic AMP generation. *J. biol. Chem.* **261**, 11456–11459.

Levi, S.N., Dix, C.J., Thomas, M.G. & Cooke, B.A. (1982) Isolation and characterization of plasma membranes containing lutropin sensitive adenylate cyclase from a Leydig cell tumour. *Int. J. Androl.* **5**, 557–569.

Metz, S.A., Fujimoto, W.Y. & Robertson, R.P. (1982) Lipoxygenation of arachidonic acid: a pivotal step in stimulus–secretion coupling in the pancreatic β-cell. *Endocrinology* **11**, 2141–2143.

Mukhopadhyay, A.K. & Schumacher, M. (1985) Inhibition of hCG-stimulated adenylate cyclase in purified mouse Leydig cells by the phorbol ester PMA. *FEBS Letters* **187**, 56–60.

Nishizuka, Y. (1984) The role of protein kinase C in cell surface signal transduction and tumour promotion. *Nature, Lond.* **308**, 693–698.

Platts, E.A., Schulster, D. & Cooke, B.A. (1988) The inhibitory GTP-binding protein (Gi) occurs in rat Leydig cells and is differentially modified by lutropin (LH) and the phorbol ester TPA. *Biochem. J.* **253**, 895–899.

Rebois, R.V. & Patel, J. (1985) Phorbol ester causes desensitization of gonadotrophin-responsive adenylate cyclase in a murine Leydig tumour cell line. *J. biol. Chem.* **260**, 8026–8031.

Reich, R., Kohen, F., Naor, Z. & Tsafriri, A. (1983) Possible involvement of lipoxygenase products of arachidonic acid pathway in ovulation. *Prostaglandins* **26**, 1011–1020.

Ribeiro-Neto, F.A.P., Maltera, R., Hildebrandt, J.D., Codina, J., Field, J.B., Birnbaumer, L. & Sekura, R.D. (1985) ADP-ribosylation of membrane components by pertussis and cholera toxin. *Methods in Enzymology* **109**, 566–572.

Rommerts, F.F.G. & Cooke, B.A. (1988) The mechanisms of action of luteinizing hormone II. Transducing systems and biological effects. In *New Comprehensive Biochemistry: Hormones and their Actions*, vol. II, pp. 163–180. Eds B. A. Cooke, R. B. J. King & H. J. van der Molen. Elsevier, Amsterdam.

Samuelsson, B. (1982) The leukotrienes: highly biologically active substances involved in allergy and inflammation. *Ang. Chemie.* **21**, 902–907.

Sibley, D.R. & Lefkowitz, R.J. (1985) Molecular mechanisms of receptor desensitization using the β-adrenergic receptor-coupled adenylate cyclase system as a model. *Nature, Lond.* **317**, 124–129.

Sibley, D.R., Nambi, P., Peters, J.R. & Lefkowitz, R.J. (1984) Phorbol diesters promote β-adrenergic receptor phosphorylation and adenylate cyclase desensitization in duck erythrocytes. *Biochem. Biophys. Res. Commun.* **121**, 973–979.

Snyder, G.D., Capdevila, J., Chacos, N., Manna, S. & Falck, J.R. (1983) Action of LHRH: involvement of novel arachidonic acid metabolites. *Proc. natn Acad. Sci. U.S.A.* **80**, 3504–3507.

Sullivan, M.H.F. & Cooke, B.A. (1985a) Effects of calmodulin and lipoxygenase inhibitors on LH- and LHRH agonist-stimulated steroidogenesis in rat Leydig cells. *Biochem. J.* **232**, 55–59.

Sullivan, M.H.F. & Cooke, B.A. (1985b) Control and production of leukotriene B$_4$ in rat tumour and testicular Leydig cells. *Biochem. J.* **230**, 821–824.

Themmen, A.P.N., Hoogerbrugger, J.W., Rommerts, F.F.G. & van der Molen, H.J. (1986) Effects of LH and an LH-releasing hormone agonist on different second messenger systems in the regulation of steroidogenesis in isolated rat Leydig cells. *J. Endocr.* **108**, 431–440.

J. Reprod. Fert., Suppl. 37 (1989), 147–153

Control of the steroidogenic machinery of the human trophoblast by cyclic AMP*

J. C. Nulsen†, S. L. Silavin†, L.-C. Kao†, G. E. Ringler†, H. J. Kliman‡ and J. F. Strauss III†‡

Departments of †Obstetrics and Gynecology and ‡Pathology and Laboratory Medicine, University of Pennsylvania, Philadelphia, PA 19104, U.S.A.

Summary. Human cytotrophoblasts express adenylate cyclase activity and possess membrane-bound regulatory proteins that bind guanine nucleotides (G proteins). Stimulation of the cyclase by forskolin or addition of 8-bromo-cAMP augments progesterone secretion by cultured cytotrophoblasts at least in part, by promoting accumulation of components of the cholesterol side-chain cleavage system. This is the consequence of increased synthesis of the proteins participating in steroidogenesis as a result of the 8-bromo-cAMP-provoked increase in their respective mRNAs. We propose that progesterone synthesis by cytotrophoblasts is up-regulated by cyclic AMP, which acts to increase expression of genes encoding the steroidogenic machinery. Paracrine or autocrine factors may initiate this cascade by stimulating the cytotrophoblast adenylate cyclase.

Keywords: placenta; steroidogenesis; progesterone; cyclic AMP; man

Introduction

The human placenta is the major source of progesterone and oestrogens during gestation (Simpson & Macdonald, 1981). The syncytial trophoblasts of the placenta, which arise from fusion of mononuclear cytotrophoblasts, are the primary site of steroidogenic activity (Kliman *et al.*, 1986, 1987). Cytotrophoblasts do not stain or stain only weakly for steroidogenic enzymes including aromatase and 17β-hydroxysteroid dehydrogenase in immunocytochemical studies, and display weak 3β-hydroxysteroid dehydrogenase activity on histochemical analyses, whereas the syncytial trophoblast layer reacts strongly for steroidogenic enzymes (Wattenberg, 1958; Fournet-Dulguerov *et al.*, 1987). These findings suggest that, in the process of differentiation leading to the formation of the syncytial trophoblast, the steroidogenic activity of the cytotrophoblasts is augmented.

In this report we will review evidence that cytotrophoblasts isolated from term placenta express adenylate cyclase and respond to cyclic AMP analogues or agents which activate adenylate cyclase with an increase in secretion of progesterone. This response to cyclic AMP is the result, at least in part, of increased synthesis of components of the steroidogenic machinery which occurs as a consequence of cyclic AMP-induced accumulation of the mRNAs which encode these proteins.

Characterization of cytotrophoblast adenylate cyclase and identification of guanine nucleotide binding regulatory proteins (G proteins) in cytotrophoblast membranes

Extracts of purified cytotrophoblasts have adenylate cyclase activity that is stimulated approximately 4-fold by the diterpene, forskolin (Fig. 1). In the presence of $10\,\text{mM-MnCl}_2$, cAMP

---

*Reprint requests to Dr J. F. Strauss III.

formation occurs at a linear rate for at least 30 min (Fig. 1a), and the formation of product is linearly related to homogenate protein up to 60 μg (Fig. 1b). In the absence of $MnCl_2$, adenylate cyclase activity is barely detectable (Fig. 2, control). $MgCl_2$ at a concentration of 10 mM stimulates activity to levels less than 50% of those achieved in the presence of 10 mM-$MnCl_2$. A combination of 10 mM-$MgCl_2$ and 100 μM-Gpp(NH)p, a GTP analogue, is as effective as 10 mM-$MnCl_2$, although both of these responses are considerably less than the response observed in the presence of 10 μM-forskolin.

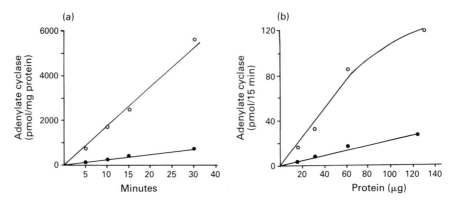

Fig. 1. Characterization of adenylate cyclase activity in isolated cytotrophoblasts. The time- and dose-dependent natures of enzyme activity are shown in (a) and (b), respectively, in the absence (●) or presence of (○) of 10 μM-forskolin. (From Nulsen *et al.*, 1988.)

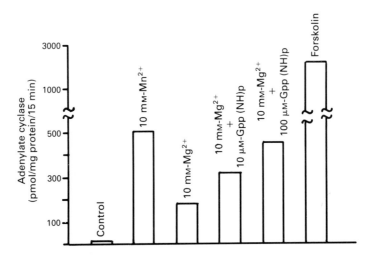

Fig. 2. Effects of $MnCl_2$, $MgCl_2$, and Gpp(NH)p on adenylate cyclase activity. Preparations of cytotrophoblasts were assayed for adenylate cyclase activity in the presence or absence of 10 mM-$MnCl_2$, 10 mM-$MnCl_2$, and 10 μM-forskolin, 10 mM-$MnCl_2$, or 10 mM-$MnCl_2$ with 10 or 100 μM-Gpp(NH)p. (From Nulsen *et al.*, 1988.)

Using cholera toxin- and pertussis toxin-mediated ADP-ribosylation, two forms of α-subunit of G_s (αs) of M_r 45 000 and 52 000 and the α-subunit of G_i (αi) of M_r 41 000 are detected in cytotrophoblast membranes (Fig. 3a). Using immunoblot analysis, molecular weight forms of

36 000 and 35 000 of the G protein β-subunit are found (Fig. 3b). The M_r 36 000 form of the β-subunit predominates, and this has been confirmed by two-dimensional gel electrophoresis studies. An antiserum raised against a peptide common to G protein α-subunits also detects the $α_i$ form of M_r 41 000 in the immunoblot analyses.

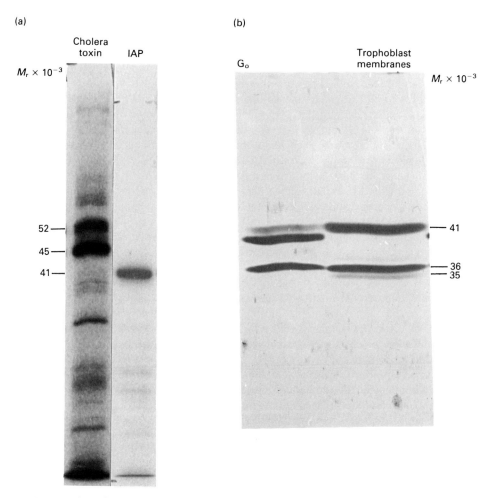

Fig. 3. Detection of G proteins in cytotrophoblast membranes. (a) Cytotrophoblast membranes (50 μg protein) were incubated with [^{32}P]NAD and cholera toxin or pertussis toxin (IAP), and then subjected to SDS–PAGE and autoradiography. (b) Cytotrophoblast membranes (50 μg protein) were reduced, alkylated, and subjected to SDS–PAGE, then to immunotransfer blotting using Antiserum 1398 (generated against a peptide common to the α-subunits of G_i, G_o and G_s) in combination with Antiserum 5357 (generated against the βγ-heterodimer obtained from brain G_o). Molecular weight forms of 35 000 and 36 000 of the β-subunit are detected as is that of $α_i$ subunit, M_r 41 000. Because G_i is generally present in greater amounts than G_s and because Antiserum 1398 has a lower affinity for $α_s$ than $α_i$, the $α_s$ subunits are not detected. Only the relevant portion of the nitrocellulose membrane is shown. (From Nulsen *et al.*, 1988.)

Effects of 8-bromo-cAMP and forskolin on progesterone secretion by cultured cytotrophoblasts

Culture of cytotrophoblasts isolated from human term placentae in the presence of 8-bromo-cAMP results in a 2-fold stimulation of progesterone secretion within 24 h (Table 1; Feinman *et al.*, 1986).

Forskolin markedly increases cyclic AMP secretion by the cells (Nulsen *et al.*, 1988) and also stimulates progesterone secretion approximately 2-fold.

Effect of 8-bromo-cAMP on synthesis and accumulation of the steroidogenic machinery in cytotrophoblasts

To examine the effects of 8-bromo-cAMP on components of the mitochondrial cholesterol side-chain cleavage system, we studied the synthesis of the iron sulphur protein, adrenodoxin. Cytotrophoblasts, cultured in the absence or presence of 8-bromo-cAMP, were pulse labelled with [^{35}S]methionine for 2 h and adrenodoxin was immunoprecipitated from cellular extracts containing equal amounts of trichloroacetic acid (TCA)-precipitable radioactivity. The immunoprecipitates were subjected to SDS–PAGE and the acrylamide gels were prepared for fluorography. Figure 4 shows a representative fluorogram which demonstrates increased de-novo synthesis of adrenodoxin in cytotrophoblasts cultured in the presence of 8-bromo-cAMP.

Immunocytochemical studies demonstrated that the newly synthesized cholesterol side-chain cleavage enzyme proteins accumulate in the cytotrophoblasts. Figure 5 is a photomicrograph of an immunocytochemical preparation detecting cytochrome P-450$_{scc}$. Exposure of the cytotrophoblasts to 8-bromo-cAMP resulted in significantly more intense immunostaining of cytoplasmic organelles (mitochondria) compared to control cells. In addition, the 8-bromo-cAMP-stimulated cells had fewer cytoplasmic lipid droplets, suggesting depletion of lipid stores, possibly sterol esters, for use in steroidogenesis.

Treatment of cultured cytotrophoblasts for 24 or 48 h with 8-bromo-cAMP causes a significant increase in the cellular content of mRNAs encoding adrenodoxin and cytochrome P-450$_{scc}$, while reducing levels of the mRNA encoding actin by 60% (Ringler *et al.*, 1988). The cytochrome P-450$_{scc}$ mRNA of ~ 2 kb increases 1·8-fold after 24 h and 2·5-fold after 48 h of treatment. The adrenodoxin mRNAs, which range in size from 1·0 to 1·75 kb as a result of multiple polyadenylation sites (Picado-Leonard *et al.*, 1988), increase 5·7-fold and 7·2-fold after 24 and 48 h of 8-bromo-cAMP treatment, respectively. The adrenodoxin mRNA increases before the cytochrome P-450$_{scc}$ mRNA, with a doubling of the adrenodoxin message being observed within 6–12 h of exposure to 8-bromo-cAMP. The inhibitor of RNA synthesis, actinomycin D, blocks the effects of 8-bromo-cAMP on these mRNAs. These findings suggest that the cyclic nucleotide acts to promote increased transcription of the P-450$_{scc}$ and adrenodoxin genes. Similar results have been obtained in studies with the JEG-3 human choriocarcinoma cell line (Picado–Leonard *et al.*, 1988).

A model for regulation of trophoblast steroidogenic activity

The observations reviewed here demonstrate that cytotrophoblast steroidogenic activity is up-regulated by cyclic AMP. The cyclic AMP-stimulated hormone production is due, at least in part, to increased levels of the mRNAs encoding proteins involved in steroidogenesis. The enhanced synthesis of these proteins results in their build up within the cells, rendering the trophoblasts capable of greater steroid formation. The accumulation of 'differentiated' cytotrophoblasts during gestation can account for the progressive increase in placental progesterone secretion.

The factor(s) which is (are) responsible for initiation of the cAMP cascade (i.e. factors which stimulate adenylate cyclase or cyclic AMP accumulation) in cytotrophoblasts are not yet known. However, we have found that several substances known to act by increasing adenylate cyclase stimulate cytotrophoblast endocrine activity (Nulsen *et al.*, 1988). These include β-adrenergic agents and corticotrophin releasing hormone (CRH). It is possible that hCG, which has been found to stimulate placental adenylate cyclase (Menon & Jaffe, 1973) could be another factor. The latter findings are of interest since both CRH and hCG are produced by the trophoblast (Robinson &

Table 1. Effect of 8-bromo-cAMP and forskolin
on human cytotrophoblast progesterone secretion

Treatment	Progesterone secretion (ng/mg protein)
Control	102 ± 15
8-Bromo-cAMP (1·5 mM)	198 ± 13[a]
Forskolin (100 μM)	204 ± 17[a]

Cytotrophoblasts were cultured for 24 h in the presence of the various treatments and progesterone secreted into the medium was quantitated by radioimmunoassay. Values presented are the means ± s.e. of triplicate cultures.
*$P < 0·01$ compared with control (Dunnett's test).

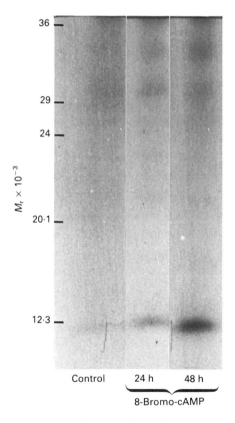

Fig. 4. Cytotrophoblasts isolated by the method of Kliman *et al.* (1986) were cultured in Dulbecco's modified Eagle's medium supplemented with 20% fetal bovine serum in the absence or presence of 1·5 mM-8-bromo-cAMP for the indicated times. The cells were incubated in methionine-free medium for 1 h before pulsing with 100 μCi[^{35}S]methionine/ml in the methionine-free medium for 2 h. The cells were then solubilized and equal quantities of TCA-precipitable radioactivity were subjected to immunoprecipitation with rabbit anti-bovine adrenodoxin antiserum. The immunoprecipitates were subjected to SDS–PAGE in 15% acrylamide gels and the gels were then processed for fluorography (Ulloa-Aguirre *et al.*, 1987).

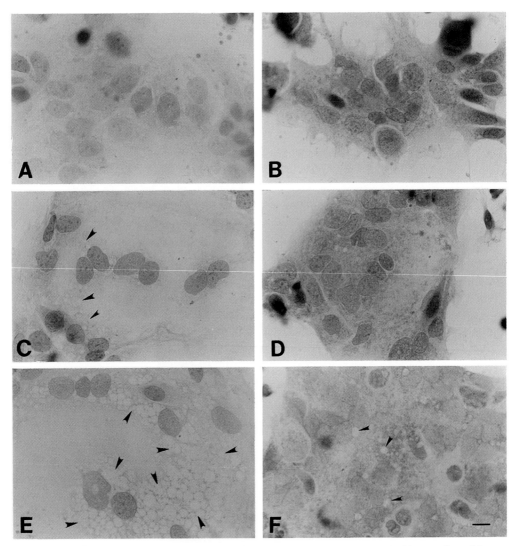

Fig. 5. Immunocytochemical detection of cytochrome P-450$_{scc}$ in cytotrophoblasts cultured for 24–72 h in the absence (A, C, E) or presence (B, D, F) of 8-bromo-cAMP (1·5 mM). The cells were cultured on glass coverslips and cytochrome P-450$_{scc}$, was detected using an antiserum raised in a rabbit against purified bovine adrenal cortex cytochrome P-450$_{scc}$, kindly provided by Dr J. David Lambeth of Emory University. Note the increased immunoperoxidase staining in mitochondria (identifiable as finely granular cytoplasmic staining) and the relative absence of lipid droplets (arrow heads) in 8-bromo-cAMP-treated cells. All micrographs are at the same magnification; bar represents 10 μm.

Mazjoub, 1987), raising the possibility that paracrine or autocrine regulation is involved in the control of cytotrophoblast function.

We thank Ms Debbie Coffin and Mrs Barbara McKenna for assistance in the preparation of this manuscript. This work was supported by USPHS Grants HD-06274 (J.F.S.) and HD-0075 (H.J.K.), AM-07409 (J.C.N.) and a grant from the Mellon Foundation.

References

Feinman, M.A., Kliman, H.J., Caltabiano, S.J. & Strauss, J.F., III (1986) 8-bromo-3′,5′-adenosine monophosphate stimulates the endocrine activity of human cytotrophoblasts in culture. *J. clin. Endocr. Metab.* **63**, 1211–1217.

Fournet-Dulguerov, N., Maclusky, N.J., Leranth, C.Z., Todd, R., Mendelson, C.R., Simpson, E.R. & Naftolin, F. (1987) Immunohistochemical localization of aromatase cytochrome P-450 estradiol dehydrogenase in the syncytiotrophoblast of the human placenta. *J. clin. Endocr. Metab.* **65**, 757–764.

Kliman, H.J., Nestler, J.E., Sermasi, E., Sanger, J.M. & Strauss, J.F., III (1986) Purification, characterization and in vitro differentiation of cytotrophoblasts from human term placenta. *Endocrinology* **118**, 1567–1582.

Kliman, H.J., Feinman, M.A. & Strauss, J.F., III (1987) Differentiation of human cytotrophoblast into syncytiotrophoblast in culture. *Trophoblast Research* **2**, 407–421.

Menon, K.M.J. & Jaffe, R.B. (1973) Chorionic gonadotropin-sensitive adenylate cyclase in human term placenta. *J. clin. Endocr. Metab.* **36**, 1104–1109.

Nulsen, J.E., Woolkalis, M.J., Kopf, G.S. & Strauss, J.F., III (1988) Adenylate cyclase in human cytotrophoblasts: characterization and its role in modulating hCG secretion. *J. clin. Endocr. Metab.* **68**, 258–265.

Picado-Leonard, J., Voutilainen, R., Kao, L.-C., Chung, B.-C., Strauss, J.F., III & Miller, W.L. (1988) Human adrenodoxin: cloning of three cDNAs and cycloheximide enhancement in JEG-3 cells. *J. biol. Chem* **263**, 3240–3244.

Ringler, G.E., Kao, L.C., Miller, W.L. & Strauss, J.F., III (1988) Molecular mechanisms underlying the effects of 8-bromo-cAMP on expression of endocrine functions by human trophoblast. *Endocrinology* **122** (Suppl.), 30, Abstr. 39.

Robinson, B. & Majzoub, J. (1987) Corticotropin releasing hormone gene expression in cultures of human placenta. *Endocrinology* **120** (Suppl.), 135, Abstr. 455.

Simpson, E.R. & Macdonald, P.C. (1981) Endocrine physiology of the placenta. *Annu. Rev. Physiol.* **43**, 163–188.

Ulloa-Aguirre, A., August, A.M., Golos, T.G., Kao, L.C., Sakuragi, N., Kliman, H.J. & Strauss, J.F., III (1987) 8-Bromo-adenosine-3′,5′-monophosphate regulates expression of chorionic gonadotropin and fibronectin in human cytotrophoblasts. *J. clin. Endocr. Metab.* **64**, 1002–1009.

Wattenberg, L.W. (1958) Microscopic histochemical demonstration of steroid 3β-OH dehydrogenase in tissue sections. *J. Histochem. Cytochem.* **6**, 225–232.

J. Reprod. Fert., Suppl. **37** (1989), 155–162

Orchestrated expression of steroidogenic side-chain cleavage cytochrome P-450 during follicular development in the rat ovary

J. Orly

Department of Biological Chemistry, Institute of Life Sciences, The Hebrew University of Jerusalem, Jerusalem, 91904, Israel

Summary. Antibody to the mitochondrial cholesterol side-chain cleavage cytochrome P-450 (P-450$_{scc}$) was used to study the expression of this key steroidogenic enzyme during follicular development. Immunofluorescence staining of tissue cryosections and isolated cells revealed unique and cell-specific patterns of P-450$_{scc}$ expressed in four cell types of the prepubertal rat ovary.

Without hormonal treatment, the interstitial gland expressed ample amounts of P-450$_{scc}$. Within 24 h after PMSG administration, theca interna acquired the cytochrome, and after an additional 24 h, the enzyme appeared also in granulosa cells. However, expression of P-450$_{scc}$ in granulosa cells was observed only in preovulatory follicles. This was in contrast to the theca interna cells which differentiated in various follicles unrelated to their stages of development. Cumulus cells were the last cell type to express P-450$_{scc}$, occurring as late as 2–3 h before ovulation. These observations indicate that the concerted expression of P-450$_{scc}$ in the different ovarian cell types is a well-timed phenomenon which is precisely co-ordinated during follicular development.

Keywords: ovarian cell types; immunofluorescence staining; cryosections; cultured cells; rat

Introduction

Follicular development in the ovary is controlled by the pituitary gonadotrophins, FSH and LH (Richards, 1980). These two gonadotrophins trigger the endocrine function of the ovarian cells, namely, the synthesis of sex steroids. The key reaction in steroidogenesis, i.e. the conversion of cholesterol to pregnenolone, is catalysed in the mitochondrial membranes by a member of the cytochrome P-450 family, the cholesterol side-chain cleavage P-450 (P-450$_{scc}$, EC 1.6.2.4). Pregnenolone is further metabolized by microsomal enzymes to yield progestagens, androgens and oestrogens.

Follicular cell types in the ovary known to participate in the synthesis of steroids are theca interna, granulosa and cumulus cells. The fourth tissue which has been suspected to be actively involved in androgen synthesis is the interstitial gland (Falck, 1959). As a result of activities of these cells, the qualitative and quantitative profiles of the sex hormones secreted into the blood stream change as the leading follicles grow and mature.

This study attempts to provide a novel approach to study the partial contribution of each functional ovarian cell type to the overall steroidogenic output of the ovary during follicular development *in vivo*. We assumed that the key regulatory event should be the expression of P-450$_{scc}$. Therefore, to monitor P-450$_{scc}$ levels directly, we raised antibodies to the rat cytochrome (Farkash *et al.*, 1986) to follow the expression of P-450$_{scc}$, with the aid of a variety of immunochemical methods.

J. Orly

Materials and Methods

Reagents. Poly-DL-lysine ($M_r > 70\,000$), hyaluronidase, collagenase type V and DNase type I, were obtained from Sigma (St Louis, MO, U.S.A.).

Hormones. PMSG (Gestyl) was purchased from Organon (Oss, The Netherlands). Ovine FSH (NIADDK oFSH 17A) was a generous gift from NIADDK (Bethesda, Maryland, U.S.A.).

Culture medium. Serum free, hormone-supplemented culture medium (4F medium) was used as previously described (Goldring *et al.*, 1986).

Animals. Immature intact female rats (Wistar-derived strain) were neither hypophysectomized nor treated with diethylstilboestrol. Animals were killed by CO_2 asphyxiation.

Cell culture. Granulosa cells were expressed by needle puncture and cultured on fibronectin-coated glass cover slips as previously described (Goldring *et al.*, 1986).
Collagenase-DNase dispersion of ovaries was performed as previously described (Goldring & Orly, 1985), and cells were cultured as described above for the granulosa cells.
Oocyte–cumulus complexes before and after ovulation were cultured on poly-lysine/fibronectin-coated glass coverslips. The latter were prepared by 10 min incubation with poly-lysine (1 mg/ml in H_2O), followed by washing with water and coating with fibronectin as above.
Dispersion of mucified post-ovulatory complexes was performed by 5 min incubation at 37°C in hyaluronidase solution (1 mg/ml in 4F medium). After washing, the cells were inoculated onto the poly-lysine/fibronectin-coated coverslips and incubated at 37°C in a humidified incubator (95% air, 5% CO_2).

Immunofluorescence staining. Polyclonal rabbit antibodies to rat cytochrome P-450$_{scc}$ were prepared as described (Farkash *et al.*, 1986). Goat anti-rabbit rhodamine-immunoglobulin G was obtained from Bio-Makor (Rehovot, Israel). Immunofluorescence staining of cultured cells was performed after fixation and permeabilization with Triton X-100 as described by Goldring *et al.* (1986). Ovarian cryostat sections were prepared and stained as described earlier (Zlotkin *et al.*, 1986). Microscopy and photography were performed as described elsewhere (Zlotkin *et al.*, 1986).

Results

The superovulated rat model served to study the expression of P-450$_{scc}$ throughout the synchronous maturation of many follicles which develop as a result of PMSG administration. One

---

Fig. 1. Cell-specific expression of P-450$_{scc}$ during follicular development after PMSG administration to immature rats. PMSG (15 i.u.) was administered (s.c.) to 25-day-old rats. At various times, ovaries were sectioned on a cryostat and immunofluorescently stained with anti-P-450$_{scc}$ serum.
(**a**) Distribution of P-450$_{scc}$ before administration of PMSG. Note expression of P-450$_{scc}$ in the secondary interstitial tissue (i); lack of P-450$_{scc}$ expression in some parts of the secondary interstitial tissues (i̲); partial expression of P-450$_{scc}$ in cells of the theca interna (ti); lack of P-450$_{scc}$ in the theca externa (te); and lack of P-450$_{scc}$ in granulosa cells (g). × 70. (**b**) Amplification of P-450$_{scc}$ expressed in secondary interstitial cells (i) and theca interna (ti), 24 h after administration of PMSG. Note lack of P-450$_{scc}$ in granulosa cells (g). × 12·5. (**c**) Non-preovulatory follicle depicted 48 h after PMSG administration. Note lack of P-450$_{scc}$ in the layers of granulosa cells (g), whereas P-450$_{scc}$ is expressed in theca interna (ti). A single layer of undifferentiated theca externa cells (te) separates the secondary interstitial cells (i) and theca interna. a, Antrum. × 90.
(**d**) Preovulatory follicle observed 48 h after PMSG administration as in (c). Note ample expression of P-450$_{scc}$ in the mural granulosa cells (g), but lack of the cytochrome in the cumulus cells (c) surrounding the oocyte (Oo). Arrows indicate the location of the follicular basement membrane; ti, theca interna; a, antrum; black asterisks indicate high P-450$_{scc}$ levels; white asterisks indicate low levels of P-450$_{scc}$. × 110. (**e**) Formation of corpus luteum 72 h after PMSG administration. Inner layers of cells contain relatively low levels of P-450$_{scc}$ (white asterisk). Outer layers (formerly theca interna) express high amounts of P-450$_{scc}$ (black asterisk). × 90. (**f**) Corpus luteum, 120 h after administration of PMSG. Note ample expression of P-450$_{scc}$ over the whole gland section. × 90.

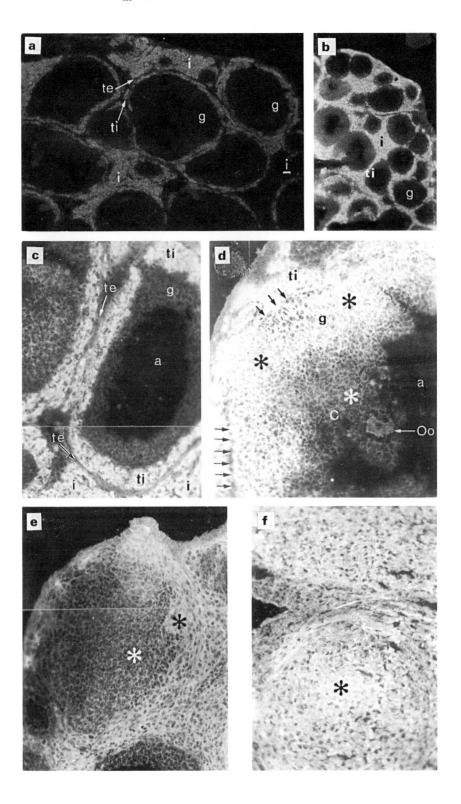

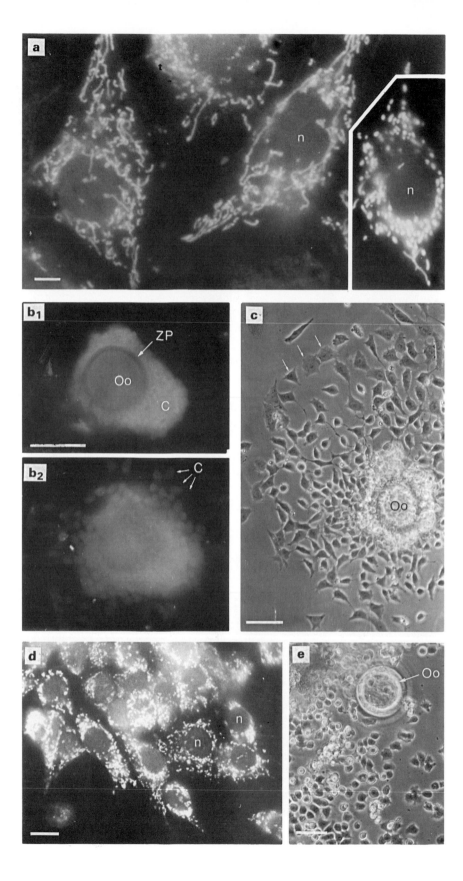

injection of PMSG (15 i.u.) was given at 10:00 h to 25-day-old rats, and the content of ovarian P-450$_{scc}$ was quantitated at various times up to 120 h after injection. Such an immuno-dot-blot assay of ovarian homogenates (Zlotkin *et al.*, 1986) revealed that the amount of P-450$_{scc}$ increased in a step-wise fashion: a 3-fold increment within 24 h after PMSG administration, a second 5-fold increase occurred between 30 and 48 h after PMSG, and the last 3-fold enrichment of the P-450$_{scc}$ content occurred after ovulation during formation of the corpus luteum.

To ascribe the first two increments of P-450$_{scc}$ to the specific cell types in the ovary, we visualized the enzyme by immunofluorescence in cryostat sections (Fig. 1). Before administration of PMSG, substantial amounts of P-450$_{scc}$ were observed in most of the interstitial tissue (Fig. 1a). No more than 30% of the theca interna cells contained the cytochrome and absolutely no traces of the enzyme were detected in the granulosa cell compartments of the follicles. We confirmed this observation by immunofluorescence staining of collagenase/DNase dispersed ovarian cells in culture. Up to 15–20% of the cultured cells, without gonadotrophin treatment, were heavily labelled in their mitochondria. The mitochondria of such cells appeared fragmented and globular (inset of Fig. 2a). These cells were typical interstitial cells. The remaining cells were negative with respect to P-450$_{scc}$ staining but the addition of an LH-free preparation of FSH (Goldring & Orly, 1985) readily induced the enzyme as shown in Fig. 2(a). We were therefore able to conclude that these FSH-inducible cells were granulosa cells.

Figure 1(b) shows that, upon administration of PMSG which contains both LH and FSH activities, a rapid expression of P-450$_{scc}$ occurred in the theca interna and the interstitial tissue, resulting in a much brighter fluorescence and completion of the contour of the stained 'belts' of cells surrounding the unstained granulosa cells.

The granulosa cells expressed P-450$_{scc}$ only after 48 h of PMSG treatment (Fig. 1d). However, only preovulatory follicles contained P-450$_{scc}$-containing granulosa, while granulosa cells in non-preovulatory follicles were not labelled at all (Fig. 1c). It should be noted that, unlike this differential expression of P-450$_{scc}$ in the granulosa compartments, the cytochrome was now expressed in the theca interna cells of all follicles, regardless of their stage of development.

Unexpectedly, the cumulus cells in the preovulatory follicles did not exhibit labelling of P-450$_{scc}$ when examined before the LH surge (Fig. 1d). On the other hand, the well known steroidogenic

---

Fig. 2. Expression of P-450$_{scc}$ in cultured follicular cells. (**a**) Granulosa cells were expressed by needle puncture from ovaries of 25-day-old intact rats. After overnight incubation, FSH (100 ng/ml) was added, and 48 h later the cells were fixed and immunofluorescently stained. Note the filamentous mitochondria containing ample amounts of P-450$_{scc}$ in three typical cells. n, nucleus. Inset shows a single secondary interstitial cell depicted in cultures of collagenase–DNase dispersed ovaries. Note the fragmented globular mitochondria bearing high content of P-450$_{scc}$. n, nucleus. Bar = 10 μm. (**b$_1$**, **b$_2$**). Two focal planes of a single oocyte–cumulus complex obtained from 25-day-old ovaries, 48 h after administration of PMSG. After overnight incubation in culture, the immunofluorescence micrograph (b$_1$) depicts the equatorial plane of the oocyte (Oo), surrounded by the cumulus cells (C) which are not stained by the P-450$_{scc}$ antibody. ZP, zona pellucida. In micrograph b$_2$ the focus plane is on the cumulus cells (C) which spread on the glass cover-slip substratum. Note lack of P-450$_{scc}$ expression, corroborating Fig. 1(d). Bar = 100 μm. (**c**) Phase-contrast micrograph of an oocyte–cumulus complex similar to that shown in b$_1$/b$_2$. After overnight incubation in culture, the oocyte (Oo) is still surrounded by 2–3 compact layers of the cumulus cells while the peripheral cells (C) have migrated onto the substratum and spread out (white arrows). Bar = 100μm. (**d**) Post-ovulatory cumulus cells obtained from the oviduct ampulla. After overnight in culture, the spread cells were fixed and immunofluorescently stained for P-450$_{scc}$. Note the fragmented mitochondria resembling those in the interstitial cells (Fig. 2a, inset). n, nucleus. Bar = 20 μm. (**e**) Phase-contrast micrograph of hyaluronidase-dispersed post-ovulatory cumulus–oocyte complex, after 60 min incubation in culture. Note the stripped oocyte (Oo) and the attached but not yet fully spread cumulus cells. Bar = 100 μm.

ability of the post-ovulatory cumulus cells was demonstrated in rat cells (Sherizly & Kraicer, 1980) and in human cells obtained from in-vitro fertilization procedures (Laufer *et al.*, 1984). Therefore, in attempts to reconcile the apparent inconsistencies between our immunofluorescence findings in cryostat sections and the previous studies mentioned above, we cultured oocyte–cumulus complexes isolated at various times between onset of the LH surge and ovulation. We also cultured post-ovulatory cumulus cells and Fig. 2(d) clearly demonstrates that these cells, obtained from the oviduct ampulla 6 h after ovulation, showed marked expression of P-450$_{scc}$. Conversely, cumulus complexes expressed before the LH surge were devoid of the cytochrome (Figs 2b$_1$ and 2b$_2$). Accumulation of newly synthesized P-450$_{scc}$ was observed only 3–4 h before ovulation (not shown).

Discussion

Preparation and use of antibody to rat P-450$_{scc}$ (Farkash *et al.*, 1986) enabled us to visualize directly, for the first time, the mitochondrial cytochrome in ovarian steroidogenic cells. The present report describes the cell-specific expression of P-450$_{scc}$ in the various ovarian cell types which comprise the functional unit of the ovary, the follicle. A unique pattern of P-450$_{scc}$ expression was revealed, schematically illustrated in Fig. 3. During ovarian development in the prepubertal rat, the interstitial tissue is the first in which measurable amounts of P-450$_{scc}$ are expressed, as early as 8 days *post partum* (T. Zlotkin & J. Orly, unpublished results). The physiological relevance of this early expression of steroidogenic capacity is as yet unclear. Our current studies indicate that, like theca interna, these cells are LH-responsive and produce 5α-reduced androgens (S. Bitzur & J. Orly, unpublished results). It is therefore tempting to speculate that these interstitial-derived unaromatizable androgens are somehow involved in maintenance of the prepubertal state of the ovary, as previously suggested by Eckstein (1985).

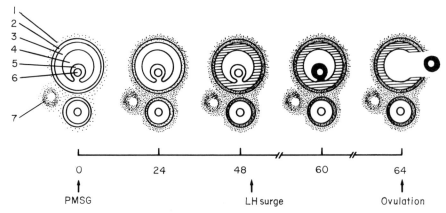

Fig. 3. Schematic representation of time-dependent expression of P-450$_{scc}$ during follicular development. Arrows indicate time of PMSG administration to the 25-day-old rat, the LH surge and ovulation. The upper large follicle represents a mature follicle destined to ovulate. The lower smaller follicle represents an immature non-preovulatory follicle in which P-450$_{scc}$ does not accumulate in the granulosa or cumulus cells. Note the time-dependent progression of P-450$_{scc}$ expression in the interstitial cells (1, dotted), theca interna (2, dotted), granulosa (3, hatched) and cumulus cells (5, solid). Antrum is designated as 4, and 7 is an atretic follicle turning into secondary interstitial tissue.

In contrast to P-450$_{scc}$ expression in granulosa cells occurring only in preovulatory follicles, synthesis of the cytochrome in the theca and interstitial cells is observed in the vicinity of any follicle in the ovarian tissue. Both tissues may therefore act as an 'all-ovarian' androgenic moiety. In other words, we feel that the current concept of follicular function, viewing theca interna cells as the major source for androgens, should be modified and include the extra-follicular interstitial cells as androgen-producing partners of no less importance. Moreover, it is well-known that androgens synergize with FSH in turning-on many granulosa cell functions (reviewed by Hsueh *et al.*, 1984). Since the present study shows that interstitial and theca cells possess P-450$_{scc}$ well before P-450$_{scc}$ is observed in granulosa cells, it is not unlikely that the androgenic environment provided at the early stages of follicular ripening is in fact the very first interplay between the two cell types. Only later, upon induction of aromatase in the FSH/androgen-primed granulosa cells, will theca–interstitial–granulosa exchange of progestagens and androgens commence, yielding oestrogen production as postulated by the 'two-cell–two-gonadotrophin theory' (Falck, 1959; Bjersing & Carstensen, 1964; Armstrong & Dorrington, 1977).

The third cell type that expresses P-450$_{scc}$, 30–48 h after PMSG administration, is the granulosa cell. As mentioned above, P-450$_{scc}$ expression in granulosa cells was confined exclusively to preovulatory follicles. Small and non-preovulatory follicles did not accumulate the cytochrome, suggesting that P-450$_{scc}$ expression in granulosa cells is a specific marker for mature preovulatory follicles. It is not clear by what mechanism the synthesis of P-450$_{scc}$ is limited in small follicles. Our in-vitro studies indicate that it is not due to a lack of functional FSH receptors (Orly *et al.*, 1982). It is also clear that this suppression of steroidogenic responsiveness is relieved when the granulosa cells are cultured (Epstein-Almog & Orly, 1985; Goldring *et al.*, 1986). However, additional experiments conducted with long-term cultures of granulosa cells demonstrated that FSH-induced P-450$_{scc}$ expression is suppressed during entry of the cultured cells into the proliferating phase during which the cell population doubled. The cells regained their steroidogenic capacity upon cessation of DNA synthesis (Epstein-Almog & Orly, 1985). We therefore postulate that a similar arrest of P-450$_{scc}$ expression occurs in non-preovulatory growing follicles exhibiting intense mitotic activity of their granulosa cells (Hirshfield, 1985).

The cumulus cells express P-450$_{scc}$ and acquire their steroidogenic capacity only a few hours before ovulation. This probably indicates the need for steroid hormones at a post-ovulatory site, most probably in the oviduct. However, it is not yet clear what these steroids are needed for. Do they participate in creating the physiologically compatible milieu for the egg to be fertilized? Alternatively, are locally high concentrations of cumulus-derived steroid hormones needed for transport of the embryo through the oviduct isthmus to the uterine horn? Neither do we understand by what mechanism expression of P-450$_{scc}$ is withheld in the cumulus cells until ovulation is due to occur.

In summary, as illustrated in Fig. 3, this study portrays a well-timed and precisely-orchestrated expression of cytochrome P-450$_{scc}$ during follicular development in the ovary. The steroidogenic capacity can be allegorized as a time-dependent tidal wave proceeding from the periphery of the follicle towards the centre where the oocyte rests. Future studies will attempt to resolve the mechanisms underlying what appears to be a programmed regulation of the P-450$_{scc}$ gene in the various follicular cell types.

I thank Mrs Devra Aaronson and Mrs Sherry Kisos for typing this manuscript; and Mrs Edith Dicker for editorial assistance. This work was supported by grant No. 3255/84 from the United States-Israel Binational Science Foundation (BSF), Jerusalem, Israel, and by the Fund for Basic Research, administered by the Israel Academy of Science and Humanities.

References

Armstrong, D.T. & Dorrington, J.H. (1977) Estrogen biosynthesis in ovaries and testes. *Adv. Sex Horm. Res.* **3**, 217–235.

Bjersing, L. & Carstensen, H. (1964) The role of granulosa in the biosynthesis of ovarian steroid hormones. *Biochim. Biophys. Acta* **86**, 639–640.

Eckstein, B. (1985) Biosynthesis and action of androgens at the onset of puberty. In *Female Adolescence*, pp. 95–116. Eds C. Flaming, S. Venturoli & J. R. Givens. Year Book Medical Publishers, Chicago.

Epstein-Almog, R. & Orly, J. (1985) Inhibition of hormone-induced steroidogenesis during cell proliferation is serum-free cultures of rat granulosa cells. *Endocrinology* **116**, 2103–2112.

Falck, B. (1959) Site of production of oestrogen in rat ovary as studied in microtransplants. *Acta physiol. scand.* **47,** *Suppl.* **163,** 1–101.

Farkash, Y., Timberg, R. & Orly, J. (1986) Preparation of antiserum to rat cytochrome P-450 cholesterol side chain cleavage, and its use for ultrastructural localization of the immunoreactive enzyme by protein A-gold technique. *Endocrinology* **118,** 1353–1365.

Goldring, N.B. & Orly, J. (1985) Concerted metabolism of steroid hormones produced by cocultured ovarian cell types. *J. biol. Chem.* **260,** 913–921.

Goldring, N.B., Farkash, Y., Goldschmit, D. & Orly, J. (1986) Immunofluorescent probing of the mitochondrial cholesterol side-chain cleavage cytochrome P-450 expressed in differentiating granulosa cells in culture. *Endocrinology* **119,** 2821–2832.

Hirshfield, A.N. (1985) Comparison of granulosa cell proliferation in small follicles of hypophysectomized, prepubertal and mature rats. *Biol. Reprod.* **32,** 979–985.

Hsueh, A.J.W., Adashi, E.Y., Jones, P.B.C. & Welsh, T.H. (1984) Hormonal regulation of the differentiation of cultured ovarian granulosa cells. *Endocrine Rev.* **5,** 76–126.

Laufer, N., De Cherney, A.H., Haseltine, F.P. & Behrman, H.R. (1984) Steroid secretion by the human egg-corona-cumulus-complex in culture. *J. clin. Endocr. Metab.* **58,** 1153–1157.

Orly, J., Farkash, Y., Hershkovitz, N., Mizrachi, L. & Weinberger, P. (1982) Ovarian substance induces steroid production in cultured granulosa cells. *In Vitro* **18,** 980–989.

Richards, J.S. (1980) Maturation of ovarian follicles: actions and interactions of pituitary and ovarian hormones on follicular cell differentiation. *Physiol. Rev.* **60,** 51–89.

Sherizly, I. & Kraicer, P.F. (1980) Progesterone secretion by the post-ovulatory rat cumulus oophorus. *Gamete Res.* **3,** 115–119.

Zlotkin, T., Farkash, Y. & Orly, J. (1986) Cell-specific expression of immunoreactive cholesterol side chain cleavage cytochrome P-450 during follicular development in the rat ovary. *Endocrinology* **119,** 2809–2820.

J. Reprod. Fert., Suppl. **37** (1989), 163–172

Regulation of side-chain cleavage enzyme and 3β-hydroxysteroid dehydrogenase by Ca^{2+} second messenger and protein kinase C systems in the placenta of the cow

M. Shemesh, W. Hansel*, J. F. Strauss† and L. S. Shore*

*Department of Hormone Research, Kimron Veterinary Institute, Bet Dagan, POB 12, Israel 50200;
*Department of Physiology, Cornell University, Ithaca, NY 14853, U.S.A.; and †Department of
Obstetrics/Gynecology, Hospital of the University of Pennsylvania, Philadelphia, PA 19104,
U.S.A.*

Summary. The steroidogenic activity of the bovine placenta is not modulated by cyclic nucleotide-mediated mechanisms. However, both translocation of intracellular Ca^{2+} and influx of extracellular Ca^{2+} activate the side-chain cleavage enzyme and 3β-hydroxysteroid dehydrogenase. Protein kinase C activation in concert with Ca^{2+} mobilization also activates the side-chain cleavage enzyme. Cholesterol availability is a rate-limiting factor. Using polyclonal antibodies against bovine adrenal cytochrome P-450$_{scc}$, the presence of P-450$_{scc}$ was demonstrated in both placental and luteal tissues. The cytochrome P-450$_{scc}$ was then localized, using gold-staining electron microscopy, in the mononuclear cells but not the binuclear cells of the placentome. The results suggest that cholesterol is metabolized by the mononuclear cell to pregnenolone, where it is further metabolized to progesterone by the mononuclear and binuclear cells.

Keywords: cow; placenta; steroidogenesis; protein kinase C; Ca^{2+}

Introduction

The placenta of the cow has been generally disregarded as a site of progesterone synthesis (Hoffmann *et al.*, 1979; Wendorf *et al.*, 1983). Nevertheless, conversion of [³H]pregnenolone to radioactive progesterone by bovine placenta preparations has been demonstrated (Ainsworth & Ryan, 1967), and our previously reported studies indicated that enzyme-dispersed bovine placentomes are capable of producing progesterone in culture (Shemesh *et al.*, 1983). The experiments described in the present paper were conducted to define further the endocrine activity of the bovine placentome with respect to progesterone production and to elucidate the mechanisms by which placental steroidogenesis is controlled.

Materials and Methods

Chemicals and reagents. 5-Cholesten-3β,25-diol (25-OH-C) was purchased from Steraloids (Wilton, NH, U.S.A.) and 12-0-tetradecanoyl-phorbol-13-acetate (TPA) was obtained from P-L Biochemicals Inc. (Milwaukee, WI, U.S.A.). Cyanoketone was kindly provided by Dr A. E. Soria (Sterling-Winthrop Res. Inst., Rennselaer, NY, U.S.A.). All other chemicals were purchased from Sigma Chemical Co. (St Louis, MO, U.S.A.). The bovine LH (USDA) was a donation from the National Hormone and Pituitary Program, Baltimore, MD, U.S.A.

Animals and tissues. Placental tissues were collected from Holstein Friesian cows at known gestational ages (N = 13) and from an abbatoir (N = 35). Fetal cotyledons were dispersed with collagenase as previously reported (Shemesh *et al.*, 1984).

Assay of progesterone and pregnenolone. Progesterone and pregnenolone were extracted or quantified directly in the media by RIA as previously described (Shemesh *et al.*, 1984, 1988).

Statistical analysis. Values presented are the means ± s.e. of 5 experiments unless otherwise stated. Each experiment included 5 replicate incubations in each treatment group. Analysis of variance followed by Dunnett's test or Student's *t* test was used to determine significant differences.

Results

Progesterone synthesis by cultured fetal and maternal cells

To define the pattern of progesterone synthesis by fetal cotyledons and maternal caruncles, placental cells derived from cows at 182–283 days of gestation were cultured in Medium 199 supplemented with 5% calf serum. Progesterone synthesis by fetal and maternal cells was greatest during the first 4 days of culture and then declined (Fig. 1). The in-vitro production of progesterone by maternal caruncle was considerably less, on a per cell basis, than by cotyledonary cells.

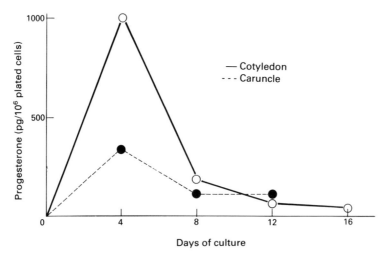

Fig. 1. Progesterone formation by cultured dispersed cotyledon and caruncle cells. Medium was changed every 4 days of culture and progesterone secretion during the subsequent 4 days was then determined. Values are means of net synthesis from 10 cows at 182–283 days of gestation. (From Shemesh *et al.*, 1984.)

Effect of LH, cyclic nucleotides and MIX on placental cell steroidogenesis

In view of this indication that placental cells produce progesterone, we decided to determine whether the steroidogenic activity of these cells could be modulated by tropic agents.

We examined the effect of addition of LH (100 ng/ml), 8Br-cAMP (0·5 mM) and 3-isobutyl-l-methylxanthine (MIX, 0·5 mM) on progesterone synthesis by fetal cotyledon and maternal caruncle cells. As indicated in Fig. 2, progesterone synthesis in fetal cotyledon cells was not elevated by LH or 8Br-cAMP. However, addition of MIX during the first and the second incubation resulted in progesterone accumulation 2–3-fold higher than was found in control cells at any given time. Addition of LH or 8Br-cAMP with MIX produced no greater progesterone synthesis than MIX alone (Fig. 3). A similar response to MIX was observed when maternal caruncle cells harvested from cows at various stages of gestation were used (Fig. 4).

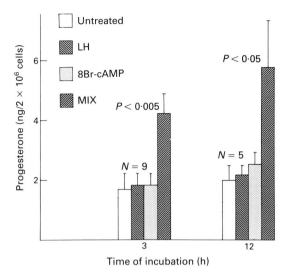

Fig. 2. Effect of agents on progesterone biosynthesis by incubated dispersed fetal cotyledon cells during incubation. Cells were washed by centrifugation and fresh medium was added after 3 h of incubation. Values are means ± s.e.m. for net synthesis by 9 animals from early and late stages of gestation. (From Shemesh *et al.*, 1984.)

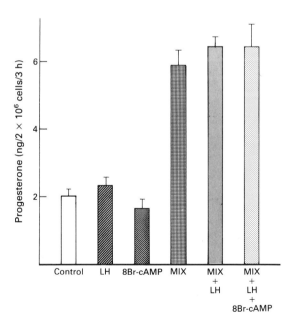

Fig. 3. Effect of LH or 8Br-cAMP with MIX on progesterone biosynthesis by incubated dispersed fetal cotyledon cells during 3 h of incubation. Values are means ± s.e.m. for net synthesis by 5 animals. (From Shemesh *et al.*, 1984.)

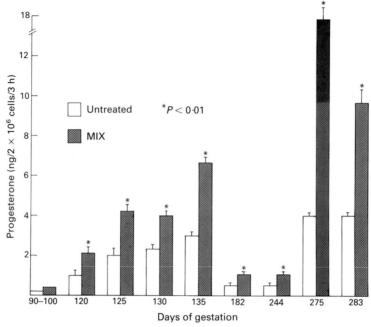

Fig. 4. Effect of MIX on progesterone biosynthesis by incubated dispersed maternal caruncle cells. Values are means ± s.e.m. for net synthesis of 5 samples from 1 animal at each stage of gestation. (From Shemesh *et al.*, 1984.)

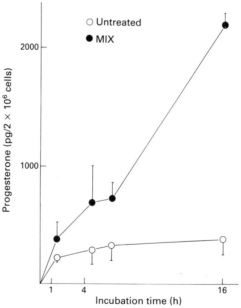

Fig. 5. Time course of basal and MIX-stimulated progesterone synthesis by dispersed bovine maternal caruncle cells. Each point is the mean ± s.e.m. of 5 replicate samples. These results are representative of 3 experiments. (From Shemesh *et al.*, 1984.)

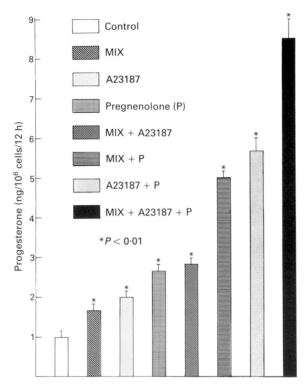

Fig. 6. Effect of pregnenolone with A23187 or MIX on progesterone biosynthesis by incubated dispersed maternal caruncle cells. Each point is the mean ± s.e.m. of 5 replicates. These results are representative of 8 experiments. (From Shemesh *et al.*, 1984.)

The time course of progesterone production by dispersed maternal caruncle cells in the presence of MIX was determined (Fig. 5). A concentration of 0·5 mM-MIX, which caused maximal stimulation, produced a 5-fold enhancement of progesterone secretion by the cells, with the steroid production being linear during the first 16 h of incubation.

We next examined the possibility that the stimulatory effect of MIX is related to translocation of extra- and intracellular calcium by studying the effect of calcium ionophore A23187 (Weissmann *et al.*, 1980) on progesterone production by the placental cells. As can be seen in Fig. 6, A23187 and MIX each produced 2-fold increases in progesterone production. Combination of A23187 and MIX resulted in an additive effect. The effect of A23187 was not potentiated by 8Br-cAMP or 8Br-cGMP. Since MIX also acts to block the receptors for adenosine, we studied the ability of adenosine to alter the stimulatory effect of MIX. However, the stimulatory effect of MIX was not altered by the addition of adenosine.

To determine whether the stimulatory effects of MIX and A23187 on progesterone synthesis are on the conversion of pregnenolone to progesterone, caruncle cells were incubated with exogenous pregnenolone, at a concentration of 100 ng per tube (found to maximally increase progesterone formation), in the presence of MIX and A23187. As can be seen from Fig. 6, pregnenolone, MIX and A23187 each caused almost 2-fold increase ($P < 0·01$) in progesterone production. An additive effect of progesterone synthesis was achieved by a combination of pregnenolone with either A23187 or MIX ($P < 0·01$), and a maximal stimulation (8-fold) ($P < 0·01$) was achieved by combination of all three additives.

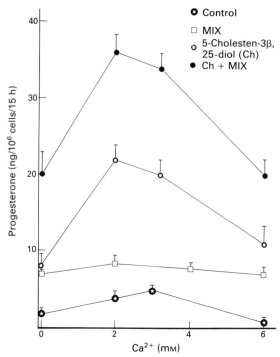

Fig. 7. Effect of medium calcium concentration on progestagen synthesis by dispersed fetal cotyledon cells incubated in the presence of 25-OH-C and MIX. Cells were incubated in the presence of various concentrations of calcium with or without MIX (0·5 mM). 25-OH-C (20 µg/ml) or 25-OH-C + MIX. Net progesterone synthesis was determined over a 15-h period. Values are the means ± s.e.m. from 4 separate experiments. (From Shemesh *et al.*, 1988.)

Effect of cholesterol on placental cell steroidogenesis

Addition of 20 µg 25-hydroxycholesterol (25-OH-C) to dispersed fetal cotyledons was optimal for augmenting progesterone formation, yielding a 5-fold stimulation of steroidogenesis ($P < 0.01$) (Shemesh *et al.*, 1988).

When the calcium concentration of the medium was increased from 0 to 3 mM, an increase in progesterone production in the presence of 25-OH-C (20 µg/ml) was observed (Fig. 7). At higher calcium concentrations, basal and 25-OH-C-stimulated progesterone production were reduced. MIX alone increased progesterone secretion and further increased the steroidogenic response to 25-OH-C at each calcium level in additive fashion ($P < 0.001$). MIX also increased pregnenolone secretion in the presence of a small amount of 25-OH-C (1 µg/ml). These effects were accentuated when an inhibitor of 3β-hydroxysteroid dehydrogenase, cyanoketone, was included in the incubation medium (Fig. 8).

Effect of TPA on placental cell steroidogenesis

Trifluoperazine (TPA: 10 ng/ml), a stimulator of protein kinase C, was tested for its ability to enhance progesterone production by fetal cotyledon cells. In most experiments the phorbol ester alone had no significant effect on progesterone secretion. However, the addition of MIX (Fig. 9) or A23187 (3 µM) (data not shown) in the presence of TPA resulted in an augmented secretion of progesterone ($P < 0.01$). The effect of TPA on progesterone was consistent during the 1st and 2nd hour of incubation in that it stimulated progesterone production in 5/7 tests. However, less consistent results were obtained in longer term incubations, i.e. after 6 h and 15 h, only 3/7 of tests were positive at either time.

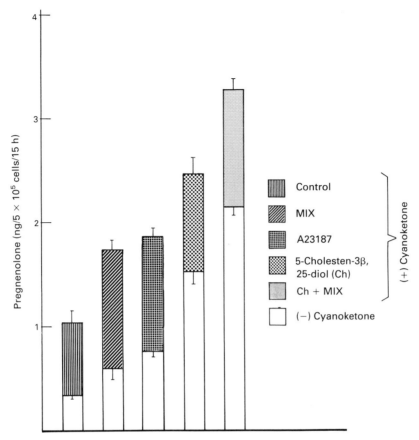

Fig. 8. Effects of MIX, A23187 and 25-OH-C on pregnenolone synthesis by dispersed fetal bovine cotyledon cells. Dispersed cells were incubated with or without MIX (0·5 mM). A23187 (3 μM) or 25-OH-C (1 μg/ml) in the absence or presence of cyanoketone (300 ng/ml) for 15 h. (From Shemesh *et al.*, 1988.)

In ongoing experiments (unpublished) we have found that TPA alone enhances the conversion of cholesterol to progestagens. Furthermore, a synergistic effect with both MIX and A23187 on pregnenolone production can be demonstrated.

Since conversion of cholesterol to progesterone requires the presence of cytochrome P-450$_{scc}$, we demonstrated the presence of P-450$_{scc}$ in fetal tissues by an immunoblotting assay. A high amount of P-450$_{scc}$ was present in the fetal cotyledon cells. Furthermore, a gold-staining reaction for P-450$_{scc}$ indicated that the cytochrome P-450$_{scc}$ was present in mononuclear but not in binuclear cells (E. Ben-David & M. Shemesh, unpublished observations).

Discussion

Our studies demonstrate that dispersed bovine fetal cotyledon and maternal caruncle cells produce progesterone *in vitro*. The ability of fetal cotyledons to secrete progesterone was evident in early as well as late pregnancy. However, appreciable progesterone synthesis by the maternal caruncles occurred only after 100–120 days of gestation.

The stimulatory effect of MIX on progesterone production by the bovine placental cells could be related to three basic actions of this compound: (i) the increased accumulation of cyclic

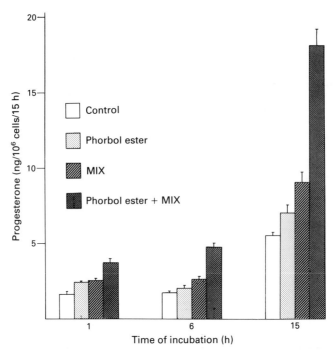

Fig. 9. Effects of TPA and TPA + MIX on progestagen synthesis by dispersed bovine fetal cotyledon cells. Dispersed cells were incubated for 1, 2, 6 or 15 h in the absence or presence of TPA (10 ng/ml) with or without MIX (0·5 mM). Values are the means ± s.e.m. from 5 replicate cultures from a representative experiment. (From Shemesh *et al.*, 1988.)

nucleotides as a result of inhibition of phosphodiesterase (Sutherland *et al.*, 1968); (ii) the translocation of intracellular calcium (Blinks *et al.*, 1972); and (iii) the blockade of receptors for adenosine (Sattin & Rall, 1970). Since neither LH, 8Br-cAMP, 8Br-cGMP, cholera toxin, or isoproterenol had effects on progesterone synthesis by themselves, nor did they potentiate the effects of LH, it is likely that MIX acted through translocation of intracellular calcium or through its effects on adenosine binding. The lack of responsiveness of the placental cells to adenosine supports the former concept. Furthermore, the calcium ionophore A23187 induced a 2-fold increase in progesterone production by the treated cells and had an additive effect when used in combination with MIX.

Calcium ions have been implicated in the steroid biosynthetic processes in testes, adrenal glands and ovaries (Veldhuis & Klase, 1982). However, in all of these tissues cAMP is thought to be the primary intracellular regulator of hormone production. The bovine placenta appears to differ from these other steroidogenic tissues and may resemble the zona glomerulosa of the adrenal cortex, a tissue in which calcium rather than cyclic nucleotides seems to be the primary intracellular signal increasing aldosterone synthesis (Fakunding & Catt, 1980).

The effects of 25-OH-C were dependent upon the extracellular calcium concentration, indicating a critical role for this ion in the steroidogenic process. MIX and the calcium ionophore, A23187, both increased pregnenolone and progesterone secretion by the dispersed fetal cotyledon cells. These findings suggest that both agents act at least in part by augmenting the conversion of cholesterol to pregnenolone. Our findings also support a role for protein kinase C, since TPA, which dramatically increases the affinity of the protein kinase C for Ca^{2+} (Ashendel, 1985), produced an enhancement of progesterone synthesis stimulated by calcium mobilization by MIX or A23187. The findings that phorbol esters stimulate bovine luteal (Hansel *et al.*, 1987) and adrenal

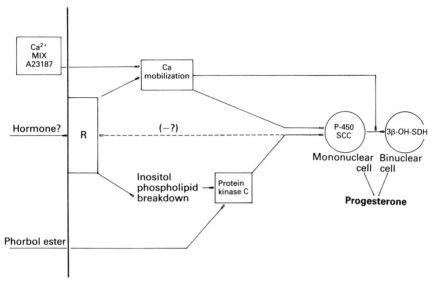

Fig. 10. Proposed model for regulation of steroidogenesis in the bovine placenta. Steroidogenesis is activated by Ca^{2+} mobilization and/or activation of protein kinase C. Both compounds act on the cytochrome $P-450_{scc}$ to increase pregnenolone production from cholesterol in the mononuclear cell. This pregnenolone may be metabolized to progesterone by mononuclear or binuclear cells. Activation of protein kinase C by phorbol ester may produce a transient inhibition in the response to phorbol ester. Ca^{2+} is the second messenger but the putative hormone pathway which stimulates it has yet to be determined. Solid lines indicate stimulation; broken lines indicate inhibition.

(Culty *et al.*, 1984) steroidogenesis, and that the cholesterol side-chain cleavage enzyme of the bovine adrenal cortex is phosphorylated by protein kinase C raise the possibility that activation of protein kinase C may increase flux through the steroidogenic pathway by phosphorylation of cytochrome $P-450_{scc}$ (Vilgrain *et al.*, 1985).

Since the synergistic effect of TPA in long-term incubations was not consistently observed, TPA activation of protein kinase C appears to be subject to a short feedback inhibition or down regulation. This is in contrast to MIX, A23187 or 25-OH-C which demonstrated a continuous augmentation of progesterone production throughout the long-term incubations.

The presence of $P-450_{scc}$ in the tissue suggests that the placentome is autonomous in that it can produce progestagens from cholesterol directly. Since Ullmann & Reimers (1989) found that binuclear cells can produce progesterone in culture, the observation that the $P-450_{scc}$ was present in the mononuclear but not the binuclear cells indicates that the pregnenolone produced by the mononuclear cells could be metabolized to progesterone by the binuclear cell through cell-to-cell communication.

We conclude that (1) both Ca^{2+} and protein kinase C enhance progesterone synthesis by the bovine placentome; (2) this activation is at the locus of the side-chain cleavage enzyme and 3β-hydroxysteroid dehydrogenase; (3) this process is cyclic nucleotide-independent; (4) Ca^{2+} is the second messenger of a putative hormone; and (5) cytochrome $P-450_{scc}$ is present in the mononuclear cells but not in the binuclear cells. Since both tissues can synthesize progesterone, this indicates that cell-to-cell communication is playing a role in progesterone synthesis in this tissue. These conclusions are summarized in Fig. 10.

This work was supported by USPHS Grant HD-16103 and BARD Grant 1-740-80.

References

Ainsworth, L. & Ryan, K.J. (1967) Steroid hormone transformations by endocrine organs from pregnant mammals. II. Formation and metabolism of progesterone by bovine and sheep placental preparations *in vitro. Endocrinology* **81,** 1349–1356.

Ashendel, C.L. (1985) The phorbol ester receptor: a phospholipid-regulated protein kinase. *Biochim. Biophys. Acta* **822,** 219–242.

Blinks, J.R., Olson, C.B., Jewell, B.R. & Braveny, P. (1972) Influence of caffeine and other methylxanthines on mechanical properties of isolated mammalian heart muscle. Evidence for a dual mechanism of action. *Circ. Res.* **30,** 367–392.

Culty, M., Vilgrain, I. & Chambaz, G.M. (1984) Steroidogenic properties of phorbol ester and Ca^{2+} ionophore in bovine adrenocortical cell. *Biochim. Biophys. Res. Commun.* **121,** 499–506.

Fakunding, J. & Catt, K.J. (1980) Dependence of aldosterone stimulation in adrenal glomerulosa cells on calcium uptake: Effects of lanthanum and Verapamil. *Endocrinology* **107,** 1345–1353.

Hansel, W., Alila, H. W., Dowd, J.P. & Yang, X. (1987) Control of steroidogenesis in small and large bovine luteal cells. *Aust. J. biol. Sci.* **40,** 331–347.

Hoffmann, B., Wagner, W.C., Hixon, J.E. & Bahr, J. (1979) Observations concerning the functional status of the corpus luteum and placenta around parturition in the cow. In *Physiology and Control of Parturition in Domestic Animals. Developments in Animal and Veterinary Sciences*, Vol. 5, pp. 253–266. Eds F. Ellendorff, M. Taverne & D. Smidt. Elsevier, Holland.

Sattin, A. & Rall, T.W. (1970) The effect of adenosine and adenine nucleotides on the adenosine 3′,5′-phosphate content of guinea pig cerebral cortex slices. *Molec. Pharmacol.* **6,** 13–23.

Shemesh, M., Hansel, W. & Strauss, J.F., III (1983) Bovine placentome contains factors which decrease progesterone secretion. *Biol. Reprod.* **29,** 856–862.

Shemesh, M., Hansel, W., & Strauss, J.F., III (1984) Calcium dependent, cyclic nucleotide-independent steroidogenesis in the bovine placenta. *Proc. natn. Acad. Sci. U.S.A.* **81,** 6403–6407.

Shemesh M., Hansel W., Strauss, J.F., III, Shore, L.S. & Izhar, M. (1988) Control of bovine placental progesterone synthesis: roles of cholesterol availability and calcium-activated systems. *J. Steroid Biochem.* **24,** 21–25.

Sutherland, E.W., Robison, G.A. & Butcher, R.W. (1968) Some aspects of the biological role of adenosine 3′5′-monophosphate (cyclic AMP) tissue particles. *Circulation* **37,** 1077–1091.

Ullmann, M.B. & Reimers, T.J. (1989) Progesterone production by bovine placental cells. *J. Reprod. Fert., Suppl.* **37,** 173–179.

Veldhuis, J.D. & Klase, P.A. (1982) Calcium ions modulate hormonally stimulated progesterone production in isolated ovarian cells. *Biochem. J.* **203,** 381–386.

Vilgrain I., DeFaye G. & Chambaz, E.M. (1985) Adrenocortical cytochrome P-450 responsible for cholesterol side chain cleavage (P-450$_{scc}$) is phosphorylated by the calcium-activated, phospholipid-sensitive protein kinase. *Biochem. biophys. Res. Commun.* **125,** 554–561.

Weissmann, G., Anderson, P., Serhan, C., Samuelsson, E. & Goodman, E. (1980) A general method, employing arsenazo III in liposomes, for study of calcium ionophores: results with A23187 and prostaglandins. *Proc. natn. Acad. Sci., U.S.A.* **77,** 1506–1510.

Wendorf, G.L., Lawyer, M.S. & First, N.L. (1983) Role of the adrenals in the maintenance of pregnancy in cows. *J. Reprod. Fert.* **68,** 281–287.

J. Reprod. Fert., Suppl. **37** (1989), 173–179

Progesterone production by binucleate trophoblastic cells of cows

Margaret B. Ullmann and T. J. Reimers

Diagnostic Laboratory, New York State College of Veterinary Medicine, Cornell University, Ithaca, NY 14853, U.S.A.

Summary. Incubation of 1×10^6 bovine binucleate trophoblastic cells (BTC) for 6 h with 0·20 and 0·30 μM-Ca^{2+} ionophore A23187 increased ($P < 0·01$) net progesterone production 49% and 111%, respectively, compared to BTC without A23187. Addition of 3 mM-8-bromo-cAMP with A23187 had no effect on the response. Trifluoperazine (40 μM), an inhibitor of calmodulin, and ethylene glycol-bis-(β-aminoethyl ether)-N,N,N',N'-tetraacetic acid (1·0 mM), a Ca^{2+} chelator, decreased ($P < 0·01$) progesterone production. Progesterone production by BTC incubated for 6 h with fetal bovine serum or lipoprotein-deficient serum (LPDS) did not differ. Addition of bovine serum low-density lipoprotein or high-density lipoprotein to LPDS did not affect progesterone production. Aminoglutethimide (100 μM) decreased ($P < 0·01$) progesterone production by BTC. These results indicate that progesterone production by bovine BTC is Ca^{2+}-dependent, cyclic nucleotide-independent, and not stimulated by bovine serum lipoproteins.

Keywords: binucleate trophoblastic cells; progesterone; calcium; cholesterol; lipoproteins; placenta

Introduction

Adenosine 3′,5′-cyclic monophosphate (cAMP) and calcium (Ca^{2+}) serve as intracellular messengers in many tissues (Rasmussen, 1970; Rasmussen *et al.*, 1984). Reimers *et al.* (1985) demonstrated that binucleate trophoblastic cells (BTC) of the bovine placenta produced progesterone *in vitro* and that progesterone production was not affected by cAMP. In contrast, Ca^{2+} was reported to be important in controlling progesterone production by heterogeneous preparations of bovine placental cells (Shemesh *et al.*, 1984). Our first study reported here was done to determine whether availability of Ca^{2+} modifies progesterone production by BTC.

Most of the cholesterol used by the human placenta for progesterone synthesis is derived from the maternal circulation (Bloch, 1945; Hellig *et al.*, 1970) and low-density lipoprotein (LDL) is a major source of cholesterol for progesterone synthesis by human trophoblastic cells in culture (Winkel *et al.*, 1980). Our second study was done to identify the source of cholesterol for progesterone synthesis by BTC. Progesterone production and de-novo sterol synthesis during incubation of bovine BTC with fetal bovine serum (FBS), bovine lipoprotein fractions, and inhibitors of de-novo sterol synthesis (aminoglutethimide and ML236B) were examined.

Materials and Methods

Role of Ca^{2+} in progesterone production. Enriched preparations of BTC (>90% purity) were obtained from trypsinized bovine cotyledons (Reimers *et al.*, 1985) and diluted to 1×10^6 BTC/ml Medium 199 (M199) containing 25 mM-Hepes (both from GIBCO, Grand Island, NY). Gestational ages of placentas based on fetal crown–rump length

(Evans & Sack, 1973) were 169, 175 and 178 days for studies with the calcium ionophore, A23187, and 156, 172, 178 and 184 days for experiments using trifluoperazine (TFP), an inhibitor of calmodulin; ethylene glycol-bis-(β-aminoethyl ether)-N,N,N,N'-tetraacetic acid (EGTA), a Ca^{2+} chelator; or 3,4,5-trimethoxybenzoic acid 8-(diethylamino)octyl ester (TMB-8), a Ca^{2+} antagonist (Sigma Chemical Co., St Louis, MO). Cells were incubated in 12 × 75-mm polystyrene culture tubes at 37°C in a humid atmosphere of 95% air and 5% CO_2.

BTC (1×10^6/tube) were incubated in triplicate for 6 h with 0, 0·05, 0·10, 0·20 or 0·30 μM-A23187 with or without addition of 3 mM-8-bromo-cAMP (Sigma). After incubation, cells and medium were stored at −20°C until progesterone was quantified using a solid-phase radioimmunoassay previously validated for measuring progesterone in medium containing Hepes, antibiotics, and disrupted BTC and their products (Reimers *et al.*, 1985). Net progesterone production was defined as the amount of progesterone measured in supernatants after samples were frozen, thawed and centrifuged and reflects intracellular progesterone plus progesterone secreted into the medium.

BTC (1×10^6/tube) also were incubated in triplicate with 40 μM-TFP, 1·0 mM-EGTA or 10 μM-TMB-8 for 6 h. In experiments with EGTA, BTC were first preincubated for 30 min in M199 containing 2 mM-EGTA. Cells were centrifuged at 150 *g* for 15 min at 4°C, supernatants were discarded, and cells were then incubated with 1 mM-EGTA. When incubations with TFP, TMB-8, and EGTA were complete, tubes were centrifuged and supernatants were decanted into culture tubes and frozen. M199 (500 μl) was added to the cells of each tube and frozen. Progesterone measured in the initial supernatants reflected progesterone secreted into the medium, whereas progesterone in supernatants after the lysed cells were thawed and centrifuged represented intracellular content.

Source of substrate for progesterone production. Low density lipoprotein (LDL; density = 1·019–1·063 g/ml) and high-density lipoprotein (HDL; density = 1·090–1·21 g/ml) were prepared from serum of normal Holstein heifers (Havel *et al.*, 1955). Lipoprotein-deficient serum (LPDS; density > 1·215 g/ml) was prepared by adjusting the density of FBS with KBr followed by ultracentrifugation (Rosenblum *et al.*, 1981). LPDS contained less than 2 μg cholesterol/ml, whereas FBS contained 350 μg cholesterol/ml.

BTC (1×10^6/tube) were incubated in triplicate for 6 h in Minimum Essential Medium (MEM; GIBCO) with 20% FBS, 20% LPDS, 20% LPDS + 100 μg LDL protein/ml, 20% LPDS + 100 μg HDL protein/ml, 20% FBS + 25 μM-ML-236B, or 20% LPDS + 25 μM-ML-236B (ML-236B is an inhibitor of 3-hydroxy-3 methylglutaryl coenzyme A reductase and was generously provided by Dr J. F. Strauss III, University of Pennsylvania). Incubations also included 25 μM-[U-^{14}C]acetate (New England Nuclear, Boston, MA) to quantify de-novo sterol synthesis. After incubation, half of the contents from each tube was used to assess de-novo sterol synthesis (Rosenblum *et al.*, 1981) while the other half was stored at −20°C until assayed for progesterone. Gestational ages of placentas were 142, 152, 156 and 165 days for this experiment.

BTC (139, 156 and 177 days of gestation) also were incubated in 20% FBS, 20% LPDS, 20% LPDS + 100 μM-aminoglutethimide (Sigma), 20% LPDS + 50 μg LDL protein/ml + 100 μM-aminoglutethimide, or 20% LPDS + 50 μg HDL protein/ml + 100 μM-aminoglutethimide. Incubations included 25 μM-[U-^{14}C]acetate. After incubation, half of the contents of tubes was assessed for de-novo sterol synthesis and the other half was centrifuged. Supernatants were stored at −20°C. MEM (500 μl) was added to the cells and frozen.

Statistical analyses. Triplicate values within treatments were averaged and results were analysed by two-way analysis of variance (Steel & Torrie, 1980). Differences among treatments were determined using Duncan's multiple range test. Results are expressed as means ± actual s.e.m. rather than error mean squares obtained from the analysis of variance.

Results

Net progesterone production increased ($P < 0.01$) 49% and 111% when 0·20 and 0·30 μM-A23187, respectively, was added to BTC incubations (Fig. 1). Addition of 8-Br-cAMP did not affect progesterone production stimulated by the Ca^{2+} ionophore alone. Progesterone secreted into medium and contained within cells both decreased ($P < 0.01$) when 40 μM-TFP was present (Fig. 2). The amount of progesterone secreted into medium, but not that contained within cells, decreased in the presence of EGTA. TMB-8 did not affect the amount of progesterone secreted into the medium nor that contained within BTC.

There was no difference ($P > 0.01$) in net progesterone production between cells incubated with FBS and LPDS (Fig. 3). Furthermore, addition of LDL or HDL to LPDS did not change net progesterone production, indicating that net progesterone production was unaffected by serum lipoproteins during a 6-h incubation.

Exposure of BTC to ML-236B in the presence of FBS did not affect net progesterone production compared to those treated with FBS alone (Fig. 3). However, cells incubated with ML-236B

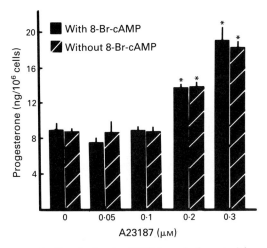

Fig. 1. Net progesterone production by bovine BTC ($n = 3$ placentas) in response to increasing doses of Ca^{2+} ionophore A23187 in the presence or absence of 8-bromo-cAMP (3 mM). *$P < 0.01$ compared to control (0 μM).

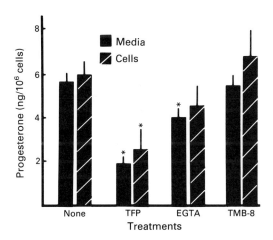

Fig. 2. Effects of TFP, EGTA and TMB-8 on progesterone synthesis and secretion by bovine BTC ($n = 4$ placentas). *$P < 0.01$ compared with no treatment.

and LPDS showed a slight but significant decrease ($P < 0.01$) in progesterone production compared to cells incubated with LPDS alone. Incorporation of [^{14}C]acetate into non-saponifiable lipids was less ($P < 0.05$) in cells incubated with FBS than in cells incubated with LPDS (Fig. 4). Therefore, the rate of de-novo sterol synthesis was greater by cells incubated without serum cholesterol. Incorporation of [^{14}C]acetate by cells incubated with FBS and ML-236B was not different ($P > 0.05$) from that by cells incubated with LPDS and ML-236B.

Progesterone concentrations in media and cells containing aminoglutethimide were different ($P < 0.01$) from concentrations in media and cells incubated without aminoglutethimide, but were not significantly different from one another (Fig. 5). Compared to cells incubated with LPDS alone, incorporation of [^{14}C]acetate by cells treated with LPDS + aminoglutethimide decreased 14%

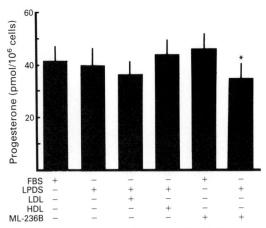

Fig. 3. Effect of bovine serum, lipoprotein fractions and ML-236B on progesterone production by bovine BTC ($n = 4$ placentas). *$P < 0.01$ compared with LPDS alone.

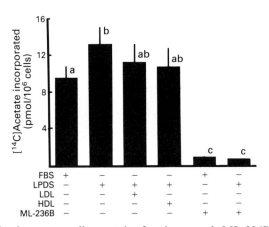

Fig. 4. Effect of bovine serum, lipoprotein fractions, and ML-236B on incorporation of [^{14}C]acetate into non-saponifiable lipids by bovine BTC ($n = 4$ placentas). Values with different superscripts differ significantly ($P < 0.05$ at least).

($P < 0.01$; Fig. 6). In addition aminoglutethimide decreased ($P < 0.01$) [^{14}C]acetate incorporation by 33% in the presence of LPDS + LDL or LPDS + HDL.

Discussion

Involvement of Ca^{2+} in steroidogenesis has been demonstrated in the adrenal gland (Fakunding & Catt, 1980, 1982; Foster *et al.*, 1981), testis (Van der Vusse *et al.*, 1976), ovary (Veldhuis & Klase, 1982a, b; Carnegie & Tsang, 1983; Tsang & Carnegie, 1983, 1984) and placenta (Shemesh *et al.*, 1984). Our results with a Ca^{2+} ionophore, an inhibitor of calmodulin, and a Ca^{2+} chelator support the conclusion of Shemesh *et al.* (1984) that progesterone synthesis by bovine placenta is dependent on Ca^{2+} but independent of cAMP. Ca^{2+} ionophore A23187 stimulated progesterone production in a dose-dependent manner indicating that Ca^{2+} is required at an intracellular locus for stimulation of progesterone production. Addition of 8-bromo-cAMP with the Ca^{2+} ionophore did not

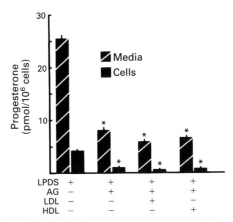

Fig. 5. Effect of aminoglutethimide (AG) on progesterone synthesis and secretion by bovine BTC (*n* = 3 placentas) in the absence or presence of serum lipoproteins. *$P < 0.01$ compared with respective control.

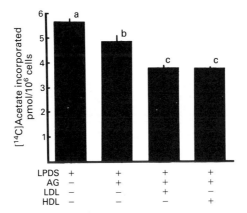

Fig. 6. Effect of aminoglutethimide (AG) on the incorporation of [^{14}C]acetate into non-saponifiable lipids by bovine BTC (*n* = 3 placentas) in the absence or presence of serum lipoproteins. Values with different superscripts differ significantly ($P < 0.01$).

increase further the response to the ionophore, suggesting that Ca^{2+} and cAMP do not interact to regulate steroidogenesis in BTC. In an earlier study, 10 mM-8-bromo-cAMP did not affect progesterone production by BTC (Reimers *et al.*, 1985).

When EGTA was added to the incubation medium, secretion of progesterone was impaired significantly and intracellular content of progesterone was also reduced, although not significantly. Therefore, the reduction in progesterone secretion caused by EGTA could not be accounted for simply by accumulation of progesterone within the cells. Hall *et al.* (1981a, b) and Tsang & Carnegie (1983) proposed a role for calmodulin in steroidogenesis. Synthesis and secretion of progesterone by BTC were inhibited by TFP, implicating involvement of high-affinity Ca^{2+}-binding protein(s).

Availability of Ca^{2+} in smooth and skeletal muscles was reduced by TMB-8 and it was proposed that TMB-8 produces its inhibitory effects on smooth and skeletal muscles by stabilizing

Ca^{2+} within cellular stores, thereby preventing release of Ca^{2+} normally associated with contractile stimuli (Chiou & Malagodi, 1975). Basal progesterone synthesis was reduced when dispersed heterogeneous caruncular cells from cows were incubated with 10 μM-TMB-8 (Shemesh *et al.*, 1984). In the current study, the same dose of TMB-8 had no effect on the quantity of progesterone secreted into medium or contained within BTC. Compensatory availability of extracellular Ca^{2+} from M199 may explain the lack of effect of TMB-8. However, this would not explain why TMB-8 had an effect on caruncular cells incubated in M199 (Shemesh *et al.*, 1984) unless there are two separate mechanisms by which the maternal and fetal portions of the placentome are controlled. There is also a possibility that TMB-8 acts at sites within mononucleate trophoblastic cells which then interact with BTC to inhibit progesterone synthesis.

Our results indicate that bovine serum lipoproteins do not affect progesterone production by BTC during a 6-h incubation. Progesterone production by cells incubated with FBS, LPDS + LDL, or LPDS + HDL was not different from production by cells incubated with LPDS alone. However, in the absence of serum cholesterol, cells showed compensatory changes in their rate of de-novo sterol synthesis. Addition of LDL and HDL to LPDS did not decrease incorporation of [^{14}C]acetate; however, these treatments contained less cholesterol than did FBS which may account for this lack of effect.

When BTC were treated with ML-236B, the rate of de-novo sterol synthesis was almost halted in the presence of both LPDS and FBS. The absence of an effect of ML-236B on progesterone production by cells incubated with FBS might be expected since [^{14}C]acetate incorporation was lower in cells treated with FBS than in those incubated with LPDS alone. This indicates that cells incubated with LPDS relied on de-novo sterol synthesis more than did cells incubated with FBS, resulting in a decrease in progesterone synthesis upon inhibition of de-novo sterol synthesis.

Treatment of BTC with aminoglutethimide decreased progesterone secretion and intracellular content indicating that cholesterol side-chain cleavage is essential for production of progesterone by BTC and that the cells do not contain a pool of pregnenolone for conversion to progesterone. Aminoglutethimide also decreased incorporation of [^{14}C]acetate into non-saponifiable lipids as opposed to cells treated with LPDS alone, and further decreased incorporation of [^{14}C]acetate into non-saponifiable lipids in the presence of lipoprotein-carried cholesterol. This indicates that, due to the reduction of cellular demands for cholesterol (i.e. treatment with aminoglutethimide), de-novo sterol synthesis was reduced. In the presence of exogenous cholesterol (i.e. LPDS + LDL or HDL aminoglutethimide), the rate of de-novo sterol synthesis was reduced further. Rosenblum *et al.*, (1981) reported similar results in cultured rat granulosa cells. However, it was noted that prolonged exposure to aminoglutethimide was required to produce this effect in rat granulosa cells, since cells treated for 6 h with the drug did not exhibit a decrease in [^{14}C]acetate incorporation into non-saponifiable lipids.

In summary, the present studies indicate that Ca^{2+} and calmodulin participate in regulation of progesterone synthesis by bovine BTC. Should a placentotrophic steroidogenic hormone exist, it most probably regulates steroidogenesis with Ca^{2+} as an intracellular messenger independently of the cyclic nucleotide messenger system. Lipoprotein-carried cholesterol had no effect on progesterone production by bovine BTC within 6 h of incubation. Binucleate trophoblastic cells exhibit compensatory changes in the rate of de-novo sterol synthesis in response to availability of exogenous sterol and the rate of sterol utilization.

This material is based upon work supported by the National Science Foundation under Grant No. PCM-8107187.

References

Bloch, K. (1945) The biological conversion of cholesterol to pregnanediol. *J. biol. Chem.* **157**, 661–666.

Carnegie, J.A. & Tsang, B.K. (1983) Follicle-stimulating hormone regulated granulosa cell steroidogenesis:

involvement of the calcium-calmodulin system. *Am. J. Obstet. Gynec.* **145**, 223–228.

Chiou, C.Y. & Malagodi, M.H. (1975) Studies on the mechanism of action of a new Ca^{2+} antagonist, 8-(*N*,*N*-diethylamino)octyl 3,4,5-trimethoxybenzoate hydrochloride in smooth and skeletal muscles. *Br. J. Pharmacol.* **53**, 279–285.

Evans, H.E. & Sack, W.O. (1973) Prenatal development of domestic and laboratory mammals: growth curves, external features and selected references. *Anat. Histol. Embryol.* **2**, 11–45.

Fakunding, J.L. & Catt, K.J. (1980) Dependence of aldosterone stimulation in adrenal glomerulosa cells on calcium uptake: effects of lanthanum and verapamil. *Endocrinology* **107**, 1345–1353.

Fakunding, J.L. & Catt, K.J. (1982) Calcium-dependent regulation of aldosterone production in isolated adrenal glomerulosa cells: effects of the ionophore A-23187. *Endocrinology* **110**, 2006–2010.

Foster, R., Lobo, M.V., Rasmussen, H. & Marusic, E.T. (1981) Calcium: its role in the mechanism of action of angiotensin II and potassium in aldosterone production. *Endocrinology* **109**, 2196–2201.

Hall, P.F., Osawa, S. & Mrotek, J. (1981a) The influence of calmodulin on steroid synthesis in Leydig cells from rat testis. *Endocrinology* **109**, 1677–1682.

Hall, P.F., Osawa, S. & Thomasson, C.L. (1981b) A role for calmodulin in the regulation of steroidogenesis. *J. Cell Biol.* **90**, 402–407.

Havel, R.J., Eder, H.A. & Bragdon, J.H. (1955) The distribution and chemical composition of ultracentrifugally separated lipoproteins in human serum. *J. clin. Invest.* **34**, 1345–1353.

Hellig, H., Gattereau, D., Lefebvre, Y. & Bolte, E. (1970) Steroid production from plasma cholesterol. I. Conversion of plasma cholesterol to placental progesterone in humans. *J. clin. Endocr. Metab.* **30**, 624–631.

Rasmussen, H. (1970) Cell communication, calcium ion, and cyclic adenosine monophosphate. *Science, N.Y.* **170**, 404–412.

Rasmusen, H., Kojima, I., Kojima, K., Zawalich, W. & Apfeldorf, W. (1984) Calcium as intracellular messenger: sensitivity modulation, C-kinase pathway, and sustained cellular response. *Adv. Cyclic Nucleotide Res.* **18**, 159–193.

Reimers, T.J., Ullmann, M.B. & Hansel, W. (1985) Progesterone and prostanoid production by bovine binucleate trophoblastic cells. *Biol. Reprod.* **33**, 1227–1236.

Rosenblum, M.F., Huttler, C.R. & Strauss, J.F., III (1981) Control of sterol metabolism in cultured rat granulosa cells. *Endocrinology* **109**, 1518–1527.

Shemesh, M., Hansel, W. & Strauss, J.F., III (1984) Calcium-dependent, cyclic nucleotide-independent steroidogenesis in the bovine placenta. *Proc. natn. Acad. Sci. U.S.A.* **81**, 6403–6407.

Steel, R.G.D. & Torrie, J.H. (1980) *Principles and Procedures of Statistics. A Biometrical Aproach.* McGraw-Hill, New York.

Tsang, B.K. & Carnegie, J.A. (1983) Calcium requirement in the gonadotropic regulation of rat granulosa cell progesterone production. *Endocrinology* **113**, 763–769.

Tsang, B.K. & Carnegie, J.A. (1984) Calcium-dependent regulation of progesterone production by isolated rat granulosa cells: effects of the calcium ionophore A23187, prostaglandin E_2, dl-isoproterenol and cholera toxin. *Biol. Reprod.* **30**, 787–794.

Van der Vusse, G.J., Kalkman, M.L., van Winsen, M.P.T. & van der Molen, H.J. (1976) Effect of Ca^{++}, ruthenium red and aging on pregnenolone production by mitochondrial fractions from normal and luteinizing hormone treated rat testes. *Biochim. Biophys. Acta* **428**, 420–431.

Veldhuis, J.D. & Klase, P.A. (1982a) Calcium ions modulate hormonally stimulated progesterone production in isolated ovarian cells. *Biochem. J.* **202**, 381–386.

Veldhuis, J.D. & Klase, P.A. (1982b) Mechanisms by which calcium ions regulate the steroidogenic actions of luteinizing hormone in isolated ovarian cells *in vitro*. *Endocrinology* **111**, 1–6.

Winkel, C.A., Macdonald, P.C. & Simpson, E.R. (1980) The role of maternal circulating low density lipoproteins in regulating placental cholesterol metabolism and progesterone biosynthesis. In *The Human Placenta: Proteins and Hormones*, pp. 401–406. Eds A. Klopper, A. Genazzani & P. G. Crosignani. Academic Press, New York.

J. Reprod. Fert., Suppl. **37** (1989), 181–187

Printed in Great Britain
© 1989 Journals of Reproduction & Fertility Ltd

Analysis of cell types in the corpus luteum of the sheep*

C. E. Farin†, H. R. Sawyer and G. D. Niswender

Animal Reproduction Laboratory, Department of Physiology, Colorado State University, Fort Collins, Colorado 80523, U.S.A.

Summary. The parenchyma of the corpus luteum of the ewe consists of two distinct steroidogenic cell types: small luteal cells and large luteal cells. Although both cell types produce and secrete progesterone, they differ with respect to morphological and bio-chemical characteristics. During the oestrous cycle, and continuing into pregnancy, the cellular composition of the corpus luteum is altered. As the oestrous cycle progresses small luteal cells increase in number but not size whereas large luteal cells remain con-stant in number but increase in size. Changes in the cellular composition of the ovine corpus luteum appear to be regulated by LH. Moreover, small luteal cells obtained from pregnant ewes were larger and lacked responsiveness to LH compared to those from non-pregnant animals. The basis of this loss of responsiveness is not clear as there is no concomitant loss of receptors for LH. The corpus luteum is a dynamic gland which changes in cellular composition and hormonal responsiveness with alterations in the reproductive state of the animal.

Keywords: corpus luteum; sheep; cell populations; oestrous cycle; pregnancy

Introduction

In domestic ruminants, the corpus luteum plays an integral role in the regulation of the oestrous cycle and is required for the establishment and maintenance of pregnancy. The corpus luteum of the ewe is composed of four major cell types which include large steroidogenic luteal cells, small steroidogenic luteal cells, fibroblasts and capillary endothelial cells. Large and small luteal cells have been identified as steroidogenic using morphological, biochemical and histochemical tech-niques (McClellan *et al.*, 1975; O'Shea *et al.*, 1979, 1980; Fitz *et al.*, 1982; Rodgers *et al.*, 1984).

Large luteal cells are the most conspicuous luteal cell type. In the ewe these cells are polyhedral in shape with a diameter of ~25–35 µm (McClellan *et al.*, 1975). They contain a spherical nucleus, a low nuclear to cytoplasmic ratio (Rodgers *et al.*, 1984), numerous mitochondria, isolated stacks of rough endoplasmic reticulum, smooth endoplasmic reticulum, lipid droplets, a prominent basal lamina, a highly folded plasma membrane with septate-like junctions and electron-dense mem-brane-bound secretory granules which are released via exocytosis (Gemmell *et al.*, 1974; McClellan *et al.*, 1975; O'Shea *et al.*, 1979; Sawyer *et al.*, 1979). In the ewe and cow, large luteal cells contain oxytocin and its associated neurophysin (Guldenaar *et al.*, 1984; Fields & Fields, 1986; Sawyer *et al.*, 1986) which is localized in the electron-dense secretory granules (Theodosis *et al.*, 1986). Concentrations of messenger RNA for oxytocin-neurophysin are greatest between ovulation and Day 6 of the oestrous cycle, peaking at approximately Day 3 (Fehr *et al.*, 1987). In contrast, the content and release of oxytocin from the corpus luteum increases from Day 5 to Day 8 and plateaus until Day 15 of the cycle (Wathes *et al.*, 1984; Ivell *et al.*, 1985). There is therefore a lag between transcription and release of oxytocin from large luteal cells.

*Reprint requests to Dr G. D. Niswender.

†Present address: Department of Animal Science, University of Missouri-Columbia, Columbia, Missouri 65211, U.S.A.

Small luteal cells of the sheep corpus luteum are stellate in shape, ranging in diameter from 12 to 22 μm (O'Shea *et al.*, 1979; Fitz *et al.*, 1982). Small luteal cells exhibit a high nuclear to cytoplasmic ratio and their cytoplasm contains abundant smooth endoplasmic reticulum, mito-chondria and lipid droplets (O'Shea *et al.*, 1979; Rodgers *et al.*, 1984). In the ewe, the population of small luteal cells appears more heterogeneous than large luteal cells since there are cells present which are intermediate in morphology between small luteal cells and fibroblasts (O'Shea *et al.*, 1979, 1980).

Although both small and large luteal cells produce progesterone, basal production by small luteal cells is 6- to 10-fold lower than that of large luteal cells. However, in response to luteinizing hormone (LH) secretion of progesterone by small luteal cells increases 6- to 20-fold (Fitz *et al.*, 1982; Harrison *et al.*, 1987). The differences in basal progesterone production between large and small luteal cells appear to be related to a difference in the volume density of mitochondria between the two cell types (Kenny *et al.*, 1988). Both small and large luteal cells contain an active adenylate cyclase system, but only in small luteal cells is this system responsive to LH and coupled to progesterone production (Hoyer & Niswender, 1985).

There are approximately 20 000–30 000 receptors for LH per small luteal cell (Fitz *et al.*, 1982; Harrison *et al.*, 1987). Receptors for LH have been found on large luteal cells obtained from corpora lutea of normally cycling ewes during the breeding season (Harrison *et al.*, 1987) and from corpora lutea of anoestrous ewes induced to superovulate in summer (Fitz *et al.*, 1982).

Cellular composition of the corpus luteum throughout the oestrous cycle

As the corpus luteum increases in mass during the early and mid-luteal phase of the oestrous cycle the volume occupied by steroidogenic luteal cells remains constant, averaging about 55% (Rodgers *et al.*, 1984; Farin *et al.*, 1986; Niswender *et al.*, 1986). Each cell type contributes to the increased luteal mass by substantially different mechanisms. Large luteal cells increase 3-fold in size between Days 4 and 12 of the oestrous cycle (Farin *et al.*, 1986), but they remain constant in number (Table 1), averaging ~ 10–12×10^6 cells per corpus luteum (Rodgers *et al.*, 1984; O'Shea *et al.*, 1986). In contrast, small luteal cells remain constant in size throughout the oestrous cycle but increase 4-fold in number between Days 4 and 8 of the cycle. Non-steroidogenic cell populations also expand in size as the corpus luteum develops. Capillary endothelial cells increase 5-fold in number between Days 4 and 12, whereas the number of luteal fibroblasts remains constant between Days 4 and 8 and increases between Days 8 and 16 of the oestrous cycle (Farin *et al.*, 1986).

The mechanism by which expansion of the small luteal cell population occurs is probably through cell division since mitotic figures have been reported in small luteal cells up to Day 6 of the oestrous cycle in both sheep and cattle (Donaldson & Hansel, 1965; McClellan *et al.*, 1975; O'Shea *et al.*, 1980). However, the majority of mitotic figures reported in the developing corpus luteum are in capillary endothelial cells and fibroblasts (Donaldson & Hansel, 1965; McClellan *et al.*, 1975; O'Shea *et al.*, 1980). It appears incongruous that the number of fibroblasts remains constant between Days 4 and 8 of the cycle (Farin *et al.*, 1986) when numerous mitotic figures within this cell type can commonly be found (Table 2). It is possible that luteal fibroblasts have a short life-span and so mitosis would be required to maintain the constant number of fibroblasts observed between Days 4 and 8. If this were the case, one would expect to find evidence of apoptosis (cell death) in luteal fibroblasts during this period. Evidence of cell death, however, is not apparent in sheep luteal tissue during the early to mid-luteal phase of the oestrous cycle (McClellan *et al.*, 1975; O'Shea *et al.*, 1986). Alternatively, it has been proposed that fibroblasts may differentiate into small luteal cells during the oestrous cycle (Niswender *et al.*, 1985a; Schwall *et al.*, 1986). In support of this hypothesis, a class of fibroblast-like cells which contain characteristics of both fibroblasts and small luteal cells is present in sheep corpora lutea (O'Shea *et al.*, 1979). Continued division of fibroblasts would then be required to replace fibroblasts which differentiate into small luteal cells. This would

Table 1. Changes in steroidogenic luteal cell populations throughout the oestrous cycle in sheep

	Day of cycle			
	4	8	12	16
No. of ewes	4	4	5	3
Luteal weight (mg)	158 ± 10^a	510 ± 31^b	649 ± 35^c	260 ± 2^d
Small steroidogenic cells				
Volume density (%)*	$14\cdot6 \pm 1\cdot1$	$17\cdot8 \pm 0\cdot8$	$22\cdot8 \pm 2\cdot4$	$18\cdot0 \pm 3\cdot5$
Number ($\times 10^{-6}$)	$10\cdot0 \pm 2\cdot7^a$	$39\cdot7 \pm 1\cdot4^b$	$46\cdot1 \pm 5\cdot8^b$	$29\cdot9 \pm 8\cdot6^{ab}$
Diameter (μm)	$16\cdot9 \pm 1\cdot0$	$16\cdot2 \pm 0\cdot3$	$18\cdot2 \pm 0\cdot8$	$14\cdot8 \pm 0\cdot8$
Large steroidogenic cells				
Volume density (%)*	$38\cdot5 \pm 3\cdot5$	$37\cdot9 \pm 1\cdot6$	$33\cdot1 \pm 3\cdot3$	$35\cdot6 \pm 0\cdot6$
Number ($\times 10^{-6}$)	$11\cdot8 \pm 1\cdot5$	$22\cdot0 \pm 5\cdot1$	$15\cdot2 \pm 3\cdot1$	$8\cdot6 \pm 1\cdot9$
Diameter (μm)	$21\cdot5 \pm 1\cdot0^a$	$26\cdot3 \pm 1\cdot7^b$	$30\cdot5 \pm 1\cdot2^b$	$28\cdot0 \pm 1\cdot1^b$

Values are mean $\pm$ s.e.

*Percentage of the corpus luteum occupied by this cell type.

[a–d]Values in rows followed by different superscripts are different ($P < 0\cdot05$).

explain the observed increase in the number of small luteal cells (Table 1) without a concomitant change in the number of fibroblasts between Days 4 and 8 of the oestrous cycle (Farin *et al.*, 1986). Based on morphological studies a similar hypothesis has been proposed for the establishment of steroidogenic cells in the testis (Jackson *et al.*, 1986). Morphological evidence therefore exists that steroidogenic cells can differentiate from a stem-cell population.

Table 2. Classification of mitotic figures by cell types found in corpora lutea on Day 4 of the oestrous cycle in sheep

Cell type	LM*	(%)	EM†	(%)
Large luteal	0	(0·0)	0	(0·0)
Small luteal	13	(5·8)	2	(10·5)
Fibroblast	134	(59·0)	12	(63·2)
Endothelial	53	(23·3)	3	(15·8)
Unidentified	27	(11·9)	2	(10·5)
Total	227	(100)	19	(100)

*Based on light microscopic examination of a total of 24 random 0·5 μm-thick sections taken from six 1–2 mm² blocks of luteal tissue from each of 4 ewes (magnification $\times 1500$).

†Based on electron microscopic examination of a total of 24 random thin sections cut from 6 tissue blocks from each of 4 ewes (magnification $\times 8000$).

Hormonal regulation of the cellular composition of the corpus luteum

Based on studies in hypophysectomized ewes, it is clear that the presence of pituitary tissue is necessary for the formation and maintenance of corpora lutea (Kaltenbach *et al.*, 1968). Attempts to define the hypophysial factors necessary for luteal development and maintenance have led to a controversy over whether prolactin is required in addition to LH (reviewed by Niswender *et al.*,

1986). Studies in which hypophysectomized and hypothalamic–pituitary stalk-disconnected ewes were treated with highly purified LH support the conclusion that LH is the only pituitary gonadotrophin required for normal luteal development and function (Niswender et al., 1986; Farin et al., 1987).

The possible mechanisms by which LH supports development and function of steroidogenic cell types includes stimulation of microtubule and microfilament formation and function, cholesterol transport, cholesterol esterase activity, and cholesterol side-chain cleavage activity (Niswender et al., 1980). In addition to the steroidogenic actions of LH, other cellular activities appear to be affected by this hormone. Treatment of cows and ewes with LH or human chorionic gonadotrophin (hCG) induces transformation of small luteal cells into large luteal cells (Table 3; Donaldson & Hansel, 1965; Alila & Hansel, 1984; Niswender et al., 1985a; Farin et al., 1988). In addition, treatment of ewes with highly purified LH promotes an increase in the size of non-steroidogenic luteal cells (Farin et al., 1988). This is particularly interesting since non-steroidogenic cells are not known to contain receptors for LH. Since steroidogenic luteal cells do have LH receptors, it is possible that these cells may produce substances which mediate the action of LH on non-steroidogenic luteal cells. In support of this proposal, corpora lutea produce fibroblast growth factor (FGF), a potent stimulator of angiogenesis (reviewed by Gospodarowicz et al., 1986). In addition, receptors for epidermal growth factor (EGF) are also present on luteal cells in the ewe (Niswender et al., 1985b). With the recent discoveries that corpora lutea of rats and women contain messenger RNA for inhibin (Davis et al., 1987), it appears likely that a variety of factors may be synthesized by luteal cells to regulate growth and development of this gland at the paracrine level.

Table 3. Effects of exogenous luteinizing hormone on the cellular composition of the corpus luteum of the sheep

	Treatment	
	Control	LH-treated
No. of ewes	4	5
Luteal weight (mg)	558 ± 85	548 ± 6.9
Small steroidogenic cells		
Volume density (%)*	20.0 ± 3.0^c	14.0 ± 1.0^d
No. per CL ($\times 10^{-6}$)	34.2 ± 11.1	22.5 ± 4.1
No. per gram CL ($\times 10^{-6}$)	58.2 ± 13.6	41.1 ± 7.5
Diameter (μm)	18.8 ± 1.2	19.3 ± 1.0
Large steroidogenic cells		
Volume density (%)*	26.0 ± 2.0^c	32.0 ± 2.0^d
No. per CL ($\times 10^{-6}$)	8.3 ± 1.6^c	17.4 ± 4.6^d
No. per gram CL ($\times 10^{-6}$)	14.6 ± 1.2^a	32.0 ± 8.6^b
Diameter (μm)	31.6 ± 1.2	28.1 ± 1.9

Values are mean $\pm$ s.e.
*Percentage of the corpus luteum occupied by this cell type.
[ab]Values in rows followed by different superscripts are different ($P < 0.05$).
[cd]Values in rows followed by different superscripts are different ($P < 0.10$).

Changes in luteal cell populations during pregnancy

As in the oestrous cycle, the corpus luteum of pregnancy contains morphologically distinct small and large steroidogenic luteal cells (O'Shea et al., 1979; Ursely & Leymarie, 1979; Fields et al., 1985).

Although there is considerable information regarding morphological and biochemical differences between small and large steroidogenic luteal cells during the oestrous cycle (reviewed by Niswender *et al.*, 1985a), comparative studies between small and large luteal cells obtained from non-pregnant and pregnant animals are limited (Harrison *et al.*, 1987; Weber *et al.*, 1987). Accordingly, we have examined the functional characteristics of corpora lutea obtained from normally cycling ewes (non-pregnant) on Day 10 after oestrus with corpora lutea obtained from pregnant ewes between Days 40 and 50 of pregnancy. As summarized in Table 4, even though no significant differences were observed in luteal weight or circulating concentrations of progesterone, the concentration of progesterone in corpora lutea obtained from pregnant ewes was higher than in corpora lutea obtained from non-pregnant ewes.

Table 4. Characteristics of corpora lutea obtained from non-pregnant and pregnant ewes

	Non-pregnant	Pregnant
No. of ewes	9	9
Wt of corpora lutea (mg)	$618·9 \pm 33·8$	$659·3 \pm 65·2$
Serum progesterone (ng/ml)	$1·7 \pm 0·2$	$2·3 \pm 0·5$
Luteal progesterone (ng/mg)	$20·6 \pm 1·1^a$	$33·8 \pm 3·5^b$
In-vitro production of progesterone (fg/cell/min)		
Small luteal cells		
Basal	$1·8 \pm 0·2^a$	$3·1 \pm 0·5^a$
LH-stimulated	$20·1 \pm 3·5^{cd}$	$7·0 \pm 0·7^a$
Large luteal cells		
Basal	$16·6 \pm 1·7^{bc}$	$13·3 \pm 1·9^{bc}$
LH-stimulated	$24·9 \pm 0·9^d$	$18·0 \pm 0·9^{bc}$

Values are mean $\pm$ s.e.
[a-d]Values within and between rows with different superscripts are different ($P < 0·01$).

Results from numerous studies have consistently shown that small and large luteal cells present in corpora lutea during the mid-luteal phase of the oestrous cycle differ with respect to basal and LH-stimulated secretion of progesterone. As summarized in Table 4, the secretion of progesterone by small luteal cells obtained from non-pregnant animals increased 9-fold in response to LH (100 ng/ml). Although the secretion of progesterone by small luteal cells obtained from pregnant animals increased 2-fold, this increase was not significant. When large luteal cells were challenged with LH there was a slight, but significant, increase in the secretion of progesterone by large luteal cells isolated from corpora lutea obtained from non-pregnant ewes. In contrast, large luteal cells from pregnant ewes failed to respond to LH. The reason for the dramatic loss of LH responsiveness by small luteal cells is not clear since the number of receptors for LH per small luteal cell was not different ($P > 0·10$) between non-pregnant and pregnant ewes. Harrison *et al.* (1987) also found similar numbers of receptors for LH when comparing small luteal cells obtained on different days of the oestrous cycle with Day 25 of pregnancy. However, in their study small luteal cells isolated from corpora lutea obtained on Day 25 of pregnancy showed a 6-fold increase in the secretion of progesterone in response to LH (100 ng/ml). Collectively, these data indicate that, between Day 25 and Days 40–50 of pregnancy, small luteal cells gradually lose their ability to respond to LH, even though there is no concomitant decrease in the number of receptors for LH. One explanation for this observation is that small luteal cells may enter a transitional phase in which they assume characteristics similar to large luteal cells. In fact, when the diameters of small and large luteal cells from non-pregnant and pregnant ewes were compared, both cell types were larger ($P < 0·01$) in pregnant animals (small luteal cells: $18\cdot8 \pm 0\cdot5$ and $23\cdot9 \pm 1\cdot1$ μm; large luteal cells: $27\cdot4 \pm 1\cdot8$ and $34\cdot3 \pm 1\cdot2$ μm). If small luteal cells do differentiate into large luteal cells, one would expect these cells to increase in size and become less responsive to LH. Thus, components of the steroidogenic pathway in small luteal cells such as adenylate cyclase may be modified during this time of transition.

Conclusions

The corpus luteum of the ewe is clearly a dynamic gland which changes in cellular composition and hormonal responsiveness with alterations in the reproductive state of the female. Although we are cognizant of alterations in the composition and function of luteal cell populations which occur during the oestrous cycle and between Days 25 and 50 of pregnancy, little is known of changes which occur during critical periods of conceptus–maternal signalling before Day 25 of gestation. Comparative studies of corpora lutea from pregnant and non-pregnant females during pre-implantation stages of gestation are needed to determine how changes in the composition and function of luteal cell populations may support the successful establishment and maintenance of pregnancy.

This research was supported by NIH Grant HD 11590.

References

Alila, H.W. & Hansel, W. (1984) Origin of different cell types in the bovine corpus luteum as characterized by specific monoclonal antibodies. *Biol. Reprod.* **31**, 1015–1025

Davis, S.R., Krozowski, Z., McLachlan, R.I. & Burger, H.G. (1987) Inhibin gene expression in the human corpus luteum. *J. Endocr.* **115**, R21-R23.

Donaldson, L & Hansel, W. (1965) Histological study of bovine corpora lutea. *J. Dairy Sci.* **48**, 905–909.

Farin, C.E., Moeller, C.L., Sawyer, H.R., Gamboni, F. & Niswender, G.D. (1986) Morphometric analysis of cell types in the ovine corpus luteum throughout the estrous cycle. *Biol. Reprod.* **35**, 1299–1308.

Farin, C.E., Nett, T.M. & Niswender, G.D. (1987) Role of LH in the cellular development of corpora lutea in hypophysectomized ewes. *Biol. Reprod.* **36** (Suppl. 1), 169, Abstr.

Farin, C.E., Moeller, C.L., Mayan, H., Gamboni, F., Sawyer, H.R. & Niswender, G.D. (1988) Effect of LH and hCG on cell populations in the ovine corpus luteum. *Biol. Reprod.* **38**, 413–421.

Fehr, S., Ivell, R., Koll, R., Schams, D., Fields, M. & Richter, D. (1987) Expression of the oxytocin gene in the large cells of the bovine corpus luteum. *FEBS Letters* **210**, 45–50

Fields, M.J. & Fields, P.A. (1986) Luteal neurophysin in the nonpregnant cow and ewe: immunocytochemical localization in membrane-bounded secretory granules of the large luteal cell. *Endocrinology* **118**, 1723–1725.

Fields, M.J., Dubois, W. & Fields, P.A. (1985) Dynamic features of luteal secretory granules: ultrastructural changes during the course of pregnancy in the cow. *Endocrinology* **117**, 1675–1682.

Fitz, T.A., Mayan, M.H., Sawyer, H.R. & Niswender, G.D. (1982) Characterization of two steroidogenic cell types in the ovine corpus luteum. *Biol. Reprod.* **27**, 703–711.

Gemmell, R.T., Stacy, B.D. & Thorburn, G.D. (1974) Ultrastructural study of secretory granules in the corpus luteum of the sheep during the estrous cycle. *Biol. Reprod.* **11**, 447–462.

Gospodarowicz, D., Neufeld, G. & Schweigerer, L. (1986). Molecular and biological characterization of fibroblast growth factor, an angiogenic factor which also controls the proliferation and differentiation of mesoderm and neuroectoderm derived cells. *Cell Differentiation* **19**, 1–17.

Guldenaar, S.E.F., Wathes, D.C. & Pickering, B.T. (1984) Immunocytochemical evidence for the presence of oxytocin and neurophysin in the large cells of the bovine corpus luteum. *Cell Tissue Res.* **237**, 349–352.

Harrison, L.M., Kenny, N. & Niswender, G.D. (1987) Progesterone production, LH receptors, and oxytocin secretion by ovine luteal cell types on Days 6, 10, and 15 of the oestrous cycle and Day 25 of pregnancy. *J. Reprod. Fert.* **79**, 539–548.

Hoyer, P.B. & Niswender, G.D. (1985) The regulation of steroidogenesis is different in the two types of ovine luteal cells. *Can. J. Physiol. Pharmacol.* **63**, 240–248.

Ivell, R., Brackett, K.H., Fields, M.J. & Richter, D. (1985) Ovulation triggers oxytocin gene expression in the bovine ovary. *FEBS Letters* **190**, 263–267.

Jackson, A.E., O'Leary, P.C., Ayers, M.M. & de Krester, D.M. (1986) The effects of ethylene dimethane sulphonate (EDS) on rat Leydig cells: evidence to support a connective tissue origin of Leydig cells. *Biol. Reprod.* **35**, 425–437.

Kaltenbach, C.C., Graber, J.W., Niswender, G.D. & Nalbandov, A.V. (1968) Effect of hypophysectomy on the formation and maintenance of corpora lutea in the ewe. *Endocrinology* 82, 735–759.

Kenny, N., Farin, C.E. & Niswender, G.D. (1988) Morphometric quantification of mitochondria in the two steroidogenic ovine luteal cell types. *Biol. Reprod.* (in press).

McClellan, M.C., Diekman, M.A., Abel, J.H., Jr & Niswender, G.D. (1975) Luteinizing hormone, progesterone and the morphological development of normal and superovulated corpora lutea in sheep. *Cell Tiss. Res.* **164**, 291–307.

Niswender, G.D., Sawyer, H.R., Chen, T.T. & Endres, D.B. (1980) Action of luteinizing hormone at the luteal cell level. In: *Advances in Sex Hormone Research*, Vol. 4, pp. 153–185. Eds J. A. Thomas & R. L. Singhi. Urban & Schwarzenberg Inc, Baltimore.

Niswender, G.D., Schwall, R.H., Fitz, T.A., Farin, C.E. & Sawyer, H.R. (1985a) Regulation of luteal function in domestic ruminants: new concepts. *Rec. Prog. Horm. Res.* **41**, 101–151.

Niswender, G.D., Roess, D.A., Sawyer, H.R., Silvia, W.J. & Barisas, B.G. (1985b) Differences in the lateral mobility of receptors for luteinizing hormone (LH) in the luteal cell plasma membrane when occupied by ovine LH versus human chorionic gonadotropin. *Endocrinology* **116**, 164–169.

Niswender, G.D., Farin, C.E., Gamboni, F., Sawyer, H.R. & Nett, T.M. (1986) Role of luteinizing hormone in regulating luteal function in ruminants. *J. Anim. Sci.* **62** (Suppl. 2), 1–14.

O'Shea, J.D., Cran, D.G. & Hay, M.F. (1979) The small luteal cell of the sheep. *J. Anat.* **128**, 239–251.

O'Shea, J.D., Cran, D.G. & Hay, M.F. (1980) Fate of the theca interna following ovulation in the ewe. *Cell Tissue Res.* **210**, 305–319.

O'Shea, J.D., Rodgers, R.J. & Wright, P.J. (1986) Cellular composition of the sheep corpus luteum in the mid- and late luteal phases of the oestrous cycle. *J. Reprod. Fert.* **76**, 685–691.

Rodgers, R.J., O'Shea, J.D. & Bruce, N.W. (1984) Morphometric analysis of the cellular composition of the ovine corpus luteum. *J. Anat.* **138**, 757–769.

Sawyer, H.R., Abel, J.H., Jr, McClellan, M.C., Schmitz, M. & Niswender, G.D. (1979) Secretory granules and progesterone secretion by ovine corpora lutea *in vitro*. *Endocrinology* **104**, 476–486.

Sawyer, H.R., Moeller, C.L. & Kozlowski, G.P. (1986) Immunocytochemical localization of neurophysin and oxytocin in ovine corpora lutea. *Biol. Reprod.* **34**, 543–548.

Schwall, R.H., Sawyer, H.R. & Niswender, G.D. (1986) Differential regulation by LH and prostaglandins of steroidogenesis in small and large luteal cells of the ewe. *J. Reprod. Fert.* **76**, 821–829.

Theodosis, D.T., Wooding, F.B.P., Sheldrick, E.L. & Flint, A.P.F. (1986) Ultrastructural localisation of oxytocin and neurophysin in the ovine corpus luteum. *Cell Tissue Res.* **243**, 129–135.

Ursely, J. & Leymarie, P. (1979) Varying response to luteinizing hormone of two luteal cell types isolated from bovine corpus luteum. *Endocrinology* **83**, 303–310.

Wathes, D.C., Swann, R.W. & Pickering, B.T. (1984) Variations in oxytocin, vasopressin and neurophysin concentrations in the bovine ovary during the oestrous cycle and pregnancy. *J. Reprod. Fert.* **71**, 551–557.

Weber, D.M., Fields, P.A., Romrell, L.J., Tumwasorn, S., Ball, B.A., Drost, M. & Fields, M.J. (1987) Functional differences between small and large luteal cells of the late-pregnant vs. nonpregnant cow. *Biol. Reprod.* **37**, 685–697.

PEPTIDES

Chairmen

J. F. Strauss III
Y. Koch

J. Reprod. Fert., Suppl. **37** (1989), 189–194

Printed in Great Britain
© 1989 Journals of Reproduction & Fertility Ltd

Characteristics of an antigonadotrophic GnRH-like protein in the ovaries of diverse mammals

H. R. Behrman, R. F. Aten, J. J. Ireland* and R. A. Milvae†‡

Reproductive Biology Section, Departments of Obstetrics/Gynecology and †Pharmacology, Yale University School of Medicine, New Haven, CT 06510, U.S.A.

Summary. A GnRH-like protein, detected with a receptor assay for GnRH in rat ovarian membranes, is present in ovarian extracts of the rat, human, cow and ewe at levels much higher than immunoreactive GnRH. This protein has been partly purified and characterized from bovine ovaries. Highest levels of this protein are found in granulosa cells, but substantial activity is present in luteal, thecal and stromal tissue. No detectable GnRH-like activity is found in follicular fluid, or in ovarian venous or jugular plasma. The GnRH-like protein is structurally and immunologically different from GnRH, but it competitively and reversibly inhibits binding of GnRH to high-affinity sites in rat ovarian membranes. The GnRH-like protein markedly inhibits the action of both LH and FSH in cultures of rat luteal and granulosa cells, respectively, to a much greater extent than GnRH. Co-elution of receptor-binding activity and anti-gonadotrophic activity occurs within and between several chromatography procedures, but the protein has not been completely purified. The presence of this antigonadotrophic GnRH-like protein in the ovaries of diverse species raises the possibility that it may represent a novel paracrine regulator of ovarian function.

Keywords: GnRH; regulatory factors; ovary; cyclic AMP; fractionation peptides; progesterone

Introduction

Gonadotrophin-releasing hormone (GnRH) has direct antigonadotrophic actions in rat granulosa and luteal cells since it inhibits the functional response of these cells to FSH and LH, respectively (Hsueh & Jones, 1981). These antigonadotrophic responses of GnRH are probably mediated by high-affinity receptors for GnRH (Hsueh & Jones, 1981). It has been suggested that GnRH is produced in the ovary and exerts its effects locally (Williams & Behrman, 1983; Birnbaumer *et al.*, 1985), because GnRH of hypothalamic origin is too diluted by systemic blood (Nett *et al.*, 1974). However, GnRH has little effect on ovarian cells of other species (Clayton & Catt, 1981; Hsueh & Jones, 1981). Moreover, ovaries of primates (Asch *et al.*, 1981; Clayton & Huhtaniemi, 1982; Bramley *et al.*, 1985) or domestic species (Brown & Reeves, 1983) do not elicit high-affinity binding of GnRH.

Our interest in the physiology of ovarian GnRH was sparked by the finding that GnRH acutely inhibits rat luteal responses to LH by a mechanism similar to, but independently of, prostaglandin F-2α (Behrman *et al.*, 1980). Our initial objectives were to determine whether GnRH is present in the ovaries of rats, humans and domestic species, and whether GnRH serves a physiological role in these tissues. These investigations led to the discovery of GnRH-like proteins, but little detectable GnRH, in ovarian tissue of all the above species. These proteins are referred to as GnRH-like

---

*Present address: Department of Animal Science, Michigan State University, East Lansing, MI 48824, U.S.A.
‡Present address: Department of Animal Science, University of Connecticut, Storrs, CT 06268, U.S.A.

because they inhibit the high-affinity binding of GnRH to rat ovarian receptors, but they are not detected by specific GnRH antisera. The characteristics of the major form of this material are summarized in this paper.

Materials and Methods

Tissue sources. Ovaries from non-pregnant cattle were placed on ice within 30 min after removal. Corpora lutea, follicular fluid and granulosa cells were obtained from some of the ovaries. Corpora lutea from sheep were obtained by dissection after surgery, and immediately frozen. Human ovaries were obtained, under an appproved protocol of the Yale University School of Medicine, from cycling, premenopausal women ranging in age from 35 to 43 years. The reason for surgery was not related to abnormal ovarian function. The ovaries were placed on ice shortly after surgical removal and either extracted immediately or retained at $-70°C$ until extracted. Rat ovaries, hypothalami and plasma were obtained from sychronized immature female rats, as previously described (Aten *et al.*, 1986).

Extraction procedure and reversed phase h.p.l.c. Tissues and fluids were extracted according to Aten *et al.* (1986). In brief, samples were homogenized in a solution containing HCl, formic acid, trifluoroacetic acid (TFA), and NaCl. The 10 000 g supernatant fractions were passed through Waters C_{18} Sep-Paks, the Sep-Paks were washed with 0·1% TFA, and the adsorbed proteins eluted with acetonitrile. The eluted material was lyophilized and stored at $-20°C$. The lyophilized extracts were fractionated by h.p.l.c. on Waters uBondaPak C_{18} columns using gradient elution with acetonitrile, as previously described (Aten *et al.*, 1986, 1987a).

Radioreceptor assay for GnRH-like activity. Before and after h.p.l.c., the lyophilized extracts were evaluated for GnRH-like activity using a receptor assay for GnRH in rat ovarian membranes. This assay is based on competition by ovarian extracts for specific binding of radiolabelled D-Ala^6, Des-Gly^{10}-GnRH ethylamide (GnRH-A), a GnRH agonist resistant to proteolytic degradation, by rat ovarian membranes (Aten *et al.*, 1986). Before assay, the rat ovarian membranes were treated with $MgCl_2$ to remove endogenous ligands. The ED_{50} for GnRH-A is 100 fmol ($K_d = 1·3 \times 10^{-10}$ M) and 1500 fmol for GnRH ($K_d = 2·8 \times 10^{-9}$ M).

GnRH radioimmunoassay. GnRH was assayed by RIA (Aten *et al.*, 1986). The GnRH-specific RIA is 40-fold more sensitive than the receptor assay for analysis of GnRH (RIA ED_{50} of 40 fmol vs receptor assay ED_{50} of 1500 fmol).

Iodination of GnRH and GnRH-A. GnRH and GnRH-A were iodinated by the chloramine-T method and purified by h.p.l.c. (Aten *et al.*, 1986). The specific radioactivities of ^{125}I-labelled GnRH and ^{125}I-labelled GnRH-A were determined by displacement in the GnRH RIA.

Protease-treatment of GnRH-like proteins. Ovarian extracts were reconstituted in 10 mM-Tris–HCl, pH 7·4, and incubated with 0·5 units of protease–cellulose, as described earlier (Aten *et al.*, 1986). After incubation, the protease–cellulose was removed by centrifugation and the supernatant fractions were assayed for GnRH-like activity by receptor assay.

Cell assays. Luteal cells were isolated from the ovaries of gonadotrophin-treated immature female rats by enzymic dispersion and enriched by density gradient centrifugation, as described previously (Hall & Behrman, 1981). Samples were dissolved in culture medium, centrifuged, and the supernatant fractions added to the luteal cell cultures. After an overnight incubation, the treatment medium was removed, fresh medium was added which contained 100 ng LH/ml, the cells were further cultured for 90 min, and the accumulation of cAMP was determined by RIA.

Granulosa cells were isolated from the ovaries of immature female rats by methods previously described (Ohkawa *et al.*, 1985). Granulosa cells were obtained by puncturing ovaries, gently pressing the ovaries against a nylon mesh, and enriching the released cells by density gradient centrifugation. Lyophilized extract was dissolved in culture medium, centrifuged, and the supernatant fractions added to the granulosa cell cultures. Ovine FSH was added to the cultures at a final concentration of 0·5 m.i.u./ml, and at 24 h the production of cAMP and progesterone were determined by RIA.

Results and Discussion

Little immunoreactive GnRH is present in ovarian extracts

Concentration of ovarian extracts showed the presence of low levels of immunoreactive GnRH in ovarian extracts of rat, human and bovine ovaries (Aten *et al.*, 1986, 1987a, b). Estimated levels of immunoreactive GnRH, based on the assumption that the water content of tissue is 90%, are similar for ovarian tissue of all species with values at about 0·1–0·3 nM. This is only a fraction of the dissociation constant (2·8 nM) of GnRH for binding to rat ovarian receptors (Aten *et al.*, 1986), and much below that necessary to inhibit LH responses in rat luteal cells (Behrman *et al.*, 1980; Aten *et al.*, 1986). Therefore it seems that GnRH may not be present in sufficient amounts to play a physiological role in the rat ovary, unless GnRH is compartmentalized within the ovary. A functional role of GnRH in ovaries of other species, such as the human and cow, is even more distant because these species do not contain high-affinity binding sites for GnRH.

Presence of receptor binding activity in ovarian extracts

Substantial GnRH-like activity is evident in extracts of rat, human, ovine and bovine ovarian tissue when assayed with the rat ovarian GnRH receptor assay (Aten *et al.*, 1986, 1987a, b). Based on equivalents of GnRH, there is several orders of magnitude more receptor binding activity than immunoreactive GnRH. Inhibition of binding by the ovarian GnRH-like activity is reversible and competitive (Aten & Behrman, 1988), and the GnRH-like activity does not degrade either the radiolabelled ligand or GnRH binding sites (Aten *et al.*, 1986, 1987a, b). In addition, this GnRH activity does not inhibit the specific binding of PGF-2α (Aten *et al.* 1987a, b), or of epidermal growth factor (unpublished observations). It therefore appears that the ovarian GnRH-like activity inhibits binding of GnRH by competing for similar sites on rat ovarian membranes.

Presence of several fractions with GnRH-like activity

After fractionation of ovarian extracts by h.p.l.c., GnRH-like activity is seen in several fractions with different retention times (Aten *et al.*, 1986, 1987a, b; Ireland *et al.*, 1988a). One of these fractions is by far the most abundant; it has the greatest retention time, and it is this fraction that we have characterized.

Protease sensitivity

Incubation of rat, human, ovine and bovine ovarian extracts with protease coupled to cellulose results in a complete loss of receptor-binding activity (Aten *et al.*, 1986, 1987a, b). Therefore, we concluded that the GnRH-like activity is a protein.

The ovarian GnRH-like protein is not GnRH

The conclusion that the ovarian GnRH-like protein is not GnRH is based on several findings. First, the ovarian GnRH-like protein is not recognized by several antisera that are specific for GnRH. Second, addition of authentic GnRH to ovarian extracts and fractionation by h.p.l.c. result in a clear separation between the GnRH-like protein and GnRH (Aten *et al.*, 1986). In addition, extraction of rat hypothalamic tissue and fractionation by h.p.l.c. show one fraction with an identical retention time to authentic GnRH (Aten *et al.*, 1987b). Another fraction shows much more GnRH-like activity; this fraction may be prepro-GnRH (Adelman *et al.*, 1986), but this fraction is not immunoreactive. However, both hypothalamic fractions have retention times different from those of the ovarian GnRH-like protein. Finally, the ovarian GnRH-like protein is much larger than GnRH (Aten *et al.*, 1986; Aten & Behrman, 1988). We do not know whether the ovarian GnRH-like protein contains the GnRH sequence which may be released upon hydrolysis. We suspect it does not because the antigonadotrophic activity of the GnRH-like protein is different from GnRH in that it is much greater than that of GnRH or its synthetic agonists (see below).

Tissue distribution

In crude extracts of rat ovarian tissue, GnRH-like activity is found in many tissues, including the ovary, kidney, liver and hypothalamus, but no activity is detectable in plasma (Aten *et al.*, 1986). After h.p.l.c. fractionation of bovine ovarian extracts, activity is found in three separate fractions, arbitrarily called A, B and C (Ireland *et al.*, 1988a). Fraction C, the most abundant form with the greatest retention time on h.p.l.c., and the fraction on which we have focussed, is 10-fold greater in granulosa cells than in any other tissue we examined. Bovine lung has detectable, but low, levels of activity associated with Fraction C. Fraction C is readily measured in luteal, thecal and stromal tissue but little detectable activity is seen in liver or kidney (Ireland *et al.*, 1988a). About the same amount of Fraction B is present in luteal, thecal, lung, liver and kidney, and variable, but low, levels of Fraction A are found in many tissues (Ireland *et al.*, 1988a). No GnRH-like activity associated with Fractions A, B or C is seen in heart, follicular fluid, or jugular and ovarian venous plasma (Ireland *et al.*, 1988a). Within the ovary, the highest amounts of GnRH-like activity are seen in granulosa cells whether normalized to DNA content or tissue weight.

It therefore appears that GnRH-like activity may be present in many different tissues and in different forms. However, one form of activity is selectively enriched in the ovary, particularly in granulosa cells. We know little about the nature of the GnRH-like activity in extraovarian tissues other than it inhibits binding of GnRH to rat ovarian membranes.

Partial purification and size

In recent studies, The bovine ovarian GnRH-like protein has been more highly purified with the use of C18 reverse-phase h.p.l.c., cation exchange chromatography, gel permeation and reverse-phase h.p.l.c. on C4 (Aten & Behrman, 1988). These procedures produce substantial, but not complete, purification of a protein which has an apparent molecular weight of about $17\,000 \pm 4000$ (Aten & Behrman, 1988). The GnRH-like protein does not appear to be disulphide cross-linked, since incubation under reducing conditions does not result in reduced receptor binding activity (Aten *et al.*, 1987a).

Antigonadotrophic activity

Partly purified bovine ovarian GnRH-like protein inhibits the action of LH in isolated rat luteal cells (Aten *et al.*, 1987a), similar to that of GnRH (Behrman *et al.*, 1980). However, unlike that of GnRH, the magnitude of inhibition by the GnRH-like protein is much greater than that of GnRH (Aten *et al.*, 1987a; Aten & Behrman, 1988). The bovine ovarian GnRH-like protein also inhibits rat granulosa cell cyclic AMP accumulation and progesterone biosynthesis in response to FSH (Aten & Behrman, 1988). Like that seen in rat luteal cells, the magnitude of inhibition by the GnRH-like protein is much greater than that produced by GnRH or synthetic agonists, and the antigonadotrophic activity is reversible upon washing the cells (Aten & Behrman, 1988).

It is possible that GnRH receptor-binding and antigonadotrophic activity may be due to different proteins in a partly purified preparation. To evaluate this possibility indirectly we compared the elution characteristics of receptor-binding activity with biological activity. Both activities co-elute on reverse-phase, ion-exchange and gel-permeation chromatography, and parallel elution of both activities during each procedure is seen (Aten & Behrman, 1988). We therefore suspect that both activities may reside in the same protein, but this has yet to be firmly established.

The ovarian GnRH-like protein of cattle also inhibits LH-stimulated progesterone production in isolated bovine luteal cells (Ireland *et al.*, 1988b). This is an interesting finding since GnRH does not elicit antigonadotrophic activity in these cells (Ireland *et al.*, 1988b), and no high-affinity binding sites for GnRH are seen in the bovine ovary (Brown & Reeves, 1983).

Uniqueness of the ovarian GnRH-like protein

The ovarian GnRH-like protein appears to be unique from other regulatory proteins that influence ovarian function, based on indirect evidence. First, the rat ovarian GnRH receptor-biding assay is not influenced by a wide concentration range of a number of proteins which include ACTH, angiotensin II, vasotocin, vasopressin, oxytocin, MSH, epidermal growth factor (EGF), bombesin, met-enkephalin, β-endorphin, neurotensin, somatostatin, TGF-β and fibroblastic growth factor (FGF) (Aten *et al.*, 1986; the results with EGF, TGF-β and FGF are unpublished). Second, other members of the TGF-β family of proteins, which include inhibin, Müllerian inhibitory substance, activin and FSH-releasing protein, have sizes different from that of the ovarian GnRH-like protein, and are disulphide cross-linked proteins (Sporn *et al.*, 1986; Vale *et al.*, 1986; Ling *et al.*, 1986). However, only purification and sequence analysis will determine whether the ovarian GnRH-like protein is unique.

Conclusions and future directions

It may be significant that the GnRH-like protein is found in the ovaries of many species and elicits antigonadotrophic activity in ovarian cells that do not respond to GnRH or contain high-affinity binding sites that recognize GnRH. The GnRH-like protein, not GnRH, may be the physiological ligand that binds to specific receptors in the ovaries of all these species. Perhaps only in the rat do these receptors also recognize GnRH. The complete characterization of purified GnRH-like protein and the evaluation of the presence of specific receptors in ovarian cells will dictate conclusions on the functional importance of this protein in the ovary.

This work was supported by NIH-HD-15403. We thank Ms Donna Wolin and Sharon Usip for expert technical assistance; Tradescript for assistance in editing; and Ms Cindy Davis for preparation of the manuscript.

References

Adelman, J.P., Mason, A.J., Hayflick, J.S. & Seeburg, P.H. (1986) Isolation of the gene and hypothalamic cDNA for the common precursor of gonadotropin-releasing hormone and prolactin release-inhibiting factor in human and rat. *Proc. natn. Acad. Sci. U.S.A.* **83**, 179–183.

Asch, R.H., Van Sickle, M., Rettori, V., Balmaceda, J.P., Eddy, C.A., Coy, D.H. & Schally, A.V. (1981) Absence of LH-RH binding sites in corpora lutea from rhesus monkeys. *J. clin. Endocr. Metab.* **53**, 215–217.

Aten, R.F. & Behrman, H.R. (1988) The ovarian GnRH-like protein: purification from bovine ovaries and characterization of biologic activity. *Endocrinology* **122** (Suppl.), 294, Abstr. 1094.

Aten, R.F., Williams, A.T. & Behrman, H.R. (1986) Ovarian gonadotropin-releasing hormone-like protein(s): demonstration and characterization. *Endocrinology* **118**, 961–967.

Aten, R.F. Ireland, H.H., Weems, C.W. & Behrman, H.R. (1987a) Presence of gonadotropin-releasing hormone-like proteins in bovine and ovine ovaries. *Endocrinology* **120**, 1727–1733.

Aten, R.F., Polan, M.L., Bayless, R. & Behrman, H.R. (1987b) A gonadotropin-releasing hormone (GnRH)-like protein in human ovaries: similarity to the GnRH-like ovarian protein in the rat. *J. clin. Endocr. Metab.* **63**, 1288–1293.

Behrman, H.R., Preston, S.L. & Hall, A.K. (1980) Cellular mechanism of the antigonadotropic action of luteinizing hormone-releasing hormone in the corpus luteum. *Endocrinology* **107**, 656–664.

Birnbaumer, L., Shahabi, N., Rivier, N. & Vale, W. (1985) Evidence for a physiological role of gonadotropin-releasing hormone (GnRH) or GnRH-like material in the ovary. *Endocrinology* **116**, 1367–1370.

Bramley, T.A., Menzies, G.S. & Baird, D.T. (1985) Specific binding of gonadotropin-releasing hormone and an agonist to human corpus luteum homogenate: characterization, properties, and luteal phase levels. *J. clin. Endocr. Metab.* **61**, 834–841.

Brown, J.L. & Reeves, J.J. (1983) Absence of specific binding of luteinizing-releasing hormone receptors in ovine, bovine and porcine ovaries. *Biol. Reprod.* **29**, 1179–1182.

Clayton, R.N. & Catt, K.J. (1981) Gonadotropin-releasing hormone receptors: characterization, physiological regulation, and relationship to reproductive function. *Endocr. Rev.* **2**, 186–209.

Clayton, R.N. & Huhtaniemi, I.T. (1982) Absence of gonadotropin-releasing hormone receptors in human gonadal tissue. *Nature, Lond.* **299**, 56–59.

Hall, A.K. & Behrman, H.R. (1981) Culture sensitization and inhibition of luteinizing hormone responsive cyclic AMP in luteal cells by luteinizing hormone, prostaglandin F2α, and D-trp6-luteinizing hormone releasing hormone. *J. Endocr.* **88**, 27–38.

Hsueh, A.J.W. & Jones, P.B.C. (1981) Extrapituitary actions of gonadotropin-releasing hormone. *Endocr. Rev.* **2**, 437–461.

Ireland, J.J., Aten, R.F. & Behrman H.R. (1988a) GnRH-like proteins in cows: concentration during corpora lutea development and selective localization in granulosal cells. *Biol. Reprod.* **38**, 544–550.

Ireland, J.J., Milvae, R.A., Aten, R.F. & Behrman, H.R. (1988b) The bovine ovarian GnRH-like protein has potent, reversible antigonadotropic effect of bovine luteal cells. *Endocrinology* **122**, (Suppl.) 294, Abstr. 1096.

Ling, N., Ying, S.Y., Ueno, N., Shimasaki, S., Esch, F., Hotta, M. & Guillemin, R. (1986) Pituitary FSH is released by a heterodimer of the b-subunits from the two forms of inhibin. *Nature, Lond.* **321,** 779–782.

Nett, T.M., Akbar, A.M. & Niswender, G.D. (1974) Serum levels of luteinizing hormone and gonadotropin-releasing hormone in cycling, castrated and anestrous ewes. *Endocrinology* **94,** 713–718.

Ohkawa, R., Polan, M.L. & Behrman, H.R. (1985) Adenosine differentially amplifies luteinizing hormone- over follicle stimulating hormone-mediated effects in rat granulosal cells. *Endocrinology* **117,** 248–254.

Sporn, M.B., Roberts, A.B., Wakefield, L.M. & Assoian, R.K. (1986) Transforming growth factor-b: biological function and chemical structure. *Science, N.Y.* **233,** 532–534.

Vale, W., Rivier, J., Vaughan, J., McClintock, R., Corrigan, A., Wilson, W., Karr, D. & Spiess, J. (1986) Purification and characterization of an FSH releasing protein from porcine follicular fluid. *Nature, Lond.* **321,** 776–779.

Williams, A.T. & Behrman, H.R. (1983) Paracrine regulation of the ovary by gonadotropin-releasing hormone and other peptides. *Sem. Reprod. Endocrinol.* **1,** 269–277.

J. Reprod. Fert., Suppl. **37** (1989), 195–204

Printed in Great Britain
© 1989 Journals of Reproduction & Fertility Ltd.

Adaptations to pregnancy in the interactions between luteal oxytocin and the uterus in ruminants

A. P. F. Flint, E. L. Sheldrick*, D. S. C. Jones*† and F. J. Auletta*‡

*Institute of Zoology, Zoological Society of London, Regent's Park, London NW1 4RY, U.K. and *AFRC Institute of Animal Physiology and Genetics Research, Babraham, Cambridge CB2 4AT, U.K.*

Keywords: corpus luteum; oxytocin; oxytocin receptor; sheep; pregnancy

Introduction

There is now a good deal of evidence indicating that oxytocin is synthesized and secreted by the corpus luteum in ruminants, and that its secretion by the ovary is involved in the control of the pulsatile release of uterine prostaglandin (PG) F-2α at the end of the non-pregnant oestrous cycle. This evidence includes the prolongation of the oestrous cycle following immunization against oxytocin, the shortening of the oestrous cycle after administration of oxytocin in some animals and the synchronous secretion of oxytocin and PGF-2α at luteolysis (see Flint & Sheldrick, 1983).

In contrast there is little evidence for any intra-ovarian role for oxytocin in the regulation of steroidogenesis. The best indication of the absence of any local effect is that obtained following hysterectomy in sheep during the oestrous cycle when, despite depletion of ovarian oxytocin after this procedure, there is no change in the circulating concentrations of progesterone (Fig. 1; Sheldrick & Flint, 1983a). This suggests that the disappearance of oxytocin from the corpus luteum has no effect on the ability of the tissue to secrete progesterone. Changes in metabolic clearance rate for progesterone are likely to be minor under these conditions, and changes in circulating concentrations may be taken as indicative of changes in secretion rate. Furthermore, under these conditions there is no change in the luteolytic action of cloprostenol on the corpus luteum (Sheldrick & Flint, 1983a), suggesting that the luteolytic action of prostaglandin is not mediated through an effect of ovarian oxytocin.

Evidence in favour of a local action of oxytocin on corpus luteum function depends heavily on in-vitro studies of corpus luteum tissue. There have been a number of studies of the effects of oxytocin carried out in this way, on bovine (Tan *et al.*, 1982a; J. Barrett, personal communication), ovine (Rodgers *et al.*, 1985) and human (Tan *et al.*, 1982b; Richardson & Masson, 1985; Bennegard *et al.*, 1987) luteal tissue. These data have described both inhibitory and stimulatory effects of oxytocin on luteal steroidogenesis, as well as indicating the absence of any effects. However, it should be noted that not all these studies were carried out with pure oxytocin; Fig. 2 shows h.p.l.c. traces of two preparations of oxytocin one of which contains substances other than oxytocin and has been used in certain of these experiments. It is possible, therefore, that impurities in the peptide preparations used are responsible for the inhibitory or activatory effects. In view of these data the contribution of ovarian oxytocin to ovarian cyclicity is most likely to be systemic, and adaptations to pregnancy involving changes in the secretion or action of luteal oxytocin may therefore involve organs other than the ovary.

---

†Present address: MRC Laboratory of Molecular Biology, Hills Rd, Cambridge CB2 2QH, U.K.
‡Present address: Department of Obstetrics & Gynecology, University of Vermont, Burlington, Vermont 05405, U.S.A.

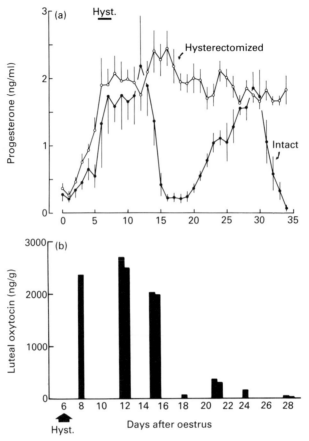

Fig. 1. Effects of hysterectomy (Hyst.) on luteal synthesis and secretion of progesterone and oxytocin. (a) Peripheral plasma concentrations of progesterone in hysterectomized (○) and sham operated (●) non-pregnant ewes during the breeding season; hysterectomy or sham hysterectomy was performed on Day 6 or 7 after oestrus. (b) Luteal concentrations of oxytocin in sheep hysterectomized as in (a). Hysterectomy results in prolonged luteal function, but maintenance of corpora lutea beyond the time at which regression normally occurs in cyclic ewes (Days 12–15) is associated with decreased luteal oxytocin concentrations. (From Sheldrick & Flint, 1983a.)

Action of oxytocin on the uterus

Induction of the oxytocin receptor in non-pregnant cycles

Evidence in favour of a systemic action of oxytocin in the control of luteolysis in non-pregnant ewes is supported by the observation that the uterus becomes increasingly sensitive to oxytocin as luteolysis proceeds. Concentrations of the oxytocin receptor in caruncular and inter-caruncular endometrium rise concomitantly with the fall in circulating progesterone concentrations at luteolysis (Sheldrick & Flint, 1985), and these results suggest either that receptor concentrations rise as a result of the fall in circulating progesterone concentration or that a rise in oxytocin receptor concentration is a cause of luteal regression. They do not allow a choice to be made between these

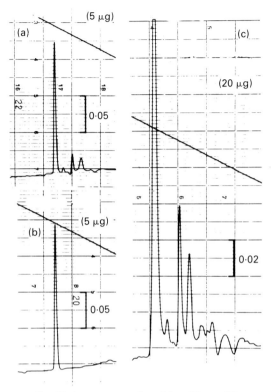

Fig. 2. High-performance liquid chromatography of 5 or 20 μg of 2 commercial preparations of oxytocin, analysed as obtained from the vendor. Note that preparation (a) contains substances other than oxytocin; this material has been used to study the effects of oxytocin on luteal function *in vitro* and *in vivo*. Trace shown in (c) was obtained using the same material in (a), at a higher sensitivity; material chromatographed in (b), from the same supplier, is pure. Vertical bars indicate detector sensitivity at 214 nm in optical density units.

hypothetical mechanisms. However, there are two experiments which suggest that the rising concentration of oxytocin receptor plays a causative role in the release of PGF-2α from the uterus which leads to luteolysis.

Effects of oestrogen administration. Administration of oestrogen in high doses during the mid-luteal phase of the oestrous cycle results in luteal regression in sheep and other ruminants (see Hixon & Flint, 1987, and references therein). In an examination of the effects of administered oestrogen on uterine PGF-2α secretion and oxytocin receptor concentrations it was shown that the appearance of the oxytocin receptor preceded prostaglandin release and the onset of luteolysis, as indicated by a decline in circulating progesterone; oxytocin receptor concentrations were raised in caruncular endometrium and myometrium within 12 h of oestrogen administration, PGF-2α secretion began at 35 h and progesterone concentrations first declined at 42 h following oestrogen (Fig. 3; Hixon & Flint, 1987). Under these conditions, therefore, it is possible that the rise in oxytocin receptor concentration in the uterus plays a causative role in the release of PGF-2α leading to luteolysis.

Effect of continuous oxytocin infusion. In a second approach to this question, Flint & Sheldrick (1985) showed that, when the rise in uterine oxytocin receptor concentration preceding oestrus was blocked by continuous infusion of oxytocin, luteal regression was prevented and the cycle prolonged. In these experiments it was shown to be necessary to begin infusion of oxytocin on Day 13

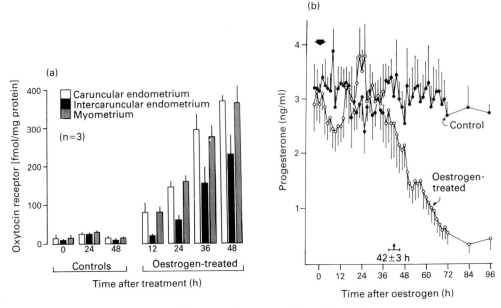

Fig. 3. Uterine concentrations of the oxytocin receptor (a) and circulating progesterone concentrations (b) in ewes treated with 750 μg oestradiol benzoate on Days 9 and 10 of the oestrous cycle. First treatment (on Day 9) was at $t = 0$ (arrow). Data of Hixon & Flint (1987).

after oestrus. That this treatment down-regulated oxytocin receptors in the uterus and blocked the rise in the receptor associated with luteolysis was demonstrated by measurement of oxytocin receptor concentrations in the tissue. Using this procedure, it has now been shown that PGF-2α concentrations remain low during oxytocin infusion (Fig. 4; Sheldrick & Flint, 1987). These results are also consistent with a causative role for the rise in oxytocin receptor concentrations at luteal regression. It should be noted that these results do not rule out the possibility of a post-receptor inhibitory effect of oxytocin on the uterus; Sheldrick & Flint (1986) showed that the transient uterine refractoriness to oxytocin caused by administration of bolus intravenous doses of oxytocin was associated with no change in oxytocin receptor concentration in any uterine compartment. It is possible therefore that oxytocin has effects in addition to those on the induction of receptor.

Phosphoinositide cycle activity and the mechanism of action of oxytocin

Many endocrine and paracrine receptors stimulate rates of phosphoinositide metabolism, and there is now evidence that several peptide hormones generate second messenger substances in this way. The evidence for an effect of vasopressin on phosphoinositide turnover is particularly strong; the action of vasopressin on the vascular receptor involved in blood pressure regulation (the V1 receptor) is mediated in this way. Oxytocin appears to stimulate phosphoinositide hydrolysis in the sheep endometrium through interaction with a receptor having characteristics similar to those of the V1 vasopressin receptor (Flint *et al.*, 1986). A similar action of oxytocin on the human decidua has also been reported (Schrey *et al.*, 1986). An effect on phosphoinositide hydrolysis might be expected to lead to prostaglandin synthesis through the provision of diacylglycerol as a product of the metabolism of phosphoinositides; the rapidity of the stimulatory effect of oxytocin on PGF-2α secretion *in vivo* can be accounted for by the effect of oxytocin on phosphoinositide hydrolysis, which occurs immediately (Fig. 5).

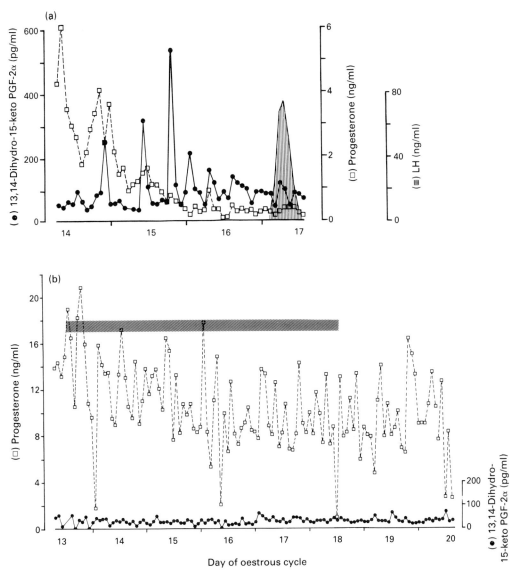

Fig. 4. Circulating concentrations of progesterone and 13,14-dihydro-15-ketoprostaglandin F-2α in non-pregnant ewes receiving oxytocin by continuous infusion. (a) Control ewe; (b) ewe treated with oxytocin (3 μg/h) between Days 13 and 18 as shown by horizontal bar. Vertical hatching indicates ovulatory LH surge.

G proteins in the uterus and the effects of steroid hormones

In the experiments reviewed above on the effect of oestrogen administration during the oestrous cycle it was shown that oestrogen activated the phosphoinositide response to oxytocin, as measured *in vitro*, in uterine tissue from treated ewes. However, there appeared to be a lag between the rise in receptor concentration and the onset of response in terms of phosphoinositide turnover; whereas receptor concentration increased within 12 h of treatment, there was no phosphoinositide response until 24 h after oestradiol administration (Hixon & Flint, 1987). This raises the possibility that administration of oestrogen affects receptor concentrations and post-receptor responses separately,

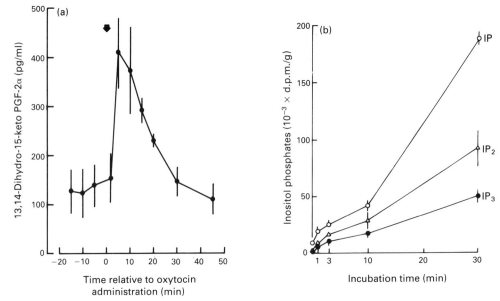

Fig. 5. Mechanism of action of oxytocin in causing uterine prostaglandin production. (a) Time course of rise in jugular venous concentrations of 13,14-dihydro-15-ketoprostaglandin F-2α after administration of a single intravenous dose of oxytocin to an ovariectomized, steroid-treated ewe. (b) Time course of effect of oxytocin *in vitro* on accumulation of inositol phosphates in slices of caruncular endometrium previously incubated with [³H]inositol to label phosphoinositides. Incubation times refer to periods following addition of oxytocin (10^{-7} M). Incubations contained 10 mM-LiCl. Increased phosphoinositide breakdown is expected to lead to increased availability of arachidonic acid for prostaglandin synthesis through the hydrolysis of diacylglycerol produced concurrently. Additional fatty acid may be released through subsequent activation, by raised intracellular calcium, of phospholipase A2.

which is consistent with the possibility that a post-receptor event is affected by acute exposure to oxytocin, as reviewed above.

In an attempt to determine the nature of the lag between induced receptor concentrations and phosphoinositide turnover, Flint (1988) investigated the possibility that a pertussis toxin-sensitive G protein might be induced in the uterus by oestrogen treatment. The phospholipase responsible for phosphoinositide hydrolysis is linked to hormone receptors through a pertussis toxin-sensitive protein in many tissues. It is possible that this protein is identical to the guanine nucleotide-binding protein (G_i) that mediates the inhibitory effects of certain agonists on adenylate cyclase (Gilman, 1984), the α subunit of which has a molecular weight of 41 000. By incubating extracts of uterine tissues with [³²P]NAD in the presence of pertussis toxin it can be demonstrated that the sheep uterus contains a protein of $M_r = 41\,000$ with the characteristics expected of the G_i protein. However, although uterine concentrations of this protein were raised 2·7- and 3·6-fold respectively by progestagen and progestagen plus oestrogen treatment of ovariectomized ewes *in vivo*, it did not appear that this protein was likely to be a candidate for an oestrogen-induced post-receptor event. Firstly, in the study of Hixon & Flint (1987) the effect of oxytocin on phosphoinositide hydrolysis was detectable only in cyclic sheep which had been treated with oestrogen, whereas the pertussis-sensitive protein was present in untreated and in progestagen-treated ovariectomized animals. Furthermore ADP-ribosylation of the major proportion of the G_i protein in tissue slices by incubation with pertussis toxin did not affect the response of the tissue to oxytocin in terms of phosphoinositide turnover (Table 1). It appears possible, therefore, that another candidate must be sought for the post-receptor event activated by oestrogen treatment.

Table 1. Effect of pertussis toxin on oxytocin-stimulated hydrolysis of phosphoinositides in slices of ovine caruncular endometrium

Tissue incubated with:	Phosphoinositide hydrolysis ($10^{-3} \times$ d.p.m./g wet wt)		
	Inositol monophosphate	Inositol bisphosphate	Inositol trisphosphate
No additions	19 ± 1.5	5.4 ± 1.6	3.0 ± 0.9
Oxytocin	145 ± 12	86 ± 18	65 ± 4.4
Pertussis toxin	12 ± 1.8	4.8 ± 0.7	3.3 ± 0.6
Pertussis toxin plus oxytocin	159 ± 27	84 ± 20	61 ± 11

Values are mean $\pm$ s.e.m. for 4 observations (data of Flint, 1988).

Oxytocin (10^{-7} M) was added 20 min before extracting the slices; pertussis toxin (1 μg/ml) was present for 2 h 40 min before adding oxytocin and thereafter. Subsequent pertussis toxin-catalysed ADP-ribosylation of membrane proteins in the presence of [^{32}P]NAD showed that 64% of available substrate had been ribosylated during incubation of slices.

Adaptations to pregnancy

Oxytocin concentrations in the corpus luteum decline in early pregnancy in a manner similar to that observed after hysterectomy (Fig. 1; Sheldrick & Flint, 1983b). It has been suggested that this decline in oxytocin concentration, which occurs despite continued secretion of progesterone and maintenance of corpus luteum weight, represents one way in which the endocrine environment of the mother is adapted to pregnancy (Sheldrick & Flint, 1983b; Flint & Sheldrick, 1986). A decrease in circulating oxytocin concentrations, which has also been noted at this time (Sheldrick & Flint, 1983b; Schams & Lahlou-Kassi, 1984), can be assumed to contribute towards the establishment of pregnancy by reducing secretion of the uterine luteolysin and reducing uterine contractility at a time when the blastocyst is becoming attached to the endometrium.

Measurement of oxytocin–neurophysin prohormone messenger RNA (mRNA) in corpora lutea of sheep during the oestrous cycle and in early pregnancy has shown that the decline in oxytocin concentration in the corpus luteum at this time reflects a drop in the luteal concentration of prohormone mRNA (Fig. 6; Jones & Flint, 1988). In the corpus luteum of cattle (Ivell *et al.*, 1985; Fehr *et al.*, 1987), the concentration of mRNA is relatively high early in the cycle; in sheep the highest level was observed on Day 3 after oestrus, after which the level declines exponentially to reach low values by Days 9 and 10. The highest concentration of oxytocin was observed in the tissue on Day 7 after oestrus. The lag between peak messenger RNA and oxytocin concentrations has been suggested to reflect the time taken for post-translational processing of the oxytocin–neurophysin prohormone. Concentrations of messenger RNA in corpora lutea from pregnant ewes on Days 13–36 were similar to those on Days 9–12 of the cycle (Fig. 6). However, luteal concentrations of oxytocin itself were lower in tissue from pregnant ewes than in that from non-pregnant animals at a comparable stage after oestrus; this difference between pregnant and non-pregnant animals could result from a reduction in translation of oxytocin–neurophysin mRNA during pregnancy or from a decrease in the storage of oxytocin. The fate of oxytocin present in the corpus luteum of pregnancy before Day 13 is not known.

Measurements of the oxytocin receptor in the uterus in early pregnancy consistently show that receptor levels remain low at a time when, in non-pregnant animals, they rise to high values (Fig. 7). It has been suggested that the maintenance of low concentrations of oxytocin receptor at this time represents one more way in which uterine responsiveness to oxytocin is reduced, in order to ensure a decreased uterine secretion of prostaglandins at this time (Sheldrick & Flint, 1985; Flint &

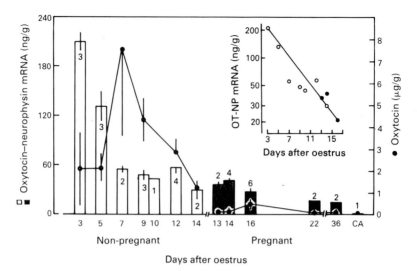

Fig. 6. Concentrations of oxytocin–neurophysin prohormone mRNA and oxytocin in corpora lutea of cyclic and pregnant sheep. CA = corpus albicans. (From Jones & Flint, 1988.) Inset shows mRNA values in the cycle (○) and pregnancy (●) as a semi-log plot.

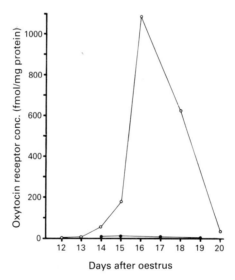

Fig. 7. Mean concentrations of oxytocin receptor in intercaruncular endometrium during the oestrous cycle (○) and in pregnancy (●) in ewes. Levels of receptor in caruncular endometrium were reduced in pregnancy to a similar extent. (Data from Flint & Sheldrick, 1986.)

Sheldrick, 1986). However, the mechanism by which the oxytocin receptor is reduced at this time is uncertain. As it is known that progesterone reduces, and oestrogen increases, uterine expression of the oxytocin receptor (see Sheldrick & Flint, 1985), it is possible that the low level of oxytocin receptor at this time reflects the maintenance of luteal progesterone secretion. However, the results reviewed above, obtained from experiments in which uterine oxytocin receptor concentrations were manipulated by oestrogen administration or continuous oxytocin infusion, suggest that the rise in receptor at the end of the non-pregnant cycle may play a causative role in luteal regression, rather than responding to it. If that is the case, then some specific mechanism must be sought to account for the low amount of receptor expressed in the pregnant uterus between Days 12 and 17 of gestation.

One possible mechanism by which this may be brought about is by blastocyst production of oxytocin. It is possible that the developing blastocyst, through secretion of oxytocin or an oxytocin-like compound, down-regulates the oxytocin receptor in a manner comparable to that observed following continuous oxytocin infusion. However, there is no evidence that the ovine blastocyst contains or secretes oxytocin; concentrations of oxytocin measured by radioimmunoassay in blastocysts flushed from uteri between Days 17 and 30 were low (E. L. Sheldrick, unpublished observations), and further work is necessary to confirm or refute this hypothesis.

A second possibility is that the reduction in oxytocin receptor is a consequence of the secretion by the blastocyst of an antiluteolytic interferon (Stewart *et al.*, 1987; Imakawa *et al.*, 1987). However, results obtained to date suggest that this is unlikely (see Stewart *et al.*, 1989).

Conclusions

The results presented here indicate that the mechanisms controlling uterine prostaglandin production in non-pregnant cycles adapt to pregnancy. The adaptations involve a reduction in the uterine concentrations of oxytocin receptor, and a decline in the concentration of oxytocin synthesized and secreted by the corpus luteum and they occur at the same time as the effects of ovine trophoblast interferon. While it is probable that these changes represent different ways in which the survival of the developing blastocyst is ensured, and that they all act to cause the prolongation of luteal function in early gestation, the exact relationships between them are uncertain. In particular, the mechanism leading to reduced endometrial oxytocin receptor concentrations is at present obscure; it may be necessary to propose the existence of a trophoblast product specifically involved in the down regulation of this receptor.

References

Bennegard, B., Hahlin, M. & Dennefors, B. (1987) Antigonadotropic effect of oxytocin on the isolated human corpus luteum. *Fert. Steril.* **47**, 431–435.

Fehr, S., Ivell, R., Koll, R., Schams, D., Fields, M. & Richter, D. (1987) Expression of the oxytocin gene in the large cells of the bovine corpus luteum. *FEBS Letters* **210**, 45–50.

Flint, A.P.F. (1988) Pertussis toxin-catalysed ADP-ribosylation of endometrial proteins in sheep. *J. Endocr.* **117**, 403–407.

Flint, A.P.F. & Sheldrick, E.L. (1983) Evidence for a systemic role for ovarian oxytocin in luteal regression in sheep. *J. Reprod. Fert.* **67**, 215–225.

Flint, A.P.F. & Sheldrick, E.L. (1985) Continuous infusion of oxytocin prevents induction of uterine oxytocin receptor and blocks luteal regression in cyclic ewes. *J. Reprod. Fert.* **75**, 623–631.

Flint, A.P.F. & Sheldrick, E.L. (1986) Ovarian oxytocin and the maternal recognition of pregnancy. *J. Reprod. Fert.* **76**, 831–839.

Flint, A.P.F., Leat, W.M.F., Sheldrick, E.L. & Stewart, H.J. (1986) Stimulation of phosphoinositide hydrolysis by oxytocin and the mechanism by which oxytocin controls prostaglandin synthesis in the ovine endometrium. *Biochem. J.* **237**, 797–805.

Gilman, A.G. (1984) G proteins and dual control of adenylate cyclase. *Cell* **36**, 577–579.

Hixon, J.E. & Flint, A.P.F. (1987) Effects of a luteolytic dose of oestradiol benzoate on uterine oxytocin receptor concentrations, phosphoinositide turnover and prostaglandin F-2α secretion in sheep. *J. Reprod. Fert.* **79**, 457–467.

Imakawa, K., Anthony, R.V., Kazemi, M., Marotti, K.R., Polites, H.G. & Roberts, R.M. (1987) Interferon-like sequence of ovine trophoblast protein secreted by embryonic trophectoderm. *Nature, Lond.* **330**, 377–379.

Ivell, R., Brackett, K.H., Fields, M.J. & Richter, D. (1985) Ovulation triggers oxytocin gene expression in the bovine ovary. *FEBS Letters* **190**, 263–267.

Jones, D.S.C. & Flint, A.P.F. (1988) Concentrations of oxytocin-neurophysin prohormone mRNA in corpora lutea of sheep during the oestrous cycle and in early pregnancy. *J. Endocr.* **117**, 409–414.

Richardson, M.C. & Masson, G.M. (1985) Lack of direct inhibitory action of oxytocin on progesterone production by dispersed cells from human corpus luteum. *J. Endocr.* **104**, 149–151.

Rodgers, R.J., O'Shea, J.D. & Findlay, J.K. (1985) Do small and large luteal cells of the sheep interact in the production of progesterone? *J. Reprod. Fert.* **75**, 85–94.

Schams, D. & Lahlou-Kassi, A. (1984) Circulating concentrations of oxytocin during pregnancy in ewes. *Acta endocr., Copenh.* **106**, 277–281.

Schrey, M.P., Read, A.M. & Steer, P.J. (1986) Oxytocin stimulates phosphoinositide hydrolysis in human uterine decidual cells. *J. Endocr., Suppl.* **108**, Abstr. 190.

Sheldrick, E.L. & Flint, A.P.F. (1983a) Regression of the corpora lutea in sheep in response to cloprostenol is not affected by loss of luteal oxytocin after hysterectomy. *J. Reprod. Fert.* **68**, 155–160.

Sheldrick, E.L. & Flint, A.P.F. (1983b) Luteal concentrations of oxytocin decline during early pregnancy in the ewe. *J. Reprod. Fert.* **68**, 477–480.

Sheldrick, E.L. & Flint, A.P.F. (1985) Endocrine control of uterine oxytocin receptors in the ewe. *J. Endocr.* **106**, 249–258.

Sheldrick, E.L. & Flint, A.P.F. (1986) Transient uterine refractoriness after oxytocin administration in ewes. *J. Reprod. Fert.* **77**, 523–529.

Sheldrick, E.L. & Flint, A.P.F. (1987) Effect of continuous oxytocin infusion on prostaglandin-$F_{2\alpha}$ secretion in the cyclic ewe. *J. Endocr., Suppl.* **115**, Abstr. 36.

Stewart, H.J., McCann, S.H.E., Barker, P.J., Lee, K.E., Lamming, G.E. & Flint, A.P.F. (1987) Interferon sequence homology and receptor binding activity of ovine trophoblast antiluteolytic protein. *J. Endocr.* **115**, R13–R15.

Stewart, H.J., Flint, A.P.F., Lamming, G.E., McCann, S.H.E. & Parkinson, T.J. (1989) Antiluteolytic effects of blastocyst-secreted interferon investigated *in vitro* and *in vivo* in the sheep. *J. Reprod. Fert., Suppl.* **37**, 127–138.

Tan, G.J.S., Tweedale, R. & Biggs, J.S.G. (1982a) Oxytocin may play a role in the control of the human corpus luteum. *J. Endocr.* **95**, 65–70.

Tan, G.J.S., Tweedale, R. & Biggs, J.S.G. (1982b) Effects of oxytocin on the bovine corpus luteum of early pregnancy. *J Reprod. Fert.* **66**, 75–78.

J. Reprod. Fert., Suppl. **37** (1989), 205–213

Printed in Great Britain
© 1989 Journals of Reproduction & Fertility Ltd

GnRH peptides and regulation of the corpus luteum

T. A. Bramley

Department of Obstetrics & Gynaecology, University of Edinburgh, Centre for Reproductive Biology, 37 Chalmers Street, Edinburgh EH3 9EW, U.K.

Keywords: LHRH; ovary; placenta; paracrine regulation

Introduction

Experiments with hypophysectomized rats have clearly demonstrated a direct effect of GnRH and its agonist analogues on the gonads *in vivo* (Rippel & Johnson, 1976; Ying *et al.*, 1981) and on rat gonadal cells *in vitro* (Sharpe, 1984; Hsueh & Jones, 1981, 1982; Knecht *et al.*, 1983a) which could be specifically reversed by GnRH antagonists. Moreover, high-affinity GnRH-binding sites similar to pituitary GnRH receptors were described in rat ovarian cells (Reeves *et al.*, 1980; Iwashita & Catt, 1984; Naor & Childs, 1985), the levels of which could be modulated by the physiological status of the animal or by hormonal manipulations (Fraser *et al.*, 1984). Both the magnitude and direction of the effects of GnRH were dependent on the end-point measured, the state of differentiation of the cells, the presence of gonadotrophins during exposure to GnRH, and the time-scale over which the response was measured (Hsueh & Jones, 1981; Fraser *et al.*, 1984; Ranta *et al.*, 1984). Acute, stimulatory actions of GnRH on rat ovarian cells generally involved a short-term increase in steroidogenesis, mediated by a complex series of changes, including a rapid mobilization of calcium ions (Eckstein *et al.*, 1986), enhanced phosphatidyl inositol turnover (Naor *et al.*, 1985), elevation of intracellular inositol phosphates (Davis *et al.*, 1986), translocation and activation of calcium-phospholipid dependent protein kinase C (Wang & Leung, 1987), and enhanced release of arachidonic acid, leukotrienes and prostaglandins (Clark, 1982; Minegishi *et al.*, 1987), processes very similar to those involved in GnRH-stimulated release of gonadotrophins from the pituitary gland (Naor, 1986; Conn *et al.*, 1987; Chang *et al.*, 1987; Morgan *et al.*, 1987). Inhibitory actions of GnRH on gonadal tissue were observed with longer-term GnRH treatment, and involved induction of a cyclic AMP-dependent phosphodiesterase (Knecht *et al.*, 1983a), changes in the synthesis of gonadotrophin receptors (Knecht & Catt, 1983; Knecht *et al.*, 1983b), steroidogenic enzymes and cell cytoskeletal proteins (Dorrington & Skinner, 1986), and the antagonism of gonadotrophin-dependent steroid secretion (Reddy *et al.*, 1980; Massicotte *et al.*, 1981; Wang & Leung, 1987) and cellular differentiation (Knecht *et al.*, 1982; Dorrington *et al.*, 1985; Amsterdam & Rotmensch, 1987). Since GnRH-like peptides (Aten *et al.*, 1986) could be isolated from rat gonadal tissues, and GnRH was rapidly inactivated by ovarian cells (Sharpe, 1984), GnRH-like peptides fully satisfied the criteria necessary to establish a role as a paracrine regulator of gonadal function in the rat (Williams & Behrman, 1983; see Table 1). These criteria were also satisfied for GnRH-like peptides in the human placenta (Siler-Khodr, 1987).

Attempts to demonstrate a similar paracrine role for GnRH-like peptides in the gonads of other species were disappointing and confusing, however. GnRH and its analogues failed to affect gonadal function *in vivo* or *in vitro*, and gonadal GnRH-binding sites could not be demonstrated in a number of species (Brown & Reeves, 1983; Clayton & Huhtaniemi, 1982; Asch *et al.*, 1981). However, despite reports of a lack of ovarian GnRH-binding sites, effects of GnRH and its analogues have been reported for some of these species (Table 1), GnRH-like peptides could be isolated from ovarian tissues (Behrman *et al.*, 1988), and specific binding sites for GnRH were

T. A. Bramley

described in human corpus luteum and a number of other human extrapituitary tissues (Bramley, 1987). It is generally held that GnRH-like peptides have no significant role as paracrine regulators of ovarian function, except in the rat. We shall outline briefly data from ourselves and others (chiefly on human luteal and placental tissue) which suggest that many of the criteria outlined in Table 1 are fulfilled by human extrapituitary sites, and indicate differences which may be significant.

Table 1. Criteria to be established for a paracrine role for GnRH: (1) local production of GnRH in close proximity to target cells; (2) termination of GnRH action requires rapid local inactivation; (3) target tissue must possess specific GnRH receptors; (4) changes in hormone/receptor levels correlate with physiology; (5) GnRH must induce a biological response

Tissue	GnRH-like factor?	GnRH inactivation?	GnRH receptors?	Physiological changes?	Response?
Ovary					
Rat	+	+	+	+	+
Pig	+		—		+
Cow	+		—		—
Sheep	+		—		—
Monkey	?		—		—
Man	+	+	+	+	?
Placenta	+	+	+	+	+

See text for references.

Local production of GnRH

The GnRH gene has been isolated and cloned from human placenta (Seeburg & Adelman, 1984), and GnRH gene expression has also been demonstrated in a human breast tumour cell line (Eidne *et al.*, 1987). The GnRH decapeptide is synthesized by and is extractable from placenta (Tan & Rousseau, 1982; Gibbons *et al.*, 1975). However, the major GnRH-like peptides extracted from placenta (Gautron *et al.*, 1981; Nowak *et al.*, 1984; Siler-Khodr, 1987) and ovary (Aten *et al.*, 1986, 1987a, b) often differed significantly from those of native GnRH in size and/or elution from h.p.l.c. and often showed little cross-reaction with antibodies raised to mammalian GnRH (Hedger *et al.*, 1987). Furthermore, attempts to extract GnRH-like peptides often begin by treatment with strong acid, followed by molecular exclusion separation, procedures which will denature larger peptides and proteins, and bias isolations towards low molecular weight peptides.

Local inactivation of GnRH

We have shown previously that human luteal and placental membrane fractions rapidly inactivated GnRH and the GnRH agonist, buserelin ([D-Ser(t Bu)^6]1–9 GnRH ethylamide) in a time- and temperature-dependent manner *in vitro* (Bramley, 1987). If, as suggested (Clayton *et al.*, 1979), low-affinity human extrapituitary binding sites represent binding of radiolabelled degradation-resistant analogues to tissue peptidases, peptidase inhibitors should prevent binding and GnRH agonist binding and degradation should behave in a parallel manner as luteal and placental membranes are purified. However, attempts to inhibit GnRH agonist binding to luteal and placental membranes with a range of inhibitors specific for the different classes of protease (including pyroglutamyl peptidase, post-proline cleaving enzyme, and endopeptidases acting at Gly^6) were unsuccessful (Bramley *et al.*, 1986). Moreover, fractionation of placental membranes on sucrose gradients (with and without perturbation with digitonin to identify cell-surface membranes) showed that binding of GnRH agonist behaved identically to two other placental surface membrane markers, epidermal growth factor (EGF) receptor and alkaline phosphatase, whereas hormone inactivation did not (Fig. 1), indicating that placental binding sites were unrelated to enzymes involved in GnRH inactivation. Similar results were also obtained for human luteal tissue (Bramley & Menzies, 1986).

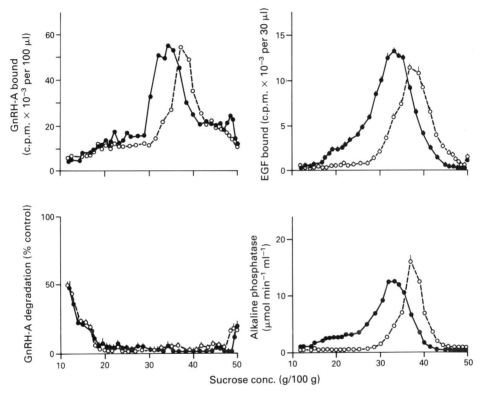

Fig. 1. Fractionation of human placental membranes on sucrose density gradients: lack of association of GnRH binding, alkaline phosphatase and EGF receptors with GnRH inactivation. ●, Control membranes; ○, membranes pretreated with digitonin to perturb the density of cell surface-membranes.

Specific binding sites for GnRH

Binding sites for GnRH and its agonist analogues have been reported in the human placenta (Currie *et al.*, 1981; Belisle *et al.*, 1984; Iwashita *et al.*, 1986) and corpus luteum (Popkin *et al.*, 1983, 1985; Bramley *et al.*, 1985, 1986). Little binding was detected in stromal (Popkin *et al.*, 1983) and follicular tissue (Bramley *et al.*, 1987). Despite their low affinity for superactive agonists of GnRH, human luteal (Bramley *et al.*, 1986) and placental (unpublished data) binding sites had an impressive specificity, in that only molecules with a structure related to GnRH could compete for binding sites. However, analogues with D-amino acid substitutions at Gly^6 showed greatly

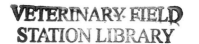

enhanced potency towards sheep and rat pituitary and rat gonadal receptors, but their potencies for human luteal and placental binding sites were enhanced only slightly (Fig. 2a). Furthermore, affinity for GnRH was similar in rat and human tissues (Fig. 2b). In addition, a number of GnRH antagonists with superactivity towards sheep and rat pituitary receptors had little or no ability to displace GnRH agonist tracers from human luteal (Fraser *et al.*, 1986) and placental (unpublished data) binding sites. The low potency of these analogues for human extrapituitary binding sites suggests that such antagonists will be of only limited use in defining GnRH effects in these tissues.

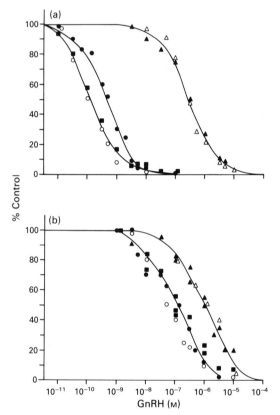

Fig. 2. Binding inhibition curves for displacement of radiolabelled GnRH agonist by (a) unlabelled agonist or (b) GnRH from membranes of rat pituitary (○), ovary (■), and testis (●), and human corpus luteum (▲) and placenta (△).

Although the mammalian preproGnRH gene was isolated from human placenta, a tissue with extrapituitary binding sites, the levels of native GnRH which can be extracted from placental tissue appear to be very low (Gibbons *et al.*, 1975; Tan & Rousseau, 1982; Mathialagan & Rao, 1986). The major GnRH-like species extracted often behave quite differently from GnRH on gel chromatography and h.p.l.c., show different reactivity to various GnRH antisera (Hedger *et al.*, 1987), and differ in their ability to release LH from pituitary cells (Siler-Khodr, 1987; Mathialagan & Rao, 1986).

Placental GnRH (hCGnRH) may arise by differential processing of preproGnRH mRNA in placental and hypothalamic tissue (Seeburg *et al.*, 1987). Indeed, placental preproGnRH mRNA differs from hypothalamic mRNA in that the first intron is not spliced out in the placenta, and hypothalamic and placental promoter regions may differ (Adelman *et al.*, 1986; Seeburg *et al.*, 1987). PreproGnRH codes for a protein, gonadotrophin-associated protein (GAP), which stimulates the release of FSH and LH from the pituitary, and inhibits prolactin release (Nikolics *et al.*, 1985), and a small region of the GAP peptide can itself release FSH and LH *in vitro* (Millar *et al.*, 1986; Milton *et al.*, 1986). However, GAP peptides failed to compete for placental membrane GnRH agonist binding sites, and a number of other substances which are known to affect pituitary gonadotrophin release, or which have significant homology to GnRH, also failed to displace placental and luteal GnRH binding (unpublished data).

Other forms of GnRH which differ in aminoacid sequence from the mammalian hormone have been isolated from other species (King & Millar, 1987), and more than one form of GnRH may be expressed in some species, with distinct anatomical distributions. Hence, pituitary and placental GnRH binding sites may recognize different GnRH molecules. We therefore compared the abilities of GnRH tracers to bind to rat and sheep pituitary and to human placental membranes (Fig. 3). Whilst the GnRH agonist buserelin bound to all three tissues, the different forms of GnRH failed to bind to pituitary membranes. Mammalian, chicken I and lamprey GnRH also failed to bind to placental membranes; however, salmon and chicken II GnRH bound as well as buserelin. Nevertheless, the affinity of binding and the specificity of displacement by a range of GnRH agonists, antagonists and truncated GnRH forms were similar for buserelin, salmon and chicken II GnRH (unpublished data).

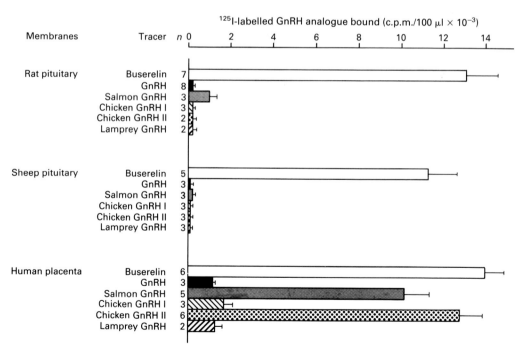

Fig. 3. Binding of radiolabelled GnRH and GnRH agonist to membranes of rat and sheep pituitary and human placenta. Bars represent means $\pm$ s.e.m. for the number of experiments shown for each tracer.

Changes in GnRH receptor or peptide levels in different physiological circumstances

Concentrations of immunoreactive GnRH in serum (Siler-Khodr et al., 1984) and placental tissue (Siler-Khodr & Khodr, 1978) have been reported which altered with changes in chorionic gonado-trophin secretion rate in vivo. Furthermore, the secretion of chorionic gonadotrophin, steroids and prostaglandins by placental explants could be stimulated by GnRH in vitro, but these responses varied markedly with gestational age (Siler-Khodr et al., 1986a, b, c, 1987). Moreover, we have described changes in the concentrations of GnRH binding sites in human corpora lutea obtained at different stages of the luteal phase which correlated with some important indices of luteal function (Bramley et al., 1987; unpublished data).

Stimulation of a physiological response by GnRH

Placental tissue explants and syncytiotrophoblast cells respond to GnRH with increased secretion of steroids, prostaglandins and chorionic gonadotrophin (but not placental lactogen) in vitro (Siler-Khodr et al., 1986a, b, c). These effects can be antagonized by high levels of some GnRH antagonist analogues (Siler-Khodr et al., 1987; but see Belisle et al., 1984), indicating that they may be exerted through stereospecific receptors.

Few direct effects of GnRH and GnRH agonists on steroidogenesis in human ovarian cells in vitro have been reported (Tureck et al., 1982; Lamberts et al., 1982). Rather, most studies have failed to show direct effects on steroid secretion in vitro (Casper et al., 1982, 1984; Tan & Biggs, 1983; Richardson et al., 1984). However, there may be differences in response to GnRH between species, individuals and cell types, and with stage of development. Methodologies used may be inappropriate with regard to length of incubation or end-point measured, or the preparation of tissue may have damaged responsiveness. Finally, the nature of the endogenous ligand for these sites is not yet known, although our observations indicate that the endogenous GnRH-like molecule differs significantly from mammalian GnRH and/or that extra-pituitary GnRH binding sites differ significantly in specificity from pituitary receptors. Should this prove to be the case, it may be possible to design analogues of GnRH which will interact specifically with luteal or placental extrapituitary binding sites and allow the manipulation of human fertility.

This work was supported by a grant (G85/2358 SB) from the Medical Research Council, U.K. I thank Garry Menzies for excellent technical assistance.

References

Adelman, J.P., Mason, A.J. Hayflick, J.S. & Seeburg, P.H. (1986) Isolation of the gene and hypothalamic cDNA for the common precursor of gonadotropin-releasing hormone and prolactin release-inhibiting factor in human and rat. Proc. natn. Acad. Sci. U.S.A. 83, 170–183.

Amsterdam, A. & Rotmensch, S. (1987) Structure-function relationships during granulosa cell differentiation. Endocrine Rev. 8, 309–337.

Asch, R.H., Van Sickle, M. Rettori, V., Balmaceda, J.P., Eddy, C.A., Coy, D.H. & Schally, A.V. (1981) Absence of LH-RH binding sites in corpora lutea from rhesus monkeys (Macaca mulatta). J. clin. Endocr. Metab. 53, 215–217.

Aten, R.F., Williams, A.T. & Behrman, H.R. (1986) Ovarian gonadotropin-releasing hormone-like protein(s): demonstration and characterization. Endocrinology 118, 961–967.

Aten, R.F., Ireland, J.J., Weems, C.W. & Behrman, H.R. (1987a) Presence of gonadotropin-releasing hormone-like proteins in bovine and ovine ovaries. Endocrinology 120, 1727–1733.

Aten, R.F., Polan, M.L., Bayless, R. & Behrman, H.R. (1987b) A gonadotropin-releasing hormone (GnRH)-like protein in human ovaries: similarity to the GnRH-like ovarian protein of the rat. J. clin. Endocr. Metab. 64, 1288–1293.

Behrman, H.R., Aten, R.F. & Ireland, J.J. (1988) Characteristics of an antigonadotrophic GnRH-like protein in the ovaries of diverse mammals. J. Reprod. Fert., Suppl. 37, 189–194.

Belisle, S., Guevin, J.-F., Bellabarba, D. & Lehoux, J.-G.

(1984) Luteinizing hormone-releasing hormone binds to enriched human placental membranes and stimulates *in vitro* the synthesis of bioactive human chorionic gonadotropin. *J. clin. Endocr. Metab.* **59**, 119–126.

Bramley, T.A. (1987) LHRH-binding sites in human tissues. In *LHRH and its Analogs: Contraceptive and Therapeutic Applications*, Part 2, pp. 123–139. Eds B. H. Vickery & J. J. Nestor. MTP Press, Lancaster.

Bramley, T.A. & Menzies, G.S. (1986) Subcellular fractionation of the human corpus luteum: distribution of GnRH agonist binding sites. *Molec. Cell. Endocrinol.* **45**, 27–36.

Bramley, T.A., Menzies, G.S. & Baird, D.T. (1985) Specific binding of gonadotrophin-releasing hormone and an agonist to human corpus luteum homogenates: characterization, properties and luteal phase levels. *J. clin. Endocr. Metab.* **61**, 834–841.

Bramley, T.A., Menzies, G.S. & Baird, D.T. (1986) Specificity of gonadotrophin-releasing hormone binding sites of the human corpus luteum: comparison with receptors of rat pituitary gland. *J. Endocr.* **108**, 323–328.

Bramley, T.A., Stirling, D., Swanston, I.A., Menzies, G.S., McNeilly, A.S. & Baird, D.T. (1987) Specific binding sites for gonadotrophin-releasing hormone, LH/chorionic gonadotrophin, low-density lipoprotein, prolactin and FSH in homogenates of human corpus luteum. II. Concentrations throughout the luteal phase of the menstrual cycle and early pregnancy. *J. Endocr.* **113**, 317–327.

Brown J.L. & Reeves, J.J. (1983) Absence of specific luteinizing hormone-releasing hormone receptors in ovine and porcine ovaries. *Biol. Reprod.* **29**, 1179–1182.

Casper, R.F., Erickson, G.F., Rebar, R.W. & Yen, S.S.C. (1982) The effect of luteinizing hormone-releasing factor and its agonist on cultured human granulosa cells. *Fert. Steril.* **37**, 406–409.

Casper, R.F., Erickson, G.F. & Yen, S.S.C. (1984) Studies on the effect of gonadotropin-releasing hormone and its agonist on human luteal steroidogenesis in vitro. *Fert. Steril.* **42**, 39–43.

Chang, J.P., Graeter, J. & Catt, K.J. (1987) Dynamic actions of arachidonic acid and protein kinase C in pituitary stimulation by gonadotropin-releasing hormone. *Endocrinology* **120**, 1837–1845.

Clark, M.R. (1982) Stimulation of progesterone and prostaglandin E accumulation by luteinizing hormone-releasing hormone (LHRH) and LHRH analogs in rat granulosa cells. *Endocrinology* **110**, 146–152.

Clayton, R.N. & Huhtaniemi, I.T. (1982) Absence of gonadotrophin-releasing hormone receptors in human gonadal tissue. *Nature, Lond.* **299**, 56–58.

Clayton, R.N., Shakespear, R.A., Duncan, J.A. & Marshall, J.C. (1979) Luteinizing hormone-releasing hormone inactivation by purified pituitary plasma membranes: effects on receptor-binding studies. *Endocrinology* **104**, 1484–1494.

Conn, P.M., McArdle, C.A., Andrews, W.V. & Huckle, W.R. (1987) The molecular basis of gonadotrophin-releasing hormone (GnRH) action in the pituitary gonadotrope. *Biol. Reprod.* **36**, 17–35.

Currie, A.J., Fraser, H.M. & Sharpe, R.M. (1981) Human placental receptors for luteinizing hormone releasing hormone. *Biochem. Biophys. Res. Commun.* **99**, 332–338.

Davis, J.S., West, L.A. & Farese, R.V. (1986) Gonadotropin-releasing hormone (GnRH) rapidly stimulates the formation of inositol phosphates and diacyglycerol in rat granulosa cells: further evidence for the involvement of Ca^{2+} and protein kinase C in the action of GnRH. *Endocrinology* **118**, 2561–2571.

Dorrington, J.H. & Skinner, M.K. (1986) Cytodifferentiation of granulosa cells induced by gonadotropin-releasing hormone promotes fibronectin secretion. *Endocrinology* **118**, 2065–2071.

Dorrington, J.H., McKeracher, H.L., Chan, A & Gore-Langton, R.E. (1985) Luteinizing hormone-releasing hormone independently stimulates cytodifferentiation of granulosa cells. In *Hormonal Control of the Hypothalamo-Pituitary-Gonadal Axis*, pp. 467–478. Eds K. W. McKerns & Z. Naor. Plenum Press, London.

Eckstein, N., Eshel, A., Eli, Y., Ayalon, D. & Naor, Z. (1986) Calcium-dependent actions of gonadotropin-releasing hormone agonist and luteinizing hormone upon cyclic AMP and progesterone production in rat ovarian granulosa cells. *Molec. cell. Endocrinol.* **47**, 91–98.

Eidne, K.A., Harris, N.S., Millar, R.P. & Wilcox, J. (1987) GnRH immunoreactivity and GnRH mRNA in two human breast cancer cell lines MDA-MB-231 and ZR-75-1. *Endocrinology* **120** (Suppl.), 184, Abstr. 653.

Fraser, H.M., Sharpe, R.M. & Popkin, R.M. (1984) Direct stimulatory actions of LHRH on the ovary and testis. In *LHRH and its Analogs: a New Class of Contraceptive and Therapeutic Agents*, pp. 181–195. Eds B. H. Vickery, J. J. Nestor & E. S. E. Hafez. MTP Press, Lancaster.

Fraser, H.M., Bramley, T.A., Miller, W.R. & Sharpe, R.M. (1986) Extra-pituitary actions of LHRH analogues in tissues of the human female and investigation of the existence and function of LHRH-like peptides. In *Gonadotropin Down-Regulation in Gynecological Practice*, pp. 29–54. Eds R. Rolland, D. R. Chadha & W. N. P. Willemsen. Alan R. Liss Inc, New York.

Gautron, J.P., Pattou, E. & Kordon, C. (1981) Occurrence of higher molecular forms of LHRH in fractionated extracts from rat hypothalamus, cortex and placenta. *Molec. cell. Endocrinol.* **24**, 1–15.

Gibbons, J.M., Mitnik, M. & Chieffo, V. (1975) *In vitro* biosynthesis of TSH- and LH-releasing factors by the human placenta. *Am. J. Obstet. Gynecol.* **121**, 127–132.

Hedger, M.P., Robertson, D.M. & de Kretser, D.M. (1987) LHRH and "LHRH-like" factors in the male reproductive tract. In *LHRH and its Analogs: Contraceptive and Therapeutic Applications*, pp. 141–160. Eds B. H. Vickery & J. J. Nestor. MTP Press, Lancaster.

Hsueh, A.J.W. & Jones, P.B.C. (1981) Extrapituitary actions of gonadotropin-releasing hormone. *Endocr. Rev.* **2**, 437–461.

Hsueh, A.J.W. & Jones, P.B.C. (1982) Regulation of ovarian granulosa and luteal cell functions by gonadotropin releasing hormone and its antagonist. In *Intraovarian Control Mechanisms*, pp. 223–262. Eds C. P. Channing & S. J. Segal. Plenum Press, London.

212   T. A. Bramley

Iwashita, M. & Catt, K.J. (1984) Photoaffinity labeling of pituitary and gonadal receptors for gonadotropin-releasing hormone. *Endocrinology* 117, 738–746.

Iwashita, M., Evans, M.I. & Catt, K.J. (1986) Characterization of a gonadotropin-releasing hormone receptor site in term placenta and chorionic villi. *J. clin. Endocr. Metab.* 62, 127–133.

King, J.A. & Millar, R.P. (1987) Phylogenetic diversity of LHRH. In *LHRH and its Analogs: Contraceptive and Therapeutic Applications*, Part 2, pp. 53–73. Eds B. H. Vickery & J. J. Nestor. MTP Press, Lancaster.

Knecht, M. & Catt, K.J. (1983) Epidermal growth factor and gonadotropin-releasing hormone inhibit cyclic AMP-dependent luteinizing hormone receptor formation in ovarian granulosa cells. *J. cell. Biochem.* 21, 209–217.

Knecht, M., Amsterdam, A. & Catt, K.J. (1982) Inhibition of granulosa cell differentiation by gonadotropin-releasing hormone. *Endocrinology* 110, 865–872.

Knecht, M., Ranta, T., Naor, Z. & Catt, K.J. (1983a) Direct effects of GnRH on the ovary. In *Factors Regulating Ovarian Function*, pp. 225–243. Eds G. S. Greenwald & P. F. Terranova. Raven Press, New York.

Knecht, M., Ranta, T., Katz, M.S. & Catt, K.J. (1983b) Regulation of adenylate cyclase activity by follicle-stimulating hormone and a gonadotropin-releasing hormone agonist in cultured rat granulosa cells. *Endocrinology* 112, 1247–1255.

Lamberts, S.W.J., Timmers, J.M., Oosterom, R., Verleun, T., Rommerts, F.F.G. & de Jong, F.H. (1982) Testosterone secretion by cultured arrhenoblastoma cells: suppression by a luteinizing hormone-releasing hormone agonist. *J. clin. Endocr. Metab.* 54, 450–454.

Massicotte, J., Borgus, J.-P., Lachance, R. & Labrie, F. (1981) Inhibition of HCG-induced cyclic AMP accumulation and steroidogenesis in rat luteal cells by an LHRH agonist. *J. Steroid Biochem.* 14, 239–242.

Mathialagan, N. & Rao, A.J. (1986) Gonadotropin releasing hormone in first trimester human placenta: isolation, partial characterisation and *in vivo* biosynthesis. *J. Biosci.* 10, 429–441.

Millar, R.P., Wormald, P.J. & Milton, R.C. de L. (1986) Stimulation of gonadotropin release by a non-GnRH peptide sequence of the GnRH precursor. *Science, N.Y.* 232, 68–70.

Milton, R.C. de L., Wormald, P.J., Brandt, W. & Millar, R.P. (1986) The delineation of a decapeptide gonadotropin-releasing sequence in the carboxyterminal extension of the human gonadotropin-releasing hormone precursor. *J. biol. Chem.* 261, 16990–16997.

Minaguchi, H., Mori, J. & Vemura, T. (1984) Partial isolation of gonadotrophin-releasing hormone (GnRH)-like substances from the porcine ovary. In *Proc. 7th Int. Congr. Endocr.* (Pittsburgh), Abstr 1560. Excerpta Medica, Amsterdam.

Minegishi, T., Wang, J. & Leung, P.C.K. (1987) Luteinizing hormone-releasing hormone (LHRH)-induced arachidonic acid release in rat granulosa cells; role of calcium and protein kinase C. *FEBS Lett.* 214, 139–142.

Morgan, R.O., Chang, J.P. & Catt, K.J. (1987) Novel aspects of gonadotropin-releasing hormone action on inositol polyphosphate metabolism in cultured pituitary gonadotrophs. *J. biol. Chem.* 262, 1166–1171.

Naor, Z. (1986) Phosphoinositide turnover, Ca²⁺

mobilization, protein kinase C activation and leukotriene action in pituitary signal transduction: effect of gonadotropin releasing hormone. *Adv. Prostagl. Thrombox. & Leukotriene Res.* 16, 225–234.

Naor, Z. & Childs, G.V. (1985) Binding and activation of gonadotropin-releasing hormone receptors in pituitary and gonadal cells. *Int. Rev. Cytol.* 103, 147–187

Naor, Z., Molcho, J., Zilberstein, M. & Zakut, H. (1985) Phospholipid turnover in gonadotropin-releasing hormone target cells: comparative studies. In *Hormonal Control of the Hypothalamo-Pituitary-Gonadal Axis*, pp. 493–508. Eds K. W. McKerns & Z. Naor. Plenum Press, London.

Nikolics, K., Mason, A.J., Szonyi, E., Ramachandran, J. & Seeburg, P.H. (1985) A prolactin-inhibiting factor within the precursor for human gonadotropin-releasing hormone. *Nature, Lond.* 316, 511–517.

Nowak, R.A., Wiseman, B.S. & Bahr, J.M. (1984) Identification of a gonadotropin-releasing hormone-like factor in the rabbit fetal placenta. *Biol. Reprod.* 31, 67–75.

Popkin, R., Bramley, T.A., Currie, A., Shaw, R.W., Baird, D.T. & Fraser, H.M. (1983) Specific binding of luteinizing hormone releasing hormone to human luteal tissue. *Biochem. Biophys. Res. Commun.* 114, 750–756.

Popkin, R.M., Bramley, T.A., Currie, A., Sharpe, R.M. & Fraser, H.M. (1985) Binding sites for LHRH in the human—does LH-RH exert extrapituitary actions in man? In *LHRH and its Analogues: Fertility and Antifertility Aspects*, pp. 61–73. Eds M. Schmidt-Gollwitzer & M. Schley. Walter de Gruyter, Berlin.

Ranta, T., Knecht, M., Baukal, A.J., Korhonen, M. & Catt, K.J. (1984) GnRH agonist-induced inhibitory and stimulatory effects during ovarian follicular maturation. *Molec. cell. Endocrinol.*, 35, 55–63.

Reddy, P.V., Azhar, S. & Menon, K.M.J. (1980) Multiple inhibitory actions of luteinizing hormone-releasing hormone agonist on luteinizing hormone/human chorionic gonadotropin receptor-mediated ovarian responses. *Endocrinology* 107, 930–936.

Reeves, J.J., Seguin, C., Lefebvre, F.-A., Kelly, P.A. & Labrie, F. (1980) Similar luteinizing hormone-releasing hormone binding sites in rat anterior pituitary and ovary. *Proc. natn. Acad. Sci. U.S.A.* 77, 5567–5571.

Richardson, M.C., Hirji, M.R., Thompson, A.D. & Masson, G.M. (1984) Effect of a long-acting analogue of LH releasing hormone on human and rat corpora lutea. *J. Endocr.* 101, 163–168./

Rippel, R.M. & Johnson, E.S. (1976) Inhibition of HCG-induced ovarian and uterine weight augmentation in the immature rat by analogs of GnRH. *Proc. Soc. exp. Biol. Med.* 152, 432–436.

Seeburg, P.H. & Adelman, J.P. (1984) Characterisation of cDNA for precursor of human luteinizing hormone releasing hormone. *Nature, Lond.* 311, 666–668.

Seeburg, P.H., Mason, A.J., Stewart, T.A. & Nikolics, K. (1987) The mammalian GnRH gene and its pivotal role in reproduction. *Recent Prog. Horm. Res.* 43, 69–98.

Sharpe, R.M. (1984) Intragonadal hormones. *Biblphy Reprod.* 44(6), C1–C16.

Siler-Khodr, T.M. (1987) Placental LHRH-like activity. In *LHRH and its Analogs: Contraceptive and Thera-*

peutic Applications, part 2, pp. 161–175. Eds B. H. Vickery & J. J. Nestor. MTP Press, Lancaster.

Siler-Khodr, T.M. & Khodr, G.S. (1978) Content of luteinizing hormone-releasing factor in the human placenta. *Am. J. Obstet. Gynecol.* **130**, 216–219.

Siler-Khodr, T.M., Khodr, G.S. & Valenzuela, G. (1984) Immunoreactive gonadotropin-releasing hormone level in maternal circulation throughout pregnancy. *Am. J. Obstet. Gynecol.* **150**, 376–379.

Siler-Khodr, T.M., Khodr, G.S., Valenzuela, G. & Rhode, J. (1986a) Gonadotropin-releasing hormone effects on placental hormones during gestation. 1. Alpha-human chorionic gonadotropin, human chorionic gonadotropin and human chorionic sommato-mammotropin. *Biol. Reprod.* **34**, 245–254.

Siler-Khodr, T.M., Khodr, G.S., Valenzuela, G. & Rhode, J. (1986b) Gonadotropin-releasing hormone effects on placental hormones during gestation. II. Progesterone, estrone, estradiol and estriol. *Biol. Reprod.* **34**, 255–264.

Siler-Khodr, T.M., Khodr, G.S., Valenzuela, G., Harper, M.J.K. & Rhode, J. (1986c) Gonadotropin-releasing hormone effects on placental hormones during gestation. III. Prostaglandin E, prostaglandin F, and 13,14-dihydro-15-keto-prostaglandin F. *Biol. Reprod.* **35**, 312–319.

Siler-Khodr, T.M., Khodr, G.S., Rhode, J., Vickery, B.H. & Nestor, J.J., Jr. (1987) Gestational age-related inhibition of placental hCG, αhCG and steroid hormone release *in vitro* by a GnRH antagonist. *Placenta* **8**, 1–14.

Tan, G.J.S. & Biggs, J.S.G. (1983) Absence of effect of LHRH on progesterone production by human luteal cells *in vitro*. *J. Reprod. Fert.* **67**, 411–413.

Tan, L. & Rousseau, P. (1982) The chemical identity of the immunoreactive LHRH-like peptide biosynthesized in the human placenta. *Biochem. Biophys. Res. Commun.* **109**, 1061–1071.

Tureck, R.W., Mastroianni, L., Blasco, L. & Strauss, J.F. (1982) Inhibition of human granulosa cell progesterone secretion by a gonadotropin-releasing hormone agonist. *J. clin. Endocr. Metab.* **54**, 1078–1080.

Wang, J. & Leung, P.C.K. (1987) Role of protein kinase C in luteinizing hormone-releasing hormone (LHRH)-stimulated progesterone production in rat granulosa cells. *Biochem. Biophys. Res. Commun.* **146**, 939–944

Williams, A.T. & Behrman, H.R. (1983) Paracrine regulation of the ovary by gonadotropin releasing hormone and other peptides. *Semin. Reprod. Endocr.* **1**, 269–277.

Ying, S.-Y., Ling, N., Bohlen, P. & Guillemin, R. (1981) Gonadocrinins: peptides in ovarian follicular fluid stimulating the secretion of pituitary gonadotropins. *Endocrinology* **108**, 1206–1215.

PEPTIDES AND PROSTAGLANDINS

Chairmen

M. Hunzicker-Dunn
U. Zor

J. Reprod. Fert., Suppl. 37 (1989), 215–223

In-vivo effect of prostaglandin F-2α treatment on secretory granules in the corpus luteum of the late pregnant cow

M. J. Fields*, W. Dubois§, K. H. Brackett*, R. F. Faulkner*, B. A. Ball†¶,
J. M. Martin†, M. Drost† and P. A. Fields‡

*Departments of *Animal Science and †Reproduction, University of Florida, Gainesville,
Florida 32611, U.S.A. and ‡Department of Anatomy, University of South Alabama, Mobile,
Alabama 36688, U.S.A.*

Summary. Electron microscopy evaluation indicated that the large luteal cells from control (saline-injected) cows were morphologically similar: 42–72% of the large luteal cells, in which the nucleus was present in the tissue section, contained secretory granules (100–300 nm diameter). From cell to cell, clustering of granules was observed in various regions of the cell cytoplasm, ranging from locations next to the nucleus to those next to the cell membrane where exocytosis was noted. The large mitochondria containing dense inclusions (500–1800 nm diameter) were uniformly distributed throughout the cytoplasm of 98% of the large luteal cells.

The morphology of large luteal cells at 2·5 and 5 min after PGF-2α treatment (25 mg) was similar to that of saline controls. However, at 15 and 30 min after PGF-2α the secretory granules were observed primarily at the cell periphery and at 15 min only 22% of the large luteal cells contained secretory granules. Exocytosis involving fusion of the granule and cell membrane was more evident at this time. At 60 min after PGF-2α few large luteal cells (0·5%) were observed with small granules. We suggest that the secretory granules represent those organelles responsible for packaging secretory proteins for transport out of the cell, and PGF-2α is an effector that will initiate cell depletion of these granules and their contents.

Keywords: secretory granules; mitochondria; pregnancy; cows; CL; PGF-2α

Introduction

Secretory granules, 100–300 nm in diameter, have been well documented in the corpus luteum of the cow (Singh, 1975; Gemmell & Stacy, 1979; Parry *et al.*, 1980; Fields *et al.*, 1985). Neurophysin (Fields, M. J., & Fields, 1986) and oxytocin (unpublished) have been localized in luteal secretory granules of the non-pregnant cow, but in the pregnant cow the content of secretory granules has not been identified. These granules have been proposed to contain relaxin since the hormone relaxin has been isolated from and immunohistochemically localized at the light microscopy level in the corpora lutea of late-pregnant cows (Fields *et al.*, 1980).

Secretory granules have also been proposed to contain progesterone since there is a close relationship between the population of luteal granules and secretion of progesterone in the cow (Quirk *et al.*, 1979). However, the failure to localize progesterone or a progesterone-binding protein in secretory granules, and the inability to release progesterone from these granules, led Rice *et al.*

---

§Present address: Department of Biology, Boston University, Boston, MA 02215, U.S.A.
¶Present address: New York State College of Veterinary Medicine, Cornell University, Ithaca, New York 14853, U.S.A.

(1986) to the conclusion that granule-associated progesterone in the ewe represented a non-specific association with granule membranes, and not the specific sequestering of a protein-bound progesterone into secretory granules. The association of progesterone secretion and granule release may reflect independent, but simultaneous biochemical and morphological events.

The corpus luteum of pregnancy in cows reportedly contains a second population of large membrane bound organelles 500–1800 nm in diameter (Sorenson & Singh, 1973; Singh, 1975; Fields *et al.*, 1985; Weber *et al.*, 1987). These organelles were believed to be formed by an increase of electron-dense material in the mitochondria during the last third of pregnancy (Fields *et al.*, 1985). Although the secretory granules are readily observed to undergo exocytosis there is a paucity of information on the large mitochondrial inclusions. The present study was designed to test the effects of PGF-2α on secretory granules and large mitochondria containing inclusions in the preparturient cow.

Materials and Methods

Angus cows (N = 20) exposed to a bull during a 70-day breeding season were treated within 1 or 2 weeks of parturition, as determined by rectal palpation of the reproductive tract. Using aseptic procedures, the reproductive tract was exposed and the ovarian pedicle ipsilateral to the corpus luteum was placed in the jaws of a large haemostatic forceps (Codman and Shurtleff Inc, Randolph, MA) without occluding its vascular supply. Ten animals were each treated with a 5-ml injection, via a jugular catheter, of 25 mg PGF-2α (Lutalyse, The Upjohn Co., Kalamazoo, MI) and ten animals each with 5 ml saline (0·15 M-NaCl, controls). At 2·5, 5, 15, 30 or 60 min after injection, the blood supply was clamped and the ovary removed.

A section from the centre of the corpus luteum was cut into fine pieces with a razor blade and fixed in 1% glutaraldehyde for processing for electron microscopy (EM) as described by Fields *et al.* (1985). From each sample, 100 cells with an observable nucleus were evaluated for the following characteristics: (1) secretory granule location, (2) percentage of cells containing secretory granules, (3) percentage of cells in which the granules were exocytosed at a blood vessel site, and (4) percentage of cells containing large mitochondria containing dense inclusions. Immunocytochemical studies evaluated the granules for the localization of relaxin, oxytocin and neurophysin as previously described (Fields, P. A. & Fields, 1985; Fields, M. J. & Fields, 1986).

Results

There were no observable ultrastructural differences for corpora lutea excised at the different times after saline treatment. The ultrastructure of small and large luteal cells observed in the periparturient cow in this study agrees with that previously described by Fields *et al.* (1985). There were two populations of electron-dense membrane-bound organelles in the large luteal cell described as small secretory granules (100–300 nm in diameter (Fig. 1a)), and large mitochondria, 500–1800 nm in diameter, with inclusions in their inner space (Figs 1b, 2). This latter material completely filled the inner areas of many mitochondria such that the cristae were not observable and 98% of the large luteal cells from saline- and PGF-2α-treated animals contained this type of mitochondrion (Table 1).

Corpora lutea removed at 2·5 and 5 min after PGF-2α treatment were similar to the saline controls. At least 50–72% of the large luteal cells from these saline- and PGF-2α-treated animals contained secretory granules (Table 1).

Only a few luteal cells contained granules in the paranuclear region of the 15 and 30 min PGF-2α-treated cows. However, secretory granules were observed around the cell periphery (Fig. 3). In addition, granules were observed more readily in canaliculi and fused with the cell membrane during exocytosis (Fig. 4). Only 23% of these large luteal cells from the 15 min PGF-2α-treated cows contained the secretory granules. At 30 min after PGF-2α the luteal cells of 1 cow were depleted of secretory granules (Table 1).

Less than 1% of the large luteal cells from the 60 min PGF-2α-treated cows contained small granules (Table 1; Fig. 5). As previously reported (Fields *et al.*, 1987) a few granules were observed occasionally at the cell periphery. As in all previous treatment times, there was no observed effect of

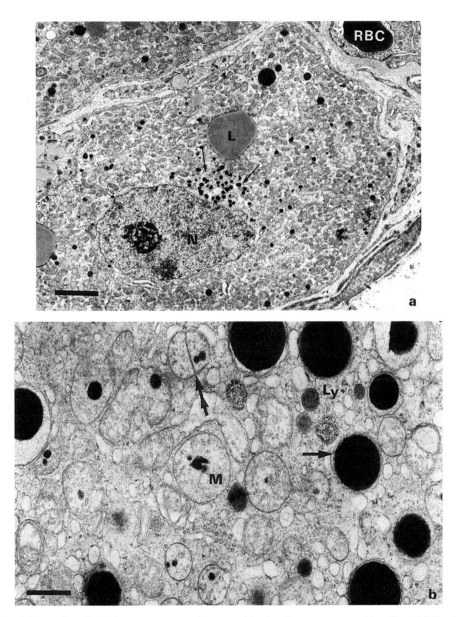

Fig. 1. Large luteal cell from a preparturient cow 15 min after treatment with saline. (**a**) Small granules are formed in a cluster next to the nucleus (N) on the nuclear side of the cell facing a blood vessel. RBC = red blood cell, L = lipid. ×8160. Bar = 2·6 μm. (**b**) Large numbers of mitochondria (M) accumulate electron-dense material (arrow) during late pregnancy. The mitochondrial cristae are evident in the early stages of the accumulation of this dense material. One mitochondrion (double arrow) appears to be in the process of dividing. ×20 000. Bar = 1·0 μm.

PGF-2α on the large electron-dense mitochondria (Fig. 5). The content of luteal secretory granules in the pregnant cow still remains a mystery, as we were unable to localize immunocytochemically oxytocin, neurophysin or relaxin within this organelle.

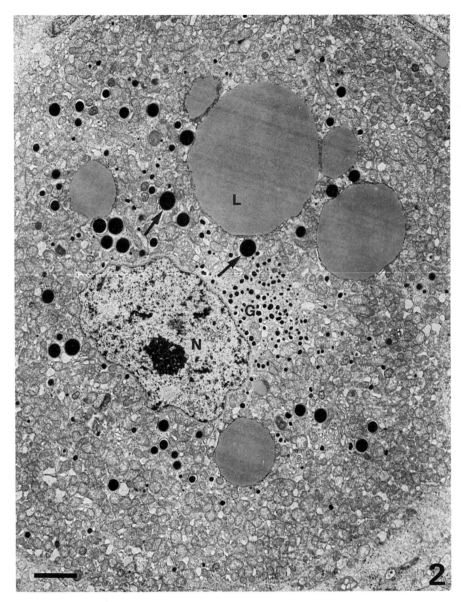

Fig. 2. A large luteal cell from a preparturient cow 5 min after treatment with PGF-2α. There were no observed morphological differences between the PGF-2α- and saline-treated cows at 5 min. Secretory granules (G) are typically found clustered together in an area devoid of mitochondria whereas the large granules (arrows) are evenly distributed throughout the cell. L = lipid. × 7500. Bar = 2·7 μm.

Discussion

The large luteal cells from the pregnant cow (Days 45–280) contain small secretory granules (100–300 nm diameter) that are not diffusely scattered throughout the cell cytoplasm, but are arranged in distinct clusters (Fields *et al.*, 1985; Chegini & Rao, 1987). The site within the cell of these polarized

Table 1. The effects of saline and PGF-2α on the percentage of large luteal cells containing the secretory granules and large electron-dense mitochondrial inclusions

Treatment* (min)	Animal no.	%Large cells† with:	
		Secretory granules	Mitochondrial inclusions
Saline			
2·5	150	54	98
	295	72	97
5·0	07	53	99
	364	52	97
15·0	429	52	98
	229/6	42	98
30·0	91	64	97
	78/4	55	99
60·0	536	62	97
	899	45	100
PGF-2α			
2·5	44/5	65	99
	739	55	99
5·0	15/2	58	98
	834	50	97
15·0	02	22	99
	711	23	98
30·0	793	1	97
	810	52	98
60·0	653	1	98
	845	0	98

*Time after treatment with saline or PGF-2α that the corpus luteum was removed.
†Only cells in which the nucleus was observed were evaluated.

clusters of granules ranged from a paranuclear to a plasma membrane location on the side of the cell towards a blood vessel. This distribution pattern indicates that each cell releases its granule content in a non-synchronous manner with other luteal cells. However, there seems to be a synchronous release of granules within a given cell since the entire cluster was located at the cell periphery during exocytosis. This lack of granule clustering in another ruminant, the ewe (Fields & Fields, 1986), with a similar luteal/uterine relationship, leaves the significance and reason for this phenomenon unexplained.

Treatment with PGF-2α resulted in a rapid (15 min) movement of secretory granules out of approximately 50% of the cells containing these granules. *In vivo*, PGF-2α treatment has previously been shown to deplete the large luteal cell of secretory granules within 1 h in non-pregnant (Heath *et al.*, 1983) and pregnant (Fields *et al.*, 1987) cows. Likewise, in the non-pregnant ewe PGF-2α-induced degranulation was reportedly obtained within 30 min of treatment (Corteel, 1975). Similar findings were reported by Chegini & Rao (1987) for the 3–4-month-pregnant cow in which in-vitro incubation of luteal slices with PGF-2α resulted in the exocytosis of clusters of secretory granules within about 2 h of treatment.

Peptide hormones are synthesized in a larger prohormone form, packaged in secretory granules where they undergo post-translational modification, and are subsequently released into the

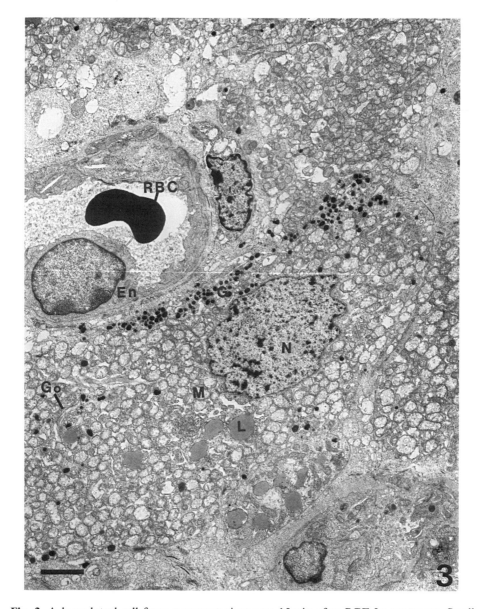

Fig. 3. A large luteal cell from a preparturient cow 15 min after PGF-2α treatment. Small granules (G) are shown palisading the cell membrane adjacent to a blood vessel. RBC = red blood cell, En = endothelial cell, N = nucleus, M = mitochondria, L = lipid and Go = Golgi complex. × 7500. Bar = 2·7 μm.

external environment of the cells via exocytosis. Consistent with PGF-2α-induced exocytosis of granules containing peptide hormones is the PGF-2α-induced release of relaxin in the pregnant pig (Nara *et al.*, 1982), pregnant rat (Gordon & Sherwood, 1983), and of oxytocin in the non-pregnant cow (Schallenberger *et al.*, 1984) and ewe (Flint & Sheldrick, 1982). However, using a pig relaxin radioimmunoassay we were unable to detect any relaxin immunoactivity in plasma taken before, during, and after PGF-2α injection.

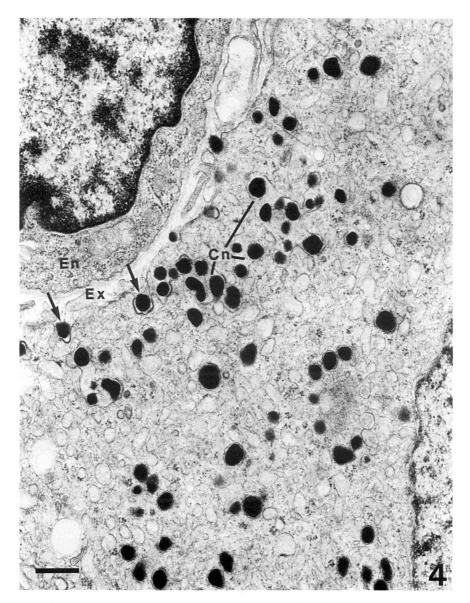

Fig. 4. A large luteal cell from a preparturient cow 30 min after PGF-2α treatment. Numerous small granules have fused with the cell membrane during exocytosis (arrows) whereas others are observed in canaliculi (Cn) which open into the extracellular space (Ex). En = endothelial cell. ×45 000. Bar = 4·4 μm.

No peptide hormone has been localized in the granules of the pregnant cow. The inability to detect relaxin in the granules from this study may reflect the poor specificity of the heterologous relaxin antiserum used for EM localization, low levels of bovine relaxin, and/or loss of the antigen during EM fixation. The absence of an oxytocin–neurophysin specific luteal mRNA in the pregnant cow (Ivell *et al.*, 1985; Fehr *et al.*, 1987) explains why these hormones are not immunohistochemically localized during pregnancy. The implication of these findings is that the content of secretory

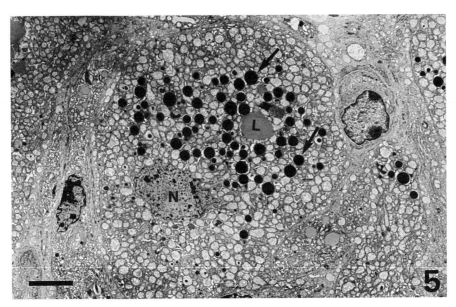

Fig. 5. Large luteal cell from a PGF-2α-treated preparturient cow in which there is a typical absence of small granules within 60 min of treatment. The large granules (arrows), although numerous, did not appear to be influenced by the PGF-2α treatment. L = lipid, N = nucleus. × 4180. Bar = 4·8 μm.

granules of the non-pregnant and pregnant cow differ as might be expected for diverging functions, i.e. new opportunity for ovulation versus maintenance of a pregnancy.

Accompanying the appearance of cytoplasmic lipid droplets during late pregnancy in the cow are electron-dense mitochondrial inclusions. These mitochondria appear distributed randomly throughout the cytoplasm and take on the appearance of large granules. Administration of PGF-2α had no effect within 1 h on the cellular distribution of these mitochondria or the apparent number of large luteal cells with mitochondria containing dense inclusions.

Several reports indicate mitochondrial inclusions are consistent with a system deficient in LH (Schwarz & Merker, 1965; Murakami & Tonutti, 1966; Chung & Hamilton, 1976). Although the content of luteal mitochondrial inclusions is unknown, the accumulation of osmiophilic substances in the matrix appears to be associated with a declining functional activity of the gland.

There is apparently a dichotomy regarding the corpus luteum of late pregnancy, with evidence of robust luteal progesterone production on the one hand, and on the other a corpus luteum in a regressed state evidenced by cytoplasmic lipid accumulation, mitochondrial inclusions and non-responsiveness to LH (Pimental *et al.*, 1986; Weber *et al.*, 1987). Although this corpus luteum has been described as regressing, a more appropriate description may be its dynamic 'involuting' nature, since it has a continual presence of secretory granules that are maintained throughout pregnancy (Fields *et al.*, 1985).

We thank Barbara M. Hyde and Dawn M. Weber for technical assistance in processing the luteal tissue; Jan Lauer and Harry H. Potter for preparation of the manuscript; and Dr Donald H. Barron for help and translation of the German papers. Supported by Grants from the National Science Foundation (PCM 8110062 and 8409304) and the National Institute of Health (RO1 HD 15773 and 18075). Florida Agriculture Experiment Station Journal Series No. 7884.

References

Chegini, N. & Rao, C.V. (1987) Dynamics of nuclear associated granules in bovine luteal cells after treatment in vitro with prostaglandin $F_{2α}$. *Endocrinology* **121**, 1870–1878.

Chung, K.W. & Hamilton, J.B. (1976) Further observations on the fine structure of Leydig cells in the testes of male pseudohermaphrodite rats. *J. Ultrastruct. Res.* **54**, 68–75.

Corteel, M. (1975) Luteolysis induced by prostaglandin $F_{2α}$ compared with natural luteolysis in the ewe. *Annls Biol. anim. Biochim. Biophys.* **15**, 175–180.

Fehr, S., Ivell, R., Koll, R., Schams, D., Fields, M.J. & Richter, D. (1987) Expression of the oxytocin gene in the large cells of the bovine corpus luteum. *FEBS Lett.* **210**, 45–50.

Fields, M.J. & Fields, P.A. (1986) Luteal neurophysin in the nonpregnant cow and ewe: immunocytochemical localization in membrane-bounded secretory granules of the large luteal cell. *Endocrinology* **118**, 1723–1725.

Fields, M.J. & Fields, P.A., Castro-Hernandez, A. & Larkin, L.H. (1980) Evidence for relaxin in corpora lutea of late pregnant cows. *Endocrinology* **107**, 869–876.

Fields, M.J., Dubois, W. & Fields, P.A. (1985) Dynamic features of luteal secretory granules: ultrastructural changes during the course of pregnancy in the cow. *Endocrinology* **117**, 1675–1682.

Fields, M.J., Dubois, W., Ball, B., Drost, M. & Fields, P.A. (1987) The effect of prostaglandin $F_{2α}$ on mitochondrial electron dense inclusions and secretory granules of the bovine large cell during late pregnancy. *Adv. exp. Med. Biol.* **219**, 677–681.

Fields, P.A. & Fields, M.J. (1985) Ultrastructural localization of relaxin in corpora lutea of nonpregnant, pseudopregnant and pregnant pigs. *Biol. Reprod.* **32**, 1169–1179.

Flint, A.P.F. & Sheldrick, E.L. (1982) Ovarian secretion of oxytocin is stimulated by prostaglandin. *Nature, Lond.* **297**, 587–588.

Gemmell, R.T. & Stacy, B.D. (1979) Ultrastructural study of granules in corpora lutea of several mammalian species. *Am. J. Anat.* **155**, 1–14.

Gordon, W.L. & Sherwood, O.D. (1983) Evidence for a role of prostaglandins in the antepartum release of relaxin in the pregnant rat. *Biol. Reprod.* **28**, 154–160.

Heath, E., Weinstein, P., Merritt, B., Shanks, R. & Hixon, J. (1983) Effects of prostaglandins on the bovine corpus luteum: granules, lipid inclusions and progesterone secretion. *Biol. Reprod.* **29**, 977–985.

Ivell, R., Brackett, K., Fields, M.J. & Richter, D. (1985) Ovulation triggers oxytocin gene expression in the bovine ovary. *FEBS Lett.* **190**, 263–267.

Murakami, V.M. & Tonutti, E. (1966) Submikroskopische veranderungen der Leydig-zellen des rattenhodens nach behandlung mit ostrogenen und nach gonadotropinzufuhr. *Endokrinologie* **50**, 231–250.

Nara, B.S., Ball, G.D., Rutherford, J.E., Sherwood, O.D. & First, N.L. (1982) Release of relaxin by a nonluteolytic dose of prostaglandin $F_{2α}$ in pregnant swine. *Biol. Reprod.* **27**, 1190–1195.

Parry, D.M. Willcox, D.L. & Thorburn, G.D. (1980) Ultrastructural and cytochemical study of the bovine corpus luteum. *J. Reprod. Fert.* **60**, 349–357.

Pimentel, S.M., Pimentel, C.A., Weston, P.G., Hixon, J.E. & Wagner, W.C. (1986) Progesterone secretion by the bovine corpora lutea to steroidogenic stimuli at two stages of gestation. *Am. J. vet. Res.* **47**, 1967–1971.

Quirk, S.J., Willcox, D.L., Parry, D.M. & Thorburn, G.D. (1979) Subcellular localization of progesterone in the bovine corpus luteum: a biochemical, morphological and cytochemical investigation. *Biol. Reprod.* **20**, 1133–1145.

Rice, G.E., Jenkin, G. & Thorburn, G.D. (1986) Comparison of particle-associated progesterone and oxytocin in the ovine corpus luteum. *J. Endocr.* **108**, 109–116.

Schallenberger, E., Schams, D., Bullermann, B. & Walters, D.L. (1984) Pulsatile secretion of gonadotrophins, ovarian steroids and ovarian oxytocin during prostaglandin-induced regression of the corpus luteum in the cow. *J. Reprod. Fert.* **71**, 493–501.

Schwarz, W. & Merker, H.J. (1965) Die hodenzwischenzellen der ratte nach hypophysektomie und nach behandlung mit choriongonadotropin und amphenon B. *Z. Zellforsch, mikrosk. Anat.* **65**, 272–284.

Singh, U.B. (1975) Structural changes in the granulosa lutein cells of pregnant cows between 61 and 245 days. *Acta anat.* **93**, 447–457.

Sorenson, V.W. & Singh, U.B. (1973) On mitochondrial inclusions in granulosa lutein cells of pregnant cows. *Experientia* **29**, 592–593.

Weber, D.M., Fields, P.A., Romrell, L.J., Tumwasorn, S., Ball, B.A., Drost, M. & Fields, M.J. (1987) Functional differences between small and large luteal cells of the late-pregnant vs nonpregnant cow. *Biol. Reprod.* **37**, 685–697.

J. Reprod. Fert., Suppl. **37** (1989), 225–231

Printed in Great Britain
© 1989 Journals of Reproduction & Fertility Ltd

Ovarian peptides in the cow and sheep

D. Schams

*Lehrstuhl für Physiologie der Fortpflanzung und Laktation, Technische Universität München,
8050 Freising-Weihenstephan, Federal Republic of Germany*

Summary. There are indications that ovarian oxytocin is involved in luteolysis and the endometrium may play a key role for the events of luteolysis. A certain priming period with progesterone is a prerequisite for the induction of luteolysis. Treatment of heifers with progesterone for 4 days beginning after the LH surge shortens the oestrous cycle length significantly. Besides an involvement in luteolysis, there are indications for an intraovarian function of oxytocin influencing steroidogenesis by inhibition of progesterone secretion. Growth factors have been identified in ovarian tissue and insulin-like growth factor-I has a very potent effect on bovine granulosa cell function. Growth factors may be involved in the growth and differentiation of follicles.

Keywords: ovary; peptides; oxytocin; growth factors; cow; sheep

Introduction

The ovary is known as a classical gland for the synthesis of steroid hormones and, as shown more recently, for prostaglandins. The central role of gonadotrophins in the regulation of ovarian function is well established. The variable fate of ovarian target cells to comparable gonadotrophin stimulation suggests the existence of additional intraovarian mechanisms. Intraovarian peptides may also have a potential for local modulation of follicular development and corpus luteum function. During the past few years evidence has accumulated that the ovary is able to produce a number of peptides which may play roles in regulation of ovarian function. There is evidence for the existence of an oocyte maturation inhibitor, luteinization inhibitor, FSH receptor binding inhibitor and gonadocrinin (GnRH-like material) in the follicular fluid. There is also an LH/hCG receptor binding inhibitor in luteal tissue and adrenocorticotrophin hormone-like material in ovarian extracts. The structure of all these factors and their physiological roles still need to be defined. There is further evidence that the corpus luteum contains large amounts of β-endorphin, α-neoendorphin/dynorphin A. Neurotransmitters (e.g. vasointestinal peptide (VIP)) are also found in ovarian tissue. Inhibin, known for over 50 years, became a reality when several laboratories reported its purification to homogeneity and others reported complementary deoxynucleic acid (cDNA) coding for the messenger ribonucleic acid (mRNA) of ovarian inhibin. Inhibin specifically suppresses secretion of FSH (follicle-stimulating hormone) by the pituitary gland without affecting release of LH (luteinizing hormone). Inhibin is a glycoprotein hormone consisting of two dissimilar, disulphide-linked subunits having a molecular weight of about 32 000 (for review see Burger *et al.*, 1988). Relaxin, another long known ovarian peptide, consists of two chains (A and B) covalently linked by two interchain disulphide bonds having a molecular weight of 6000. It is produced in luteal cells. Our knowledge of relaxin in ruminants is rather limited due to the lack of specific and sensitive assays. Vasopressin has been extracted from corpora lutea (CL) of non-pregnant cows (Wathes *et al.*, 1983a, 1984) and the mRNA has been demonstrated (Ivell & Richter, 1984).

Ovarian oxytocin

The presence of oxytocin has been confirmed in sheep and cow ovaries (for review Wathes *et al.*, 1983b; Schams, 1987). Oxytocin is localized in large luteal cells which seem not be be under the direct control of gonadotrophins. Luteinization appears to be the main trigger for production of ovarian oxytocin. Synthesis of luteal oxytocin seems to occur during the early luteal phase according to measurements of oxytocin mRNA. Under in-vitro and in-vivo conditions, oxytoxin is secreted concomitantly with neurophysin and progesterone, and there appears to be some form of communication between small and large luteal cells for the secretion of progesterone and oxytocin under in-vivo conditions. There is evidence that oxytocin may be involved in controlling luteolysis and may have intraovarian effects influencing steroidogenesis.

Luteolysis

For details see review by Schams (1987). Exogenous oxytocin in heifers and goats given during the first days of the oestrous cycle leads to a significant decrease in oestrous cycle length, but does not appear to cause luteal regression in ewes. Exogenous oxytocin also stimulated the release of prostaglandin (PG) F-2α from the endometrium around the time of luteolysis in heifers, sheep and goats. It appears that the luteolytic action of oxytocin is normally mediated by this response, since it can be prevented by hysterectomy in the cow and by simultaneous treatment with a PG synthetase inhibitor in the goat. The best evidence that oxytocin may be involved in controlling luteal regression comes from the active immunization of cyclic ewes and goats in which luteal regression was delayed. However, passive immunization of heifers did not prolong the oestrous cycle (D. Schams, unpublished observations).

At the time of luteolysis a positive feedback loop between ovarian oxytocin and endometrial PGF-2α exists in ruminants. It is suggested that the massive discharge of PGF-2α from the uterus towards the end of the luteal phase is stimulated by oxytocin release. Pulses of ovarian oxytocin induced by infusion of PGE-2 at 12-h intervals on Day 13 and 14 of the oestrous cycle failed to stimulate release of PGF-2α (N = 5 heifers, D. Schams & J. Kotwica, unpublished observations). One example is given in Fig. 1. Luteolysis with a parallel increase of oxytocin and PGF-2α occurred at the normal time on Days 17–18, as during the previous control cycle (Fig. 2).

The parallel surge-like secretion pattern of oxytocin and PGF-2α at the time of luteolysis seems to be not absolutely necessary for stimulation of PGF-2α release in cattle. Constant infusion of oxytocin from Day 15 of the oestrous cycle did not influence luteolytic events significantly (Kotwica *et al.*, 1988), unlike the sheep in which constant infusion of oxytocin between Day 13 and 21 blocked the rise in uterine oxytocin receptor concentrations and prolonged the length of the oestrous cycle (Flint & Sheldrick, 1985). The results suggest that the timing of luteolysis is regulated by the endometrium to be ready for the surge-like release of PGF-2α. The interaction of the endometrium with steroid hormones and changes in receptor concentrations for steroids and oxytocin seem to play a key role. Oestradiol induced and progesterone reduced the formation of receptors for oxytocin (for review see McCracken *et al.*, 1984). However, after about 10 days the action of progesterone in the uterus begins to diminish, and so oestradiol is able to induce synthesis of oxytocin receptors again and permits oxytocin-induced secretion of PGF-2α. The profile of receptors for oxytocin, cytosolic progesterone and oestrogen in the endometrium of heifers slaughtered at defined times of the oestrous cycle supports the findings in ewes (Meyer *et al.*, 1988). Further evidence for the important role of luteal progesterone on the endometrium and length of the oestrous cycle was found in heifers (J. Kotwica, D. Schams & E. Schallenberger, unpublished data). Treatment of heifers (N = 5) with exogenous progesterone (30 mg/100 kg body weight/day) for 4 days (Days 1–4) beginning after the preovulatory LH surge reduced length of the cycle significantly from $20{\cdot}7 \pm 0{\cdot}8$ to $14{\cdot}4 \pm 2{\cdot}7$ days.

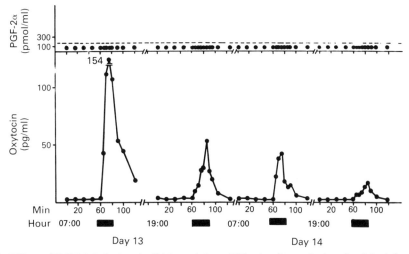

Fig. 1. Effect of PGE-2 infusion (solid bar, 1·5 mg/200 ml saline solution for 15 min) at 12-h intervals on Days 13 and 14 of the oestrous cycle on secretion of ovarian oxytocin and PGF-2α in a heifer. Blood samples were collected from the vena cava.

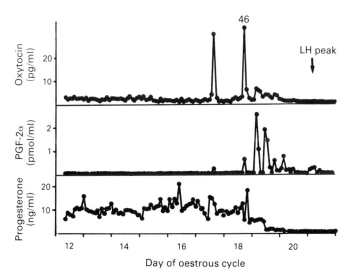

Fig. 2. Secretion pattern of progesterone, PGF-2α and oxytocin in the vena cava around the time of luteolysis in a cow after infusion of PGE-2 on Days 13 and 14.

Measurement of progesterone after frequent bleeding on Days 6 and 9 showed that exogenous progesterone did not disturb the development of the corpus luteum. The period of progesterone concentrations above 2 ng/ml plasma was very similar in the control and experimental cycles. At the time of luteolysis more or less the same events were measured as during the control cycle (one example is given in Fig. 3).

It is suggested that the massive discharge of PGF-2α from the uterus towards the end of the luteal phase is stimulated by oxytocin release, thereby initiating luteolysis. However, it has been

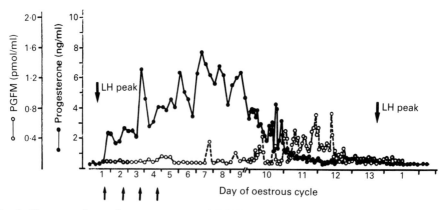

Fig. 3. Concentrations of progesterone and PGFM in the vena cava of a heifer during the oestrous cycle after daily treatment on Days 1–4 with progesterone (↑), 30 mg/100 kg body weight in sesame oil.

shown by Moore *et al.* (1986) that concentrations of PGF-2α in utero-ovarian vein samples in ewes begin to increase before the concentrations of oxytocin and oxytocin-associated neurophysin. This suggests that uterine PGF-2α initiates the release of ovarian oxytocin and oxytocin-associated neurophysin pulses during luteolysis in ewes. This is consistent with the inhibition of pulsatile oxytocin-associated neurophysin release in ewes (Watkins *et al.*, 1984) and oxytocin release in goats (Cooke & Homeida, 1984) after systemic treatment with indomethacin. Pulsatile release of oxytocin was also absent in hysterectomized cows bearing a persistent corpus luteum (Schams *et al.*, 1985). It appears therefore that basal concentrations of oxytocin interact with uterine oxytocin receptors, thus initiating PGF-2α release which induces further release of oxytocin and hence amplifies the release of PGF-2α from the uterus.

Ovarian oxytocin seems to be not absolutely necessary for the pulsatile release of PGF-2α. A pulsatile release of PGFM was observed in ovariectomized ewes primed with progesterone and treated with oestrogen (Lye *et al.*, 1983). A permissive action of oxytocin on luteolysis seems to be more likely than a direct one.

Intra-ovarian effects of oxytocin on steroidogenesis

The function of oxytocin in the ovary is an area of considerable interest and several groups have investigated the effect of oxytocin on luteal progesterone synthesis. The first evidence for a direct action of oxytocin on steroidogenesis was obtained by Tan *et al.* (1982). We proved the effect of oxytocin and vasopressin in a series of experiments on bovine luteal cells dispersed by means of collagenase digestion. Corpora lutea were obtained at different stages of the oestrous cycle (Days 2–3, 4–6 and 10–12). Tissue culture was performed for 4 h with 2–5 × 10⁵ cells/dish/ml in Medium 199 at 37°C. Four parallel dishes were used for each dose. The effect of oxytocin on unstimulated and LH-stimulated cells is shown in Fig. 4. Significant effects were seen in stimulated cells with 100 pg oxytocin. As shown in Fig. 5, arginine-vasopressin also showed an inhibitory effect on secretion of progesterone by bovine luteal cells. A significant effect was achieved with 1 pg/ml. A high variability between the experiments (corpora lutea) in our study indicates differences in receptivity. Oxytocin inhibited secretion of progesterone by dispersed pig luteal cells at doses similar to those in our experiments (Einspanier *et al.*, 1986), but oxytocin added to large and small luteal cell fractions obtained from fully developed sheep corpora lutea did not affect progesterone production by either fraction (Rodgers *et al.*, 1985). The results suggest a paracrine action of the neurohormones in the ovary but further clarification is still needed.

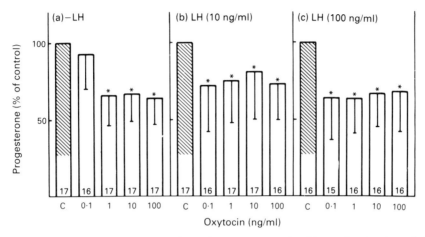

Fig. 4. Effect of oxytocin on production of progesterone by (a) unstimulated, and (b, c) LH-stimulated bovine luteal cells in culture (4 h). Values are mean $\pm$ s.d. for the no. of observations indicated. Absolute concentrations (ng/10^5 cells) for progesterone were (a) $11\cdot0 \pm 10\cdot7$, (b) $15\cdot6 \pm 13\cdot0$ and (c) $19\cdot1 \pm 14\cdot9$. *$P < 0\cdot05$ compared with control (c).

Ovarian growth factors

There is clear evidence that a number of growth factors are produced by ovarian tissue as shown in Table 1. Most of the growth factors combine replicative and in some instances cyto-differentiative properties. EGF and FGF are the most potent mitogens for granulosa cells. FGF may act as an angiogenic factor in the bovine corpus luteum: it is very active in triggering the proliferation of vascular endothelial cells.

In bovine granulosa cells EGF has a stimulating effect *in vitro* on growth of granulosa cells and inhibits production of inhibin and progesterone (Franchimont *et al.*, 1986). EGF binding has been demonstrated in bovine granulosa and luteal cells. EGF under in-vitro conditions stimulated secretion of oxytocin only and not of progesterone from bovine granulosa cells. IGF-I was the most potent stimulator of granulosa cells for production of oxytocin and progesterone. However, dispersed luteal cells did not respond to IGF-I, EGF or FGF in secretion of oxytocin or progesterone (Schams *et al.*, 1988). As shown in Table 2 bovine follicular fluid contains concentrations of IGF-I which are comparable with those in peripheral blood. Furthermore, large follicles seem to contain higher concentrations. There is a correlation with oestradiol-17β but not with the progesterone content in follicular fluid. Large follicles collected during early pregnancy (E. Schallenberger, R. Koll & D. Schams, unpublished data) have the lowest IGF-I and oestradiol values. Surprisingly, concentrations are highest in cysts. More evidence for the important role of IGF-I in ovarian function has been accumulated from rats and pigs, i.e. gene expression and secretion of IGF-I by granulosa cells, receptors for IGF-I in granulosa cells and the stimulating effect of trophic hormones (LH, FSH) in synergism with oestradiol on IGF-I secretion by pig granulosa cells (Adashi *et al.*, 1985; Veldhuis *et al.*, 1986; Hernandez *et al.*, 1988). Furthermore, IGF-I raised not

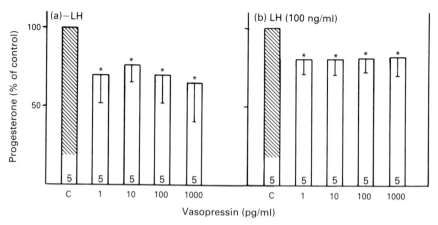

Fig. 5. Effect of arginine-vasopressin on production of progesterone by (a) unstimulated and (b) stimulated bovine luteal cells. Values are mean ± s.d. for the no. of observations indicated. Absolute concentrations for progesterone were (a) 10.2 ± 4.2 and (b) 16.9 ± 4.3 ng/10^5 cells. *$P < 0.05$ compared with control (c).

Table 1. Growth factors in ovarian tissue

	Tissue	Receptors
Fibroblast growth factor (FGF)	Corpus luteum	+
Transforming growth factor-β (TGF-β)	Follicle	+
Epidermal growth factor (EGF)	Corpus luteum; theca	+
Insulin-like growth factor-I (IGF-I)	Granulosa cells	+
Insulin-like growth factor-II (IGF-II)	Granulosa cells	+

Table 2. Concentrations (mean ± s.d.) of IGF-I, progesterone and oestradiol in bovine follicular fluid

Follicle	n	IGF-I (ng/ml)	Progesterone (ng/ml)	Oestradiol (ng/ml)
<5 mm (pooled)	11	335 ± 147	74 ± 55	$9 \pm 5,7$
5–9 mm (pooled)	10	353 ± 216	113 ± 117	187 ± 188
10–20 mm	38	469 ± 178	73 ± 87	433 ± 642
Early pregnancy 10–15 mm	10	293 ± 142	105 ± 114	76 ± 77
Cysts	7	1087 ± 242	438 ± 375	201 ± 299

only FSH-stimulated inhibin levels, but basal levels as well, in rat granulosa cells (Bicsak *et al.*, 1986). In conclusion, the results suggest the relevance of growth factors for ovarian physiology and possible importance for growth and differentiation of follicles.

References

Adashi, E.Y., Resnick, E., D'Ercole, J., Svoboda, M.E. & Van Wyk, J.J. (1985) Insulin-like growth factors as intraovarian regulators of granulosa cell growth and function. *Endocrine Reviews* **6**, 400–420.

Bicsak, T.A., Tucker, E.M., Cappel, S., Vaughan, J., Rivier, J., Vale, W. & Hsueh, A.J.W. (1986) Hormonal regulation of granulosa cell inhibin biosynthesis. *Endocrinology* **119**, 2711–2719.

Burger, H.G., Findlay, J.K. & de Kretser, D.M. (Eds) (1988) *Inhibin—Non-Steroidal Regulation of Follicle Stimulating Hormone.* Raven Press, New York.

Cooke, R.G. & Homeida, A.M. (1984) Delayed luteolysis and suppression of the pulsatile release of oxytocin after indomethacin treatment in the goat. *Res. vet. Sci.* **36**, 48–51.

Einspanier, R., Pitzel, L., Wuttke, W., Hagendorff, G., Preuß, K.D., Kardalinou, E. & Scheitt, K.H. (1986) Demonstration of messenger-RNA for oxytocin and prolactin in porcine granulosa and luteal cells. Effect of these hormones on progesterone secretion in vitro. *FEBS Letters,* **204**, 37–40.

Flint, A.P.F. & Sheldrick, E.L. (1985) Continuous infusion of oxytocin prevents induction of uterine oxytocin receptor and blocks luteal regression in cyclic ewes. *J. Reprod. Fert.* **75**, 623–631.

Franchimont, P., Hazee-Hagelstein, M.T., Charlet-Renard, Ch. & Jaspar, J.M. (1986) Effect of mouse epidermal growth factor on DNA and protein synthesis, progesterone and inhibin production by bovine granulosa cells in culture. *Acta endocr., Copenh.* **111**, 122–127.

Hernandez, E.R., Resnick, C.E., Svoboda, M.E., Van Wyk, J.J., Payne, D.W. & Adashi, E. (1988) Somatomedin-C/Insulin-like growth factor I as an enhancer of androgen biosynthesis by cultured rat ovarian cells. *Endocrinology* **122**, 1603–1612.

Ivell, R. & Richter, D. (1984) The gene for the hypothalamic peptide hormone oxytocin is highly expressed in the bovine corpus luteum: biosynthesis, structure and sequence analysis. *EMBO J.* **3**, 2351–2354.

Kotwica, J., Schams, D., Meyer, H.H.D. & Mittermeier, Th. (1988) Effect of continuous infusion of oxytocin on length of the oestrous cycle and luteolysis in cattle. *J. Reprod. Fert.* **83**, 287–294.

Lye, S.J., Sprague, C.L. & Challis, J.R.G. (1983) Modulation of ovine myometrial activity by estradiol-17β. The possible involvement of prostaglandins. *Can. J. Physiol. Pharmacol.* **61**, 729–735.

McCracken, J.A., Schramm, W. & Okulicz, W.C. (1984) Hormone receptor control of pulsatile secretion of PGF2α from the ovine uterus during luteolysis and

its abrogation in early pregnancy. *Anim. Reprod. Sci.* **7**, 31–55.

Meyer, H.H.D., Mittermeier, Th. & Schams, D. (1988) Dynamics of oxytocin, estrogen and progestin receptors in the bovine endometrium during the estrous cycle. *Acta endocr., Copenh.* **118**, 96–104.

Moore, L.G., Choy, V.J., Elliot, R.L. & Watkins, W.B. (1986) Evidence for the release of PGF-2α inducing the release of ovarian oxytocin during luteolysis in the ewe. *J. Reprod. Fert.* **76**, 159–166.

Rodgers, R.J., O'Shea, J.D. & Findlay, J.K. (1985) Do small and large cells of the sheep interact in the production of progesterone? *J. Reprod. Fert.* **75**, 85–94.

Schams, D. (1987) Luteal peptides and intercellular communication. *J. Reprod. Fert.* **34**, 87–99.

Schams, D., Schallenberger, E., Meyer, H.H.D., Bullermann, B., Breitinger, H.-J., Enzenhöfer, G., Koll, R., Kruip, T.A.M., Walters, D.L. & Karg, H. (1985) Ovarian oxytocin during the estrous cycle in cattle. In *Oxytocin, Clinical and Laboratory Studies,* pp. 317–334. Eds J. A. Amico & A. G. Robinson. Elsevier Biomedical, Amsterdam.

Schams, D., Koll, R. & Li, C.H. (1988) Insulin-like growth factor-I stimulates oxytocin and progesterone production by bovine granulosa cells in culture. *J. Endocr.* **116**, 97–100.

Tan, G.J.S., Tweedale, R. & Biggs, J.S.G. (1982) Effects of oxytocin on the bovine corpus luteum of early pregnancy. *J. Reprod. Fert.* **66**, 75–78.

Veldhuis, J.D., Rodgers, R.J. & Furlanetto, R.W. (1986) Synergistic actions of estradiol and the insulin-like growth factor somatomedin-C on swine ovarian (granulosa) cells. *Endocrinology* **119**, 530–538.

Wathes, D.C., Swann, R.W., Birkett, S.D., Porter, D.G. & Pickering, B.T. (1983a) Characterization of oxytocin, vasopressin and neurophysin from the bovine corpus luteum. *Endocrinology* **113**, 693–698.

Wathes, D.C., Swann, R.W., Hull, M.G.R., Drife, J.O., Porter, D.G. & Pickering, B.T. (1983b) Gonadal sources of the posterior pituitary hormones. *Prog. Brain Res.* **60**, 513–520.

Wathes, D.C., Swann, R.W. & Pickering, B.T. (1984) Variation in oxytocin, vasopressin and neurophysin concentrations in the bovine ovary during the oestrous cycle and pregnancy. *J. Reprod. Fert.* **71**, 551–557.

Watkins, W.B., Moore, L.G., Fairclough, R.J., Peterson, A.J. & Tervit, H.R. (1984) Possible role for ovarian prostaglandin $F_{2\alpha}$ in stimulating luteal oxytocin release in ewes at luteolysis. *J. Steroid Biochem.* **20**, 15–7, Abstr.

J. Reprod. Fert., Suppl. **37** (1989), 233–240

Mechanism of the luteolytic action of prostaglandin F-2α in the rat

M. Lahav, J. S. Davis* and H. Rennert

*Faculty of Medicine, Technion—Israel Institute of Technology, Haifa 31096, Israel; and *James A. Haley Veterans Administration Hospital and Department of Internal Medicine, University of South Florida, Tampa, FL 33612, U.S.A.*

Summary. PGF-2α suppresses the LH-induced accumulation of cyclic AMP in young and mature corpora lutea (CL) of pseudopregnant rats, with mature CL being more sensitive. Calcium ions, and later phospholipase C activation, are believed to mediate this effect. In isolated CL of 2 and 10 days of age, depletion of extracellular calcium, or addition of calmodulin inhibitors or of 8-(N,N-diethylamino)-octyl-3,4,5-trimethoxy-benzoate (TMB-8), did not prevent the suppressive effect of PGF-2α. Phorbol 12-myristate 13-acetate augmented, rather than inhibited, the LH-induced cAMP accumulation in young and mature CL. Polyphosphoinositide turnover was stimulated by PGF-2α in young, but not in mature CL. The suppression by PGF-2α of luteal cAMP is therefore apparently not mediated by phospholipase C activation but two phosphodiesterase inhibitors, 3-isobutyl-1-methylxanthine and Ro-20-1724, abolished the inhibitory effect of PGF-2α.

Keywords: rat; corpus luteum; luteolysis; PFG-2α; phorbol ester; calcium ions

Introduction

Prostaglandin (PG) F-2α was shown to trigger luteal regression in many species (Rothchild, 1981). Some years ago we reported that, in corpora lutea (CL) of pregnant rats incubated *in vitro*, PGF-2α prevented, or reversed within 15 min, the luteinizing hormone (LH)-induced cyclic AMP (cAMP) accumulation (Lahav *et al.*, 1976). This effect was later confirmed in isolated CL (Khan *et al.*, 1979) and luteal cell suspensions (Dorflinger *et al.*, 1983) from pseudopregnant rats. Treatment with PGF-2α of rats, or of isolated CL, resulted in impaired luteal adenylate cyclase activity in cell-free preparations; PGF-2α added directly to the enzyme assay had no effect (Khan & Rosberg, 1979; Lindner *et al.*, 1980). It has been proposed that calcium ions mediate the action of PGF-2α in the rat corpus luteum, based on the ability of ionophores and ouabain to inhibit cAMP accumulation in intact luteal cells, and of calcium ions at micromolar concentrations to inhibit adenylate cyclase in luteal cell membranes (Dorflinger *et al.*, 1984; Gore & Behrman, 1984).

Apparent support for this suggestion has come from studies by Leung *et al.* (1986) who showed that PGF-2α added to rat luteal cells after 3 days in culture stimulated polyphosphoinositide metabolism. The causal relationship between phosphatidylinositol bisphosphate turnover and elevation of cytosolic calcium is well established (Berridge & Irvine, 1984).

We have studied the mode of action of PGF-2α in isolated rat CL of pseudopregnancy incubated *in vitro*. Very young CL, known to be relatively resistant to the luteolytic effect of PGF-2α (Khan *et al.*, 1979), were compared to mature CL, the physiological target of PGF-2α as a luteolytic agent.

Materials and Methods

The sources for most materials, as well as the experimental procedures, have been described (Lahav *et al.*, 1983, 1987). Briefly, the formation of CL (20–35/rat) was induced in immature rats by 15 i.u. PMSG; these CL remain functional for 11 days, and so 2- and 10-day-old CL were studied. In some experiments, CL (10–20/rat) with a functional life-span of 9 days were induced by 8 i.u. PMSG, and 2- and 7-day-old CL were compared. Isolated CL were pooled and incubated in defined, oxygenated medium. After a preincubation period of 90 min, CL were distributed in test tubes (9–14 CL/2 ml medium) and incubated with hormones and drugs for 90 min, unless specified otherwise. In each experiment, there were duplicate or triplicate incubations per treatment. The medium was then removed, and sometimes saved for progesterone determination (Bauminger *et al.*, 1974). cAMP was extracted from the CL by rapidly bringing them to the boil in acetate buffer (pH 4). In the experiments in which phospholipid metabolism was examined, incubation conditions and determination of labelled phospholipids and inositol phosphates were as described by Davis *et al.* (1984, 1987).

In many experiments, cAMP and progesterone are presented in normalized units; for each sample, the absolute concentration of cAMP (pmol/mg protein) or progesterone (ng/mg protein) was normalized to the mean cAMP, or progesterone, concentration in the LH-treated samples of the same experiment. Values from several experiments were combined, and means ± s.e.m. are presented. Student's *t* test was used to determine statistical significance.

Results

Role of calcium ions in the action of PGF-2α in mature (Day-10) CL

In rats in which pseudopregnancy had been induced by 15 i.u. PMSG, Day-10 CL were still functional, as indicated by the high concentration of plasma progesterone and the negligible 20α-hydroxysteroid dehydrogenase. LH (5 µg/ml) increased the concentration of cAMP from 2·9 ± 0·4 ($n = 25$) to 37·4 ± 0·3 ($n = 66$) pmol/mg protein. In LH-treated samples, PGF-2α at 0·01, 0·1, 1 and 10 µM reduced the cAMP level by 27% (n.s.), 54% ($P < 0·001$), 62% ($P < 0·001$) and 55% ($P < 0·001$), respectively ($n = 14$). PGF-2α had no effect on basal cAMP (Lahav *et al.*, 1983).

Effect of extracellular calcium deprivation. In Day-10 CL incubated in calcium-depleted medium, the inhibitory effect of PGF-2α on LH-induced cAMP accumulation was not impaired (Lahav *et al.*, 1983, 1987). The concentration of free calcium ions in this medium was 30 nM, i.e. less than the basal level of cytosolic calcium. The whole luteal mass was presumably effectively exposed to the calcium-depleted medium, since total calcium content in the tissue (measured by atomic absorption) was reduced by 64% (Lahav *et al.*, 1987).

Table 1. Effect of phorbol 12-myristate 13-acetate (PMA) on cAMP accumulation in rat Day-10 corpora lutea incubated with LH for 120 min

Additions			
PMA (nM)	LH (µg/ml)	*n*	Cyclic AMP (normalized)†
0	5	16	100 ± 10
20	5	6	119 ± 15
50	5	6	115 ± 14
100	5	10	128 ± 23
1000	5	14	147 ± 19*
10 000	5	14	144 ± 14**

Values are mean ± s.e.m.; *n* is the total number of incubated samples, collected in several experiments (2–3 incubations per experiment, 9–14 CL per incubation).
*$P < 0·05$, **$P < 0·02$ compared to LH alone.
†100 normalized units of cAMP = 32·0 ± 8·6 pmol/mg protein.

Table 2. Effect of PGF-2α on polyphosphoinositide metabolism in Day-2 and Day-7 rat corpora lutea

Fraction†	PGF-2α (μM)	Radioactivity (c.p.m. × 10^{-3}/mg protein)‡	
		Day-2 CL	Day-7 CL
(a) $H_3{}^{32}PO_4$			
Phosphatidic	0	15·7 ± 1·6	29·5 ± 5·9
acid	10	39·1 ± 6·0*	32·8 ± 7·4
Phosphatidyl-	0	23·6 ± 1·3	35·2 ± 8·2
inositol	10	55·8 ± 3·8**	29·6 ± 7·0
(b) [^{3}H]Inositol			
Inositol	0	15·8 ± 3·1	64·9 ± 6·2
monophosphate	10	89·6 ± 9·6*	69·1 ± 8·2
Inositol	0	0·57 ± 0·18	3·51 ± 1·48
bisphosphate	10	8·17 ± 1·09**	4·66 ± 0·61
Inositol	0	0·31 ± 0·10	0·58 ± 0·09
trisphosphate	10	1·99 ± 0·05***	0·80 ± 0·10

*$P < 0·02$, **$P < 0·005$, ***$P < 0·001$ compared to the respective controls.

†In (a), isolated, halved CL were incubated with $H_3{}^{32}PO_4$ (100 μCi/ml) for 60 min, and PGF-2α was sometimes present during the last 30 min.
In (b), isolated, halved CL were preincubated for 3 h with [^{3}H]inositol (50 μCi/ml), washed, and incubated in the presence of LiCl (10 mM) with and without PGF-2α for 15 min.

‡There were triplicate incubations per experiment (2–4 CL per incubation); experiments were repeated 5 times (Day-7 CL, $H_3{}^{32}PO_4$ labelling) or 3 times (the other three series). For each experiment, and each fraction, the average of the triplicate incubations was calculated, and the presented results are means ± s.e.m. of these averages.

Table 3. Effect of TMB-8 on cAMP concentration and progesterone secretion in rat Day-2 corpora lutea incubated with LH (5 μg/ml) and PGF-2α (10 μM)

Additions		Cyclic AMP (normalized)‡	Progesterone (normalized)§
TMB-8	Hormones		
0	None	2 ± 0****	35 ± 7****
	LH	100 ± 9	100 ± 8
	LH + PGF-2α	62 ± 9**	97 ± 9
30 μM	None	2 ± 0***	37 ± 4
	LH	121 ± 27	60 ± 12†
	LH + PGF-2α	58 ± 7*	67 ± 13

Values are mean ± s.e.m.; the total number of incubated samples, collected in several experiments, was 5–7 (2–3 incubations per experiment, 9–14 CL per incubation).

*$P < 0·05$, **$P < 0·02$, ***$P < 0·005$, ****$P < 0·001$ compared to LH-treated samples with same concentration of TMB-8.

†$P < 0·02$ compared to samples treated with LH alone.

‡100 normalized units of cAMP = 247 ± 63 pmol/mg protein.

§100 normalized units of progesterone = 267 ± 31 ng/mg protein.

Table 4. Effect of trifluoperazine on cAMP concentration and progesterone secretion in rat Day-2 corpora lutea incubated with LH (5 µg/ml) and PGF-2α (10 µM)

Additions			Cyclic AMP	Progesterone
Trifluoperazine	Hormones	n	(normalized)‡	(normalized)§
0	None	9	2 ± 0****	44 ± 6***
	LH	10	100 ± 8	100 ± 13
	LH + PGF-2α	10	59 ± 7***	92 ± 11
30 µM	None	9	2 ± 0****	52 ± 5***
	LH	9	113 ± 19	95 ± 11
	LH + PGF-2α	9	66 ± 9*	92 ± 9
300 µM	None	6	2 ± 0****	27 ± 3**
	LH	6	143 ± 30	47 ± 5†
	LH + PGF-2α	6	70 ± 11*	46 ± 3†

Values are mean ± s.e.m.; n is the total number of incubated samples, collected in several experiments (2–3 incubations per experiment, 9–14 CL per incubation).
*P < 0·05, **P < 0·01, ***P < 0·005, ****P < 0·001 compared to LH-treated samples with same concentration of trifluoperazine.
†P < 0·01 compared to samples with same hormones but no trifluoperazine.
‡100 normalized units = 169 ± 19 pmol/mg protein.
§100 normalized units = 187 ± 25 ng/mg protein.

Table 5. Effect of phorbol 12-myristate 13-acetate (PMA) on cAMP accumulation and progesterone secretion in rat Day-2 corpora lutea

Additions			
PMA (nM)	LH (µg/ml)	Cyclic AMP (normalized)‡	Progesterone (normalized)§
0	0	2 ± 0	65 ± 7
	5	100 ± 8	100 ± 6††
100	0	2 ± 0	71 ± 5
	5	98 ± 13	103 ± 6†††
1000	0	2 ± 0	77 ± 6
	5	133 ± 11*	117 ± 5†††
10 000	0	2 ± 0	76 ± 6
	5	105 ± 11	113 ± 12†

Values are mean ± s.e.m.; the total number of incubated samples, collected in several experiments, was 9 (2–3 incubations per experiment, 9–14 CL per incubation).
*P < 0·025 compared to LH alone.
†P < 0·02, ††P < 0·005, †††P < 0·001 compared to samples without LH and same concentration of PMA.
‡100 normalized units = 120·9 ± 10·0 pmol/mg protein.
§100 normalized units = 162 ± 15 ng/mg protein.

Verapamil (100 µM) did not attenuate the inhibitory effect of PGF-2α on cAMP (Lahav *et al.*, 1983). However, mature rat CL may lack voltage-dependent calcium channels, since $^{45}Ca^{2+}$ uptake was unaffected by verapamil, but blocked by lanthanum ions, which inhibit general calcium movement across the plasma membrane (Lahav *et al.*, 1988a).

Effect of TMB-8 and calmodulin inhibitors. TMB-8 (8-(N,N-diethylamino)-octyl-3,4,5-trimethoxybenzoate) was shown to interfere with intracellular calcium by inhibiting its release from intracellular stores and possibly by blocking its action (Donowitz *et al.*, 1986; see also Lahav *et al.*, 1987). In Day-10 CL, TMB-8 at 30 or 150 μM did not prevent the inhibitory action of PGF-2α on cAMP accumulation; the combination of 150 μM-TMB-8 and calcium-depleted medium was similarly ineffective (Lahav *et al.*, 1987). None of the three calmodulin inhibitors examined, trifluoperazine (30 or 300 μM), pimozide (25 or 50 μM) and W-7 (15 or 45 μM), abolished the suppressive effect of PGF-2α on cAMP accumulation (Lahav *et al.*, 1983, 1987).

Effect of PGF-2α on the uptake of $^{45}Ca^{2+}$. In Day-10 CL, PGF-2α (10 μM) added simultaneously with, or 150 min after, $^{45}Ca^{2+}$ for up to 18 min did not affect calcium uptake (Lahav *et al.*, 1983, 1988a). In mature (Day 7) CL from rats pretreated with 8 i.u. PMSG, PGF-2α had no effect when added 90 min after $^{45}Ca^{2+}$ for exposure periods of 30, 60 or 90 min (M. Lahav, unpublished).

Effect of phorbol 12-myristate 13-acetate (PMA). Day-10 CL were exposed to LH and to PMA (20–10 000 nM), a phorbol ester known to activate protein kinase C. As shown in Table 1, PMA at 1 and 10 μM augmented the effect of LH on cAMP accumulation; at no concentration was PMA inhibitory.

Effect of PGF-2α on polyphosphoinositide metabolism

When Day-2 CL were isolated from rats pretreated with 8 i.u. PMSG, exposure to PGF-2α (10 μM) for 30 min resulted in a 2-fold increase in $^{32}PO_4$ incorporation into phosphatidic acid and phosphatidylinositol (PI) (Table 2). A GnRH agonist (GnRHa), but not LH, had a similar effect. Results were the same when agents were added simultaneously with $^{32}PO_4$ at 0, 30, or 150 min after $^{32}PO_4$. Moreover, PGF-2α (Table 2) and GnRHa, but not LH, increased inositol lipid hydrolysis, as reflected by increased formation of inositol phosphates in Day-2 CL prelabelled with [^{3}H]inositol (Lahav *et al.*, 1988b).

In Day-7 CL, which are much more sensitive to the luteolytic action of PGF-2α *in vivo* and *in vitro* (Khan *et al.*, 1979), neither PGF-2α (Table 2) nor GnRHa increased $^{32}PO_4$ incorporation into phosphatidic acid and PI, or the formation of inositol phosphates. Basal phosphoinositide turnover, however, was much higher in mature, compared to young CL (Table 2). There was therefore no correlation between the effectiveness of PGF-2α in suppressing luteal cAMP and in stimulating phospholipase C, suggesting that the latter is not the only mechanism of PGF-2α action in the rat corpus luteum.

Role of calcium ions in PGF-2α action in young (Day-2) CL

In Day-2 CL from rats pretreated with 15 i.u. PMSG, basal cAMP level (3·5 ± 0·4 pmol/mg protein, $n = 37$) was similar to that found on Day 10; however, in the presence of LH, much higher cAMP levels were attained (184 ± 15 pmol/mg protein, $n = 41$). PGF-2α was less effective in Day-2 than in Day-10 CL: at 0·1, 1 and 10 μM it inhibited cAMP accumulation by 13% (n.s.), 36% ($P < 0·01$) and 50% ($P < 0·001$) ($n = 7$), respectively, in LH-treated CL. Basal progesterone secretion was lower on Day 2, compared to Day 10; however, only in young CL was progesterone secretion stimulated by LH (~3-fold).

Although in young CL PGF-2α stimulated phospholipase C, again this mechanism does not seem to underlie the PGF-2α-induced suppression of cAMP accumulation. Incubation in calcium-depleted medium did not impair this inhibitory effect of PGF-2α (unpublished). TMB-8 at 30 μM abolished the LH-induced progesterone secretion, but not the suppression of cAMP by PGF-2α (Table 3). Similarly, trifluoperazine, which inactivates calmodulin, and, at higher concentrations, also inhibits protein kinase C, inhibited steroidogenesis (at 300 μM), but not the effect of PGF-2α on cAMP (Table 4). PMA added simultaneously with LH augmented the effect of LH on cAMP (at 1 μM), or had no effect. Progesterone secretion was not influenced by PMA (Table 5).

Table 6. Effect of IBMX on the action of LH (5 μg/ml) and PGF-2α (10 μM) on cAMP concentration in rat Day-2 and Day-10 corpora lutea

Additions		Cyclic AMP (normalized)‡	
IBMX	Hormones	Day 2	Day 10
0	None	3 ± 1**	—
	LH	100 ± 10	100 ± 6
	LH + PGF-2α	55 ± 7*	42 ± 5**
0·5 mM	None	5 ± 1**	—
	LH	163 ± 25†	227 ± 22††
	LH + PGF-2α	159 ± 18††	204 ± 27††

Values are mean ± s.e.m. for $n = 6$ on Day 2 and $n = 21$ on Day 10; n is the total number of incubated samples, collected in several experiments (2–3 incubations per experiment, 9–14 CL per incubation).

*$P < 0.01$, **$P < 0.001$ compared to LH-treated samples with same concentration of IBMX.

†$P < 0.05$, ††$P < 0.001$ compared to samples with same hormones but no IBMX.

‡100 normalized units (in pmol/mg protein) = 131 ± 27 on Day 2 and 40·7 ± 4·2 on Day 10.

Table 7. Effect of Ro-20-1724 on the action of LH (5 μg/ml) and PGF-2α (10 μM) on cAMP accumulation in Day-2 and Day-10 corpora lutea of rats

Additions		Cyclic AMP (normalized)‡	
Ro-20-1724	Hormones	Day 2	Day 10
0	None	2 ± 1*	—
	LH	100 ± 6	100 ± 13
	LH + PGF-2α	45 ± 5*	36 ± 6*
0·1 mM	None	4 ± 1*	—
	LH	183 ± 25†	363 ± 54†††
	LH + PGF-2α	144 ± 19†††	316 ± 79††
0·5 mM	None	5 ± 1*	—
	LH	230 ± 25†††	366 ± 37†††
	LH + PGF-2α	180 ± 22†††	292 ± 42†††

Values are mean ± s.e.m. for $n = 8$–9 on Day 2 and $n = 12$ on Day 10; n is the total number of incubated samples, collected in several experiments (2–3 incubations per experiment, 9–14 CL per incubation).

*$P < 0.001$ compared to samples treated with LH and same concentration of Ro-20-1724.

†$P < 0.01$, ††$P < 0.005$, †††$P < 0.001$ compared to samples with same hormones but no Ro-20-1724.

‡100 normalized units (in pmol/mg protein) were 118 ± 14 on Day 2 and 31·8 ± 6·0 on Day 10.

Effect of phosphodiesterase inhibitors in young and mature CL

The inhibitory effect of PGF-2α on LH-induced cAMP accumulation persisted in the presence of 0·1 mM-3-isobutyl-1-methylxanthine (IBMX) in isolated CL (Khan *et al.*, 1979) and in luteal cell suspensions (Dorflinger *et al.*, 1983). However, this concentration of IBMX is probably suboptimal (Khan *et al.*, 1979; Dorflinger *et al.*, 1983; Lahav *et al.*, 1983). At 0·5 mM, IBMX abolished the effect of PGF-2α in Day-2 as well as in Day-10 CL (Table 6). The same was found with another phosphodiesterase inhibitor, Ro-20-1724 (Table 7). With both inhibitors, the percentage augmentation of the LH-stimulated cAMP production was greater in Day-10 than in Day-2 CL. LH-induced progesterone secretion, estimated in Day-2 CL, was not affected by 0·1 mM-Ro-20-1724, but was inhibited by each drug at 0·5 mM (unpublished).

Discussion

The inhibition of LH-induced cAMP accumulation in luteal tissue is a very early effect of PGF-2α, and is considered relevant to luteolysis. During the past few years, calcium ions and protein kinase C have been proposed to mediate this effect (Dorflinger *et al.*, 1984; Gore & Behrman, 1984; Sender-Baum & Rosberg, 1987), and PGF-2α was indeed shown to activate phospholipase C in some luteal cells (Leung *et al.*, 1986; Davis *et al.*, 1987). However, several lines of evidence led us to believe that a mechanism other than phospholipase C activation underlies the suppression of cAMP accumulation by PGF-2α.

We found that PGF-2α stimulated polyphosphoinositide hydrolysis in young, but not in mature, CL (Table 2), although the latter are much more sensitive to PGF-2α with regard to cAMP suppression *in vitro* and *in vivo*. Faulty uptake of the labelled precursors ($^{32}PO_4$ and [^{3}H]inositol) cannot explain these results, since basal phosphoinositide turnover was much higher in the mature CL; total $^{32}PO_4$ incorporation into phospholipids was similar in CL of both ages (Lahav *et al.*, 1988b).

Depletion of extracellular calcium, which also led to a reduction in intracellular calcium, did not prevent the inhibitory effect of PGF-2α on cAMP. Also without influence were TMB-8 and 3 calmodulin inhibitors; these drugs, although not entirely specific, are very effective inhibitors of processes in which elevated intracellular calcium and activated calmodulin, respectively, are involved. One such process is steroidogenesis (see Lahav *et al.*, 1983, 1987, for references), and, indeed, we found that progesterone production was inhibited by TMB-8 and trifluoperazine (Tables 2 & 3). Dorflinger *et al.* (1984) demonstrated inhibition by Ca^{2+} of adenylate cyclase activity in luteal membranes, but the concentrations required were much higher than those attained by activation of phospholipase C in a variety of cell types.

PMA augmented, rather than inhibited, LH-induced cAMP accumulation (Tables 1 & 4), as it is reported to do for luteal cells of cattle (Budnik & Mukhopadhyay, 1987); in such cells, PGF-2α stimulated phospholipase C and did not inhibit steroidogenesis (Davis *et al.*, 1987). Sender-Baum & Rosberg (1987) reported that, in rat luteal cell suspensions incubated with LH, PMA inhibited cAMP and progesterone accumulation. However, high concentrations of PMA were required, and the effect had a delayed onset. In steroidogenic cells, inhibitory as well as stimulatory effects of PMA were observed (see Budnik & Mukhopadhyay, 1987; Sender-Baum & Rosberg, 1987, for references).

An unexpected finding was the reversal by phosphodiesterase inhibitors of the suppressive effect of PGF-2α on cAMP. A number of phosphodiesterase types have been described, and all are inhibited by IBMX; Ro-20-1724 is apparently selective for the 'cAMP-specific' low-K_m enzyme (Beavo *et al.*, 1982). Pretreatment of intact luteal tissue with PGF-2α *in vivo* and *in vitro* resulted in impaired adenylate cyclase stimulation in luteal homogenates (see 'Introduction'). This stable inhibition of adenylate cyclase may therefore be secondary to the effect of PGF-2α on phosphodiesterase. Alternatively, IBMX and Ro-20-1724 may act at a site other than phosphodiesterase. At present, no known effect of the two drugs can explain a stimulatory effect on cAMP production.

We suggest that the difference between rat CL of the two ages regarding the magnitude of the responses to LH and phosphodiesterase inhibitors may be partly due to higher levels of phosphodiesterase in the mature CL.

This study was supported by the Fund for Basic Research Administered by the Israel Academy of Science and Humanities, and by the Dario and Mathilde Beraha Fund for Hormones and Cancer Research (M.L.) and by NIH HD 22248 and the Veterans Administration (J.S.D.).

References

Bauminger, S., Kohen, F. & Lindner, H.R. (1974) Steroids as haptens: optimal design of antigens for the formation of antibodies to steroid hormones. *J. Steroid Biochem.* **5**, 739–749.

Beavo, J.A., Hansen, R.S., Harrison, S.A., Hurwitz, R.L., Martins, T.J. & Mumby, M.C. (1982) Identifications and properties of cyclic nucleotide phosphodiesterases. *Molec. cell. Endocr.* **28**, 387–410.

Berridge, M.J. & Irvine, R.F. (1984) Inositol trisphosphate, a novel second messenger in cellular signal transduction. *Nature, Lond.* **312**, 315–321.

Budnik, L.T. & Mukhopadhyay, A.K. (1987) Desensitisation of LH-stimulated cyclic AMP accumulation in isolated bovine luteal cells—effect of phorbol ester. *Molec. cell. Endocr.* **54**, 51–61.

Davis, J.S., West, L.A. & Farese, R.V. (1984) Effects of luteinizing hormone on phosphoinositide metabolism in rat granulosa cells. *J. biol. Chem.* **259**, 15028–15034.

Davis, J.S., Weakland, L.L., Weiland, D.A., Farese, R.V. & West, L.A. (1987) Prostaglandin $F_2\alpha$ stimulates phosphatidylinositol 4,5-bisphosphate hydrolysis and mobilizes intracellular Ca^{2+} in bovine luteal cells. *Proc. natn. Acad. Sci. U.S.A.* **84**, 3728–3732.

Donowitz, M., Cusolito, S. & Sharp, G.W.G. (1986) Effects of calcium antagonist TMB-8 on active Na and Cl transport in rabbit ileum. *Am. J. Physiol.* **250**, G691–G697.

Dorflinger, L.J., Luborsky, J.L., Gore, S.D. & Behrman, H.R. (1983) Inhibitory characteristics of prostaglandin $F_2\alpha$ in the rat luteal cell. *Molec. cell. Encocr.* **33**, 225–241.

Dorflinger, L.J., Albert, P.J., Williams, A.T. & Behrman, H.R. (1984) Calcium is an inhibitor of luteinizing hormone-sensitive adenylate cyclase in the luteal cell. *Endocrinology* **114**, 1208–1215.

Gore, S.D. & Behrman, H.R. (1984) Alteration of transmembrane sodium and potassium gradients inhibit the action of luteinizing hormone in the luteal cell. *Endocrinology* **114**, 2020–2031.

Khan, M.I. & Rosberg, S. (1979) Acute suppression by $PGF_2\alpha$ on LH, epinephrine and fluoride stimulation of adenylate cyclase in rat luteal tissue. *J. cyclic Nucleotide Res.* **5**, 55–63.

Khan, M.I., Rosberg, S., Lahav, M., Lamprecht, S.A.,

Selstam, G., Herlitz, H. & Ahrén, K. (1979) Studies on the mechanism of action of the inhibitory effect of prostaglandin $F_2\alpha$ on cyclic AMP accumulation in rat corpora lutea of various ages. *Biol. Reprod.* **21**, 1175–1183.

Lahav, M., Freud, A. & Lindner, H.R. (1976) Abrogation by prostaglandin $F_2\alpha$ of LH-stimulated cyclic AMP accumulation in isolated rat corpora lutea of pregnancy. *Biochem. Biophys. Res. Commun.* **68**, 1294–1300.

Lahav, M., Weiss, E., Rafaeloff, R. & Barzilai, D. (1983) The role of calcium ion in luteal function in the rat. *J. Steroid Biochem.* **19**, 805–810.

Lahav, M., Rennert, H., Sabag, K. & Barzilai, D. (1987) Calmodulin inhibitors and 8-(N,N-diethylamino)-octyl-3,4,5-trimethoxybenzoate (TMB-8) do not prevent the inhibitory effect of prostaglandin $F_2\alpha$ on cyclic AMP production in rat corpora lutea. *J. Endocr.* **113**, 205–212.

Lahav, M., Shariki-Sabag, K. & Rennert, H. (1988a) Lack of effect of prostaglandin $F_2\alpha$ and verapamil on calcium uptake by isolated corpora lutea from pseudopregnant rats. *Biochem. Pharmacol.* (in press).

Lahav, M., West, L.A. & Davis, J.S. (1988b) Effect of prostaglandin $F_2\alpha$ and a gonadotropin-releasing hormone agonist on inositol phospholipid metabolism in isolated rat corpora lutea of various ages. *Endocrinology* **123**, 1044–1052.

Leung, P.C.K., Minegishi, T., Ma, F., Zhou, F. & Ho-Yuen, B. (1986) Induction of polyphosphoinositide breakdown in rat corpus luteum by prostaglandin $F_2\alpha$. *Endocrinology* **119**, 12–18.

Lindner, H.R., Zor, U., Kohen, F., Bauminger, S., Amsterdam, A., Lahav, M. & Salomon, Y. (1980) Significance of prostaglandins in the regulation of cyclic events in the ovary and uterus. *Adv. Prostaglandin Thromboxane Res.* **8**, 1371–1390.

Rothchild, I. (1981) The regulation of the mammalian corpus luteum. *Recent Progr. Horm. Res.* **37**, 183–298.

Sender-Baum, M. & Rosberg, S. (1987) A phorbol ester, phorbol 12-myristate 13-acetate, and a calcium ionophore, A23187, can mimic the luteolytic effect of prostaglandin $F_2\alpha$ in isolated rat luteal cells. *Endocrinology* **120**, 1019–1026.

ENVIRONMENT OF THE EARLY EMBRYO

Chairmen

F. W. Bazer
G. Somme
W. W. Thatcher
M. J. Fields

J. Reprod. Fert., Suppl. **37** (1989), 241–244

Printed in Great Britain
© 1989 Journals of Reproduction & Fertility Ltd

Progesterone and the development of the early embryo

R. B. Heap, M.-W. Wang, M. J. Sims, S. T. Ellis and M. J. Taussig

AFRC Institute of Animal Physiology and Genetics Research, Babraham, Cambridge CB2 4AT, UK

Keywords: progesterone; embryo; pregnancy

Central to the maternal recognition of pregnancy is the secretion of progesterone for without it embryonic signals fail to achieve their function of either protecting the corpus luteum from uterine luteolytic mechanisms, as in certain ungulates, or prolonging luteal life-span and function by luteotrophic stimulation, as in the human female. Antibodies to progesterone have been used as a non-surgical means to investigate further its physiological actions during the earliest stages of gestation. Special attention has been given to the mechanisms by which anti-progesterone monoclonal antibodies block the establishment of pregnancy in terms of effects on the early embryo, the uterine luminal environment and cellular responses of the preimplantation uterus. These topics have been the subject of recent reviews (Wilmut *et al.*, 1986; Heap *et al.*, 1986, 1988a, b; Hahn *et al.*, 1989). In this paper we present a brief synopsis of our recent published work and of studies in progress.

Anti-progesterone monoclonal antibodies were prepared and those of high affinity selected (Wright *et al.*, 1982; Ellis *et al.*, 1988). Intraperitoneal or intravenous injection of antibody at 32 h after mating consistently prevented implantation in BALB/c mice (Wright *et al.*, 1982; Wang *et al.*, 1984). Studies in F1/C hybrid mice (BALB/c female × CBA male, fast rate of embryo development) showed that the antibody was less efficacious than in inbred females (BALB/c or CBA, slow rate of embryo development), indicating that efficacy is influenced by genotype and the rate of early embryo development. Antibody was more effective, however, when injected in F1/C hybrid mice at 8 h rather than 32 h after mating (Rider *et al.*, 1986). These findings suggest that perturbation of progesterone action by passive immunization is more detrimental at certain times of the preimplantation period than at others.

The ability of one anti-progesterone antibody, designated DB3, to block implantation was not due to embryotoxicity according to experiments carried out *in vitro* (Rider *et al.*, 1987). Evidence obtained in early studies indicated that there was an arrest of cleavage probably as a result of changes in the uterine environment which were detrimental to embryonic development (Wang *et al.*, 1984). In later experiments, however, we were unable to confirm that this was the underlying cause of the consistent pregnancy block (Heap *et al.*, 1988a). The block was reversed by the administration of a large dose of progesterone provided treatment was started within 48 h after passive immunization (Rider *et al.*, 1985).

Efficacy studies have shown that the anti-implantation action of antibody depends on progesterone binding: purified anti-progesterone immunoglobulin or the $F(ab')_2$ fragment of the antibody molecule both prevented implantation. The latter result shows that efficacy is not dependent on binding of antibody to F_c receptors (Ellis *et al.*, 1988). Experiments with 5 other high-affinity anti-progesterone antibodies gave comparable values for efficacy ($ED_{50} \sim 0.05 \, \mu mol/kg$). The finding that efficacy was similar for antibodies that were IgG or IgM molecules indicated a lack of class specificity and a common mechanism of action (Ellis *et al.*, 1988).

Further information about the specificity of the effect was derived from studies of the antibody itself. The Fab' fragment of DB3 has now been crystallized in its native form and co-crystallized with 7 different, but structurally related, steroids (Stura *et al.*, 1987). X-ray crystallographic studies are in progress in order to define the structural requirements for progesterone–DB3 binding. The primary structure of DB3 and other high-affinity anti-progesterone antibodies has been obtained from nucleotide and amino acid sequencing showing up to 88% identity in heavy chain variable (V_H) region sequences and no more than 50% homology with any of the 8 other mouse V_H gene families (Deverson *et al.*, 1987; Stura *et al.*, 1987; M. J. Sims & M. J. Taussig, unpublished results). The heavy chains are encoded by a rarely used family of V_H genes now designated V_HIX (or V_H GAM 3–8), while the light chain sequences are encoded by a V_K1 gene (Deverson *et al.*, 1987; Stura *et al.*, 1987). The heavy chain of two anti-arsenate monoclonal antibodies have also been found to be encoded by the V_HIX family of genes. When tested for anti-implantation efficacy the anti-arsenate antibodies were found to be without effect (Table 1), confirming the requirement for progesterone binding.

Table 1. Effect on pregnancy in BALB/c mice after a single i.p. injection of monoclonal antibodies (mAb) in which the heavy chain variable region is encoded by a family of genes designated V_HIX

Group	Treatment	Dose (nmol)	No. of corpora lutea	No. of mice pregnant/ no. treated	No. of implantation sites	% Pregnancy
1	9A5	9·0	9·4 ± 0·3	10/12	6·3 ± 1·2	83
2	22B5	9·0	9·5 ± 0·7	8/10	6·3 ± 1·4	80
3	3665 IgG	9·0	8·7 ± 0·6	8/10	6·3 ± 1·3	80
4	DB3	9·0	9·9 ± 0·5	0/10	0	0
5	Saline	250 μl	9·6 ± 0·7	8/10	6·5 ± 1·2	80

Mature female mice were injected i.p. at 32 h after mating with 9 nmol monoclonal antibody (mAb, ascitic fluid diluted in saline up to 250 μl). Control animals received a similar volume of saline. Autopsies were performed on Day 10 of pregnancy. Anti-arsenate mAbs 9A5 and 22B5 (V_HIX) were prepared from BALB/c mice (Meek *et al.*, 1984); anti-arsenate mAb 3665 IgG (non-V_HIX) from A/J mice (Capra *et al.*, 1982); and anti-progesterone mAb, DB3 (V_HIX) from BALB/c mice (Deverson *et al.*, 1987).

Returning to the question of the time when passive immunization is most effective, results in rats show that efficacy is most marked when antibody is given (i.p.) on Days 1 and 2 of pregnancy. Treatment was less effective on either Day 1 or Day 2, while the same treatment on Day 3 or Day 4 was ineffective. The same antibody was found to be equally effective in a second pregnancy and there was no evidence for anti-mouse or anti-idiotypic antibody production (Phillips *et al.*, 1988). Experiments in ferrets also demonstrated an anti-implantation effect when antibody was injected (i.p.) on Day 3 and/or Day 4 after mating. In this species there was a striking arrest of cleavage probably mediated through changes in the uterine environment. Embryos failed to undergo cavitation and remained distributed throughout the uterine lumen even at Day 14 after mating, 2 days after the expected time of implantation (Rider & Heap, 1986).

Passive immunization against progesterone in the preimplantation period of the mouse has a considerable impact on target cell responses normally associated with early pregnancy. Oviducal glycosylation in the ampullary region was affected (Whyte *et al.*, 1987). The changing pattern of mitotic activity in the endometrium was disrupted (Rider *et al.*, 1986), the increase in uterine sensitization was prevented and decidualization induced by oil instillation into the uterine lumen was inhibited (Rider *et al.*, 1985). In addition, the expected alteration in uterine protein synthesis was interrupted (Heap *et al.*, 1988a). Tubal transport of fertilized eggs was unaffected in all mouse stocks examined (Rider *et al.*, 1987) and in this respect the action of antibody differed from that of progesterone antagonists, RU 38486 and ZK 98734, competitive inhibitors of progesterone action. When injected into mice 32 h after mating RU 38486 and ZK 98734 increased the rate of tubal transport of fertilized eggs, unlike DB3 (S. T. Ellis, unpublished observations). When given to rats, RU 38486 was most efficacious when administered orally on Days 3 and 4, whereas DB3 was most effective (i.p.) on Days 1 and 2. The results imply that the action of anti-progesterone antibody differs from that of antagonists since the mechanism of action and period of efficacy differ between antibody and antagonists.

Recent evidence points to a local action of anti-progesterone antibody within the uterus. A method has been developed to localize anti-progesterone immunoglobulin with affinity-purified anti-idiotypic polyclonal antibodies (Wang *et al.*, 1988). Antibody DB3 has been localized on the surface of the uterine luminal and glandular epithelia about 36 h after injection at 32 h *p.c.* The results indicate that an unknown determinant recognized by DB3 is expressed transiently within the uterus, possibly affecting uterine uptake of progesterone. The fact that this determinant is found in pregnant, but not in pseudopregnant, mice provides a new example of uterine recognition of the presence of the developing embryo *in utero* approximately 20 h before the onset of implantation.

We gratefully acknowledge the supply of monoclonal antibodies 9A5, 22B5 and 3665 IgG provided by Dr K. Meek, Dr J. Urbain and Dr J. D. Capra.

References

Capra, J.D., Slaughter, C., Milner, E.C.B., Estess, P. & Tucker, P.W. (1982) The cross-reactive idiotype of A-strain mice: Serological and structural analyses. *Immunol. Today* **3**, 332–339.

Deverson, E., Berek, C., Feinstein, A. & Taussig, M.J. (1987) Monoclonal BALB/c anti-progesterone antibodies use family IX variable region heavy chain genes. *Eur. J. Immunol.* **17**, 9–13.

Ellis, S.T., Heap, R.B., Butchart, A.R., Rider, V., Richardson, N.E., Wang, M.-W. & Taussig, M.J. (1988) Efficacy and specificity of monoclonal antibodies to progesterone in preventing the establishment of pregnancy in the mouse. *J. Endocr.* **118**, 69–80.

Hahn, D.W., Capetola, R.J., McGuire, J.L., Wang, M.-W., Taussig, M.J. & Heap, R.B. (1989) Anti-implantation effects of monoclonal anti-progesterone antibody. In *Development of Pre-implantation Embryos and their Environment*, (in press).

Heap, R.B., Rider, V., Wooding, F.B.P. & Flint, A.P.F. (1986) Molecular and cellular signalling and embryonic survival. In *Embryonic Mortality in Farm Animals*, pp. 46–73. Eds J. M. Sreenan & M. G. Diskin. Martinus Nijhoff, Dordrecht.

Heap, R.B., Fleet, I.R., Finn, C., Ellis, S.T., Yang, C.-B., Whyte, A. & Brigstock, D.R. (1988a) Maternal reactions affecting early embryogenesis and implantation. *J. Reprod. Fert., Suppl.* **36**, 83–97.

Heap, R.B., Davis, A.J., Fleet, I.R., Goode, J.A., Hamon, M., Nowak, R.A., Stewart, H.J., Whyte, A. & Flint, A.P.F. (1988b) Maternal recognition of pregnancy. *Proc. 11th Int. Congr. Anim. Reprod. & A.I., Dublin,* vol. 5, pp. 55–60.

Meek, K., Jeske, D., Slaoui, M., Leo, O., Urbain, J. & Capra, J.D. (1984) Complete amino acid sequence of heavy chain variable regions derived from two monoclonal anti-p-azophenylarsonate antibodies of BALB/c mice expressing the major cross-reactive idiotype of the A/J strain. *J. exp. Med.* **160**, 1070–1086.

Phillips, A., Hahn, D.W., McGuire, J., Wang, M.-W., Heap, R.B., Rider, V. & Taussig, M.J. (1988) Inhibition of pregnancy before and after implantation in rats with monoclonal antibody against progesterone. *Contraception* **38**, 109–116.

Rider, V. & Heap, R.B. (1986) Heterologous anti-progesterone monoclonal antibody arrests early embryonic development and implantation in the ferret (*Mustela putorius*). *J. Reprod. Fert.* **76**, 459–470.

Rider, V., McRae, A., Heap, R.B. & Feinstein, A. (1985) Passive immunization against progesterone inhibits endometrial sensitization in pseudopregnant mice and has antifertility effects in pregnant mice which are reversible by steroid treatment. *J. Endocr.* **104**, 153–158.

Rider, V., Wang, M.-Y., Finn, C., Heap, R.B. & Feinstein, A. (1986) Antifertility effect of passive immunization against progesterone is influenced by genotype. *J. Endocr.* **108**, 117–121.

Rider, V., Heap, R.B., Wang, M.-Y. & Feinstein, A. (1987) Anti-progesterone monoclonal antibody affects early cleavage and implantation in the mouse by mechanisms that are influenced by genotype. *J. Reprod. Fert.* **79**, 33–43.

Stura, E.A., Arevalo, J.H., Feinstein, A., Heap, R.B., Taussig, M.J. & Wilson, I.A. (1987) Analysis of an anti-progesterone antibody: variable crystal morphology of the Fab' and steroid-Fab' complexes. *Immunology* **62**, 511–521.

Wang, M.-Y., Rider, V., Heap, R.B. & Feinstein, A. (1984) Action of anti-progesterone monoclonal antibody in blocking pregnancy after postcoital administration in mice. *J. Endocr.* **101**, 95–100.

Wang, M.-W., Heap, R.B., King, I., Taussig, M.J. & Whyte, A. (1988) Anti-idiotypic antibody used for the localisation of parenterally administered monoclonal antiprogesterone antibody in mice. *Scand. J. Immunol.* **28**, 367–376.

Whyte, A., Yang, C.-B., Rutter, F. & Heap, R.B. (1987) Lectin-binding characteristics of mouse oviduct and

uterus associated with pregnancy block by auto-
logous antiprogesterone monoclonal antibody. *J.
Reprod. Immunol.* **11,** 209–219.

Wilmut, I., Sales, D.I. & Ashworth, C.J. (1986) Maternal
and embryonic factors associated with prenatal loss
in mammals. *J. Reprod. Fert.* **76,** 851–864.

Wright, L.J., Feinstein, A., Heap, R.B., Saunders, J.C.,
Bennett, R.C. & Wang, M.-Y. (1982) Progesterone
monoclonal antibody blocks pregnancy in mice.
Nature, Lond. **295,** 415–417.

J. Reprod. Fert., Suppl. **37** (1989), 245–252

Printed in Great Britain
© 1989 Journals of Reproduction & Fertility Ltd

Corpus luteum function in dairy cows and embryo mortality

G. E. Lamming, A. O. Darwash and H. L. Back

AFRC Research Group on Hormones and Farm Animal Reproduction, University of Nottingham, Faculty of Agricultural Science, Sutton Bonington, Loughborough LE12 5RD, U.K.

Keywords: corpus luteum; embryo mortality; pregnancy recognition; cattle

Introduction

High rates of embryo and fetal mortality continue to be a major cause of reproductive failure particularly in milked cows. Approximately 90% of ova are fertilized following either artificial or natural insemination (see Sreenan & Diskin, 1985), but on average only about 55% of dairy cows in U.K. herds calve to first insemination. These figures imply that about 35% of fertilized eggs are lost, the majority (in about 28% of cows) occurring before Day 25 after mating, the remainder occurring as late embryo or early fetal loss. The majority of embryo loss is sufficiently early (i.e. before Day 17) not to affect the initiation of the next phase of follicular growth and ovulation. The possible reasons for this loss include failure of normal embryo development, a failure of embryo-derived signals initiating the maternal recognition of pregnancy, or luteal dysfunction which could reflect inadequate preovulatory follicle development and maturation. Detailed studies are required to indicate the nature of embryo loss and thereby aid the development of remedial treatment.

The objective of this study was to examine the possibility that abnormal luteal function causes embryo and fetal loss in the cow and, following an earlier study (Bulman & Lamming, 1978), we have measured progesterone concentrations in whole milk from a substantial number of dairy cows maintained under natural farm conditions to examine the pattern of luteal function during early pregnancy for assessing the extent of progesterone synthesis and release. A clear relationship has previously been established between plasma and milk progesterone concentrations (Lamming & Bulman, 1976), milk progesterone levels at a given milking generally reflecting the plasma progesterone concentrations experienced during the inter-milking interval. Therefore, examination of milk concentrations over time gives an indication of the progesterone pattern of the individual animal and permits analysis, under field conditions, of factors associated with pregnancy failure without the stress of manually restraining the animal or subjecting it to frequent venepuncture.

Methods

Milk samples were collected 3 times weekly at the same milking from all cows in 21 dairy herds located in the East Midlands area of the U.K. (latitude 52·5°N). In addition, the University's experimental herd at Sutton Bonington was sampled to provide information on daily changes in milk progesterone concentrations and to provide data to authenticate the thrice weekly sampling approach. Animals were sampled from about 10 days *post partum* for 225 days and the study spanned at least 3 years.

Progesterone concentrations were measured in aliquants of whole milk as described by Lamming & Bulman (1976) and Bulman & Lamming (1978), using antiserum BT465 No. 6 (Furr, 1973). The intra- and inter-assay coefficient of variation was 8·9% and 10·3% respectively and the limit of sensitivity, defined as twice the standard deviation of blank values, was 0·3 ng/ml. Data from 2093 cows were available for analysis, but for this paper 446 animals, which exhibited early abnormal ovarian cycles and were allocated for specific remedial veterinary drug treatments or remained as untreated control animals, were specifically excluded from this analysis. This left a data base of 1647 cow post-partum profiles. The data were stored using a main-frame computer and subsequently analysed by a Fortran program. Statistical analysis of possible differences in milk progesterone concentrations between various categories of animals was made by interpolation within the selected time spans involved. Comparisons of regressions used standard least-squares methods provided by the GENSTAT program, produced by the Lawes Agricultural Trust, Rothamsted.

This discussion contains an analysis of two sections of the data concerning progesterone patterns in relation to (1) 'early embryo loss' before Day 25 and (2) 'late embryo and early fetal loss' between Days 25 and 125 after mating. The milk progesterone patterns of cows were used to study potential luteal dysfunction before or during the period of embryo or fetal loss. In Section 1 the progesterone profiles of animals subsequently calving to a given insemination are compared with those of unmated cyclic animals and with inseminated animals which failed to maintain a pregnancy. In Section 2 a further analysis is presented for animals considered pregnant as a result of an elevated milk progesterone concentration on Days 23–25 after insemination, but which subsequently experienced, by Day 125, a decline in milk progesterone value of a type usually associated with embryo loss.

Results

Section 1: early embryo loss

Out of 1647 cows, 1103 exhibited extended luteal function following artificial or natural insemination and were therefore assumed pregnant, while 759 showed a decline in milk progesterone value by Day 21–23 after insemination and were designated 'inseminated non-pregnant'. The mean milk progesterone data from this large data base have to be handled appropriately in that different animals were sampled on different days. Single readings from such assays have such a high variation that the prospect of detecting, from milk progesterone values, whether any individual animal is pregnant has to be regarded as negligible. The combined un-transformed data also showed an increasing variation with increasing value of the mean and this is traditionally treated by a transformation to stabilise it; in this case the logarithmic transformation (Log_e) of the values plus 1·0 proved appropriate. The graphs of the 'inseminated pregnant' (N = 1103) and the 'inseminated non-pregnant' (N = 759) groups shown in Fig. 1 illustrate a major separation of the two milk progesterone curves after Day 9. The curves are appropriately described by parallel quadratic equations and because of the apparent differences between the curves, especially after Day 9, these have been calculated for Days 7–16 and Days 10–16 respectively. This is particularly helpful in the overall analysis because it allows data from the fitted curves to be compared with observed values which then permits a more precise analysis for significant deviations in the pattern of change in milk progesterone concentrations. The relevant fitted, observed and residual values are given in Table 1.

Cows in the pregnant group showed a consistent daily rise in milk progestrone concentrations to Day 24, with significantly higher levels from Day 10–16 when compared to the equivalent phase of mated non-pregnant cows. However, the data for the pregnant group do show a lower than expected progesterone rise solely on Day 11 (residual −0·43, s.e. = 0·032) with a subsequent recovery on Day 12, possibly the first indication of the initial anti-luteolytic protective effect due to the presence of the embryo. This may be important in comparison with the inseminated non-pregnant group in which there was a major depression of milk progesterone concentration on Day 8 with a substantial recovery on Day 9. We believe that these were an authentic fall (residual error −0·069) and rise (residual error of +0·097) which were more than double their own standard errors. The progesterone concentration falls again on Day 10 and thereafter continues below that of the pregnant group. Based on this statistical analysis we can conclude that the increase in milk progesterone in the non-pregnant group Day 9 following the decline on Day 8 is probably a real phenomenon, not observed at the equivalent period in the 'pregnant' group.

From Day 7 to 16 the curves which produce the lowest r.s.d., and explain 96·4% of the total variation, are given by divergent quadratic curves which have the same quadratic term but differ in both the constant and linear coefficients required. For pregnant cows, Log milk progesterone (ng + 1) = $2·305 + 0·0682t − 0·00793 (t − 11·5)^2$ and, for inseminated not pregnant cows, Log milk progesterone (ng + 1) = $2·298 + 0·0588t − 0·00793 (t − 11·5)^2$ where t = time in days from insemination and residual standard deviation = $±0·0397$.

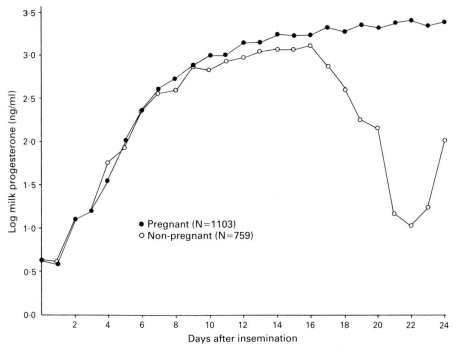

Fig. 1. Log$_e$ milk progesterone concentrations in inseminated pregnant dairy cows and inseminated non-pregnant cows sampled 3 times weekly.

Table 1. Daily Log milk progesterone values (ng +1) in milked dairy cows from Days 7 to 16 after insemination

Day from insemination	Pregnant (N = 1103)			Non-pregnant (N = 759)		
	Observed	Fitted	Residual	Observed	Fitted	Residual
7	2·61	2·62	−0·008	2·57	2·55	0·017
8	2·74	2·75	−0·019	2·60	2·67	−0·069*
9	2·89	2·87	0·025	2·88	2·78	0·097*
10	3·00	2·97	0·028	2·84	2·87	−0·028
11	3·01	3·05	−0·043*	2·94	2·94	−0·003
12	3·15	3·12	0·026	2·98	3·00	−0·020
13	3·16	3·17	−0·016	3·05	3·05	0·008
14	3·24	3·21	0·029	3·07	3·07	−0·006
15	3·22	3·23	−0·012	3·05	3·08	−0·032
16	3·23	3·24	−0·009	3·12	3·08	0·036

*Residual values of special note, see text.

Neither the difference between the constant terms nor that between the linear coefficients are significant ($P > 0.05$). The r.s.d. is relatively large compared to the errors derived for each datum point.

However, using the same comparison, from Days 10–16 to the curves are best described by the following equations. For pregnant cows, Log milk progesterone (ng + 1) = $2·632 + 0·0416t - 0·00743 (t - 13)^2$ and, for inseminated not pregnant cows, Log milk progesterone (ng + 1) = $2·598 + 0·0416t - 0·00743 (t - 13)^2$ where residual standard deviation = $\pm 0·0267$.

Over this period there is a significant difference between the constant terms ($P < 0.001$) and the r.s.d. of the pair of curves is relatively small compared to the errors given with each datum point, i.e. the fit of the data to the curves is good.

Such curves are best analysed by tabulating the fitted values and the deviations of each point as given in Table 1. The oscillations in the 'non-pregnant curve', including the dramatic increase on Day 9, increase the r.s.d. and therefore decreases the power to detect the difference in the two curves over the total period from Days 7 to 16. This means we cannot prove a significant divergence before Day 9. Nevertheless from Days 10 to 16 the two curves are clearly separated and significantly different. These conclusions are supported by a similar analysis on the single farm where daily progesterone values were recorded, albeit with fewer cows.

Finally, in this context we were able to exploit the data base further by analysing data derived from cows following observed oestrus. This generated three sets of data, a 'not-inseminated' group (i.e. cows with normal oestrous cycles): an 'inseminated pregnant' group and an 'inseminated non-pregnant' group. The data for observed, fitted and residual values from Days 7 to 16 are given in Table 2 and the observed and fitted curves are illustrated in Figs 2 and 3. Only the data for 'not-inseminated' and 'inseminated non pregnant' groups have been included in this part of the statistical analysis since clearly the analyses in Table 1 and Fig. 1 described previously involved data for more animals in the pregnant group.

Table 2. Daily Log milk progesterone values (ng/ml +1) in milked cows from Days 7 to 16 after oestrus for inseminated and non-inseminated cows

Day from service	Non-pregnant (N = 149)			Not served (N = 617)		
	Observed	Fitted	Residual	Observed	Fitted	Residual
7	2·41	2·40	0·008	2·42	2·44	−0·022
8	2·53	2·57	−0·036	2·66	2·62	0·043
9	2·71	2·71	0·005	2·79	2·77	0·018
10	2·87	2·82	0·043	2·86	2·90	−0·039
11	2·91	2·91	−0·002	2·98	3·00	−0·013
12	2·94	2·97	−0·029	3·10	3·07	0·030
13	3·02	3·01	0·012	3·08	3·12	−0·035
14	3·02	3·02	−0·002	3·12	3·14	−0·020
15	3·01	3·00	0·010	3·19	3·14	−0·056
16	2·95	2·96	−0·011	3·09	3·11	−0·017

The relevant quadratic equations are:

For not-inseminated cows, Log milk progesterone (ng + 1) $= 2.229 + 0.0621t - 0.0129 (t - 11.5)^2$ and, for inseminated non-pregnant cows, Log milk progesterone (ng + 1) $= 2.183 + 0.0742t - 0.0129 (t - 11.5)^2$ where t = time in days from oestrus.

Analysis of this section of data reveals a significant difference ($P < 0.05$) between the 'non-inseminated' group (i.e. normal pre-insemination cycles) and the 'inseminated non-pregnant' animals, indicating that animals which lose embryos early have significantly lower concentrations of milk progesterone from Days 7 to 16 when compared both to the pregnant group and to normally cyclic pre-inseminated animals. This finding suggests that early embryo loss is probably associated with a complex endocrine syndrome, one feature of which is manifestly a lower capacity to synthesize and/or release luteal progesterone. There was, however, no difference between any group in milk progesterone concentrations before Day 9.

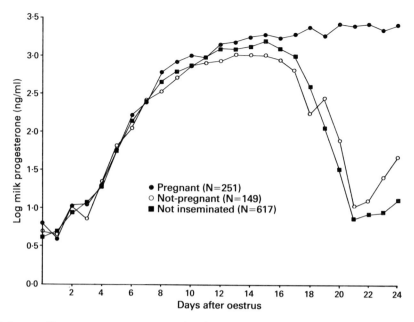

Fig. 2. Log$_e$ milk progesterone concentration in non-inseminated, inseminated pregnant and inseminated non-pregnant cattle from day of oestrus, sampled 3 times weekly.

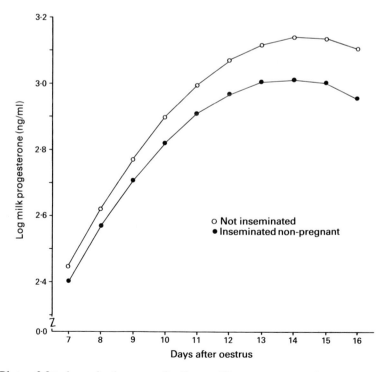

Fig. 3. Plots of fitted quadratic curves for Log$_e$ milk progesterone of non-inseminated and inseminated non-pregnant cows for Days 7 to 16 from time of oestrus.

Section 2: late embryo and early fetal loss

A decline in milk progesterone concentrations after a previously recorded high level at Day 25 after insemination occurred in 160 of the 2093 cows (7·7%) providing profiles. Spontaneous extension of luteal activity in non-inseminated animals is estimated to have accounted for no more than 0·5% of this (unpublished observations), and so the estimated late embryo and early fetal loss occurred in 7·2% of this population. Collectively they exhibited a milk progesterone concentration of > 10 ng/ml for a period 47·0 ± 1·1 days.

To determine whether embryo loss between 25 and 125 days after insemination is associated with abnormal progesterone patterns, the profiles of those cows which lost embryos were examined retrospectively. In summary we could observe no features of the pre-insemination or post-insemination progesterone patterns which were suggestive that abnormal luteal function or deficient placental progesterone synthesis at this stage of pregnancy was a causal factor in embryo mortality. Using a similar classification of pre-inseminated progesterone patterns as outlined by Bulman & Lamming (1978), 115 of the 160 animals (71·8%) losing embryos had 'normal' progesterone profiles before insemination, a figure comparable to that of the total data set. Immediately before the period of embryo loss (i.e. before the typically precipitous decline in milk progesterone concentrations), there were no differences in milk progesterone concentration between cows losing embryos and those completing normal pregnancies. This finding may explain why the administration of exogenous progesterone had no effect on embryo loss when given to groups of cows exhibiting normal levels of fertility (Diskin & Sreenan, 1986), although this procedure will improve the conception rate of sub-fertile animals which have lower plasma progesterone concentrations (Wiltbank *et al.*, 1956; Johnson *et al.*, 1958; Shemesh *et al.*, 1981). Subsequent to embryo loss the progesterone patterns of 110/115 animals (96%) showed that there was a normal resumption of ovarian activity, and the remaining 5 cows showed evidence of ovarian cysts. Altogether, 20 animals had more than one embryo loss during the same lactation. After the embryo loss conception occurred in 107/160 cows (66·9%) at 168 ± 3·6 days after calving and required 2·9 ± 0·1 services per conception, compared with 1811/2093 (86·5%) conceiving at 87·8 ± 0·7 days *post partum* and requiring 1·45 ± 0·02 services per conception for the total data set.

Discussion

The early recognition of pregnancy in cattle involves a series of embryo-generated signals to the mother which are believed to prevent the onset of luteolysis and thereby permit the continued development of the corpus luteum of pregnancy. In view of the heavy losses due to embryo mortality in the cow it is necessary to investigate how these signals are generated and whether they occur in the correct sequence in animals which lose embryos. This study involved an analysis of progesterone concentrations of a large number of dairy cows in relation to two distinct phases of early embryo development, i.e. the period from ovulation to Day 8 when hatching occurs, and the period from Day 8 until the onset of the precipitous decline in progesterone on Day 16–17 due to luteolysis.

We can find no evidence by retrospective analysis that cows losing fertilized ova or embryos have any deficiency of progesterone production before Day 7 and indeed there was uniformity in progesterone profiles in all cows irrespective of pregnancy status. It appears that ovulation is followed by normal development of the corpora lutea in terms of progesterone production up to Day 8 irrespective of whether the cow is inseminated or whether pregnancy is maintained. When sheep are induced to ovulate out of season by GnRH injections without progesterone pretreatment initial development is normal for up to 4 days after mating but the CL then declines prematurely (Southee *et al.*, 1988a; Hunter *et al.*, 1988). The demise is prevented by hysterectomy, a result implicating a role for the uterus for this mechanism (Southee *et al.*, 1988b). It is possible that the oscillations of the milk progesterone concentrations shown in cows losing early embryos in this study could be due to luteal sensitivity to low levels of PGF-2α, not manifest before Day 8 but present thereafter, since Lafrance & Goff (1988) have shown that a period of priming of the uterus with progesterone (about 7 days) is required in the cow before an oxytocin-induced release of PGF-2α can occur. This may explain the appearance of a significant depression in milk progesterone in the inseminated non-pregnant cows after Day 7. Day 8 in the inseminated non-pregnant cows or indeed in the normal oestrous cycle may therefore indicate the initiation of a pattern of events leading to luteolysis, which then causes a significant depression in milk progesterone concentrations as revealed by the present analyses. Because of the consistency of the data with low standard errors, the decline of milk progesterone on Day 9 and the subsequent increase on Day 10 in the mated, non-pregnant group is a real phenomenon although at this stage we have no established biological explanation for its occurrence, except that it might signal the onset of a sustained luteolytic effect in animals which are failing to maintain the pregnancy. However, the causal factors associated with the divergence of milk progesterone patterns remain to be clarified. High vena caval concentrations of both oestradiol-17β and oxytocin have been measured during the period Days 4–7 after oestrus in non-pregnant compared to pregnant animals (E. Schallenberger, personal communication), and this may influence the subsequent development of oxytocin receptors in the uterus of these animals, thereby increasing the release of small episodes of PGF-2α which may depress luteal progesterone synthesis.

In the inseminated pregnant cows there was a steady rise in milk progesterone concentrations over the whole period up to Day 24 after insemination, with the exception of Day 11 when a lower than expected rise occurred. However, this was followed by a compensatory rise on Day 12, which could indicate the initial appearance and effect of embryo-derived antiluteolysin (designated bTP-1) (Helmer *et al.*, 1988a, b; see also Thatcher *et al.*, 1989). The smooth progressive increase in milk progesterone concentration over the whole period in the inseminated pregnant group does not give support for a major change in embryo-generated luteotrophic support during this stage, although the possibility that the embryo contributes to luteal activity cannot be ruled out. The results therefore indicate that, during pregnancy, suppression of luteolysis is more important than the generation of embryo-derived luteotrophic support. It is significant, however, that the milk progesterone concentrations of the 'inseminated non-pregnant' cows are significantly lower than those of the non-inseminated and the inseminated pregnant cows, implying that the less fertile animals are those which exhibit a depressed milk progesterone concentration over the period 8–16 days after insemination. These results coincide with those previously presented for plasma progesterone concentrations in mated and unmated experimental heifers by Hansel (1981) which also show a depression of plasma progesterone concentration in the pregnant group on Day 12 after insemination.

Conclusions

(1) There is a steady increase in luteal progesterone synthesis during the early phase of pregnancy which continues up to Day 25 after insemination leading to higher milk progesterone concentrations from Days 10 to 16 when compared to the equivalent phase of the oestrous cycle. The development of the CL of pregnancy represents the norm which implies an inbuilt ability to maintain progesterone synthesis and the 'not inseminated' and 'inseminated non-pregnant' cows which have lower rates of progesterone production after Day 10 deviate from this norm. The results provide circumstantial evidence for the appearance of the embryo-derived anti-luteolytic trophoblastin (bTP-1) at least by Day 12 after mating.

(2) Inseminated cows subsequently shown to be not pregnant by a dramatic decline in milk progesterone concentrations on Days 21–23 after insemination have retrospectively significantly ($P < 0.001$) lower milk progesterone values from Days 10 to 16 after insemination, but with progesterone curves parallel on a log basis (equivalent to a difference of ∼4 ng/ml) when compared

with both pre-inseminated cows with normal oestrous cycles and with inseminated pregnant cows. Animals which fail to maintain the early embryos therefore have a small but measurable depression in progesterone output although the differences between the pregnant and non-pregnant groups do not appear sufficient to provide a valid explanation of why such animals fail to maintain the pregnancy. This finding may indicate a decreased competence of the preovulatory follicle or post-ovulatory luteal structure which might be associated with the loss of the embryo and which additionally contributes to a depressive effect on luteal progesterone production. Alternatively, Day 8 may signify the termination of a critical period of progesterone activity required before PGF-2α can be released and the oscillation of progesterone in the inseminated non-pregnant cows on Days 9 and 10 may indicate the onset of luteolysis which then results in embryo mortality.

(3) It is not possible from analysis of this large data base to implicate abnormal progesterone concentrations as a causal factor and it is therefore necessary to examine other potential factors.

It is our contention that pregnancy in the cow is the normal condition, and therefore the corpus luteum does not require to be 'rescued' via embryo-derived luteotrophic activity.

We thank the Milk Marketing Board of England and Wales, and the AFRC for financial support.

References

Bulman, D.C. & Lamming, G.E. (1978) Milk progesterone levels in relation to conception, repeat breeding and factors influencing acyclicity in dairy cows. *J. Reprod Fert.* **54**, 447–458.

Diskin, M.G. & Sreenan, J.M. (1986) Progesterone and embryo survival in the cow. In *Embryonic Mortality in Farm Animals*, pp. 142–158. Eds J. M. Sreenan & M. G. Diskin. Martinus Nijhoff, Dordrecht.

Furr, B.J.A. (1973) Radioimmunoassay of progesterone in peripheral plasma of the domestic fowl in various physiological states and in follicular venous plasma. *Acta endocr., Copenh.* **72**, 89–100.

Hansel, W. (1981) Plasma hormone concentrations associated with early embryo mortality in heifers. *J. Reprod. Fert., Suppl.* **30**, 231–239.

Helmer, S.D., Hansen, P.J., Thatcher, W.W., Johnson, J.W. & Bazer, F.W. (1988a) Intrauterine infusion of purified bovine trophoblast protein-1 (bTP-1) extends corpus luteum (CL) livespan in cyclic cattle. *J. Anim. Sci.* **67**, (Suppl. 1) 415, Abstr.

Helmer, S.D., Gross, T.S., Hansen, P.J. & Thatcher, W.W. (1988b) Bovine conceptus secretory proteins (bCSP) and bovine trophoblast protein-1 (bTP-1) a component of bCSP, alter endometrial prostaglandin (PG) secretion and induce an intracellular inhibitor of PG synthesis in vitro. *Biol. Reprod.* **38**, Suppl. 1, 153, Abstr.

Hunter, M.G., Southee, J.A. & Lamming, G.E. (1988) Function of abnormal corpora lutea *in vitro* after GnRH-induced ovulation in the anoestrous ewe. *J. Reprod. Fert.* **84**, 139–148.

Johnson, K.R., Ross, R.H. & Fourt, D.L. (1958) Effect of progesterone administration on reproductive efficiency. *J. Anim. Sci.* **17**, 386–390.

Lafrance, M. & Goff, A.K. (1988) Effects of progesterone and oestradiol-17β on oxytocin-induced release of prostaglandin F-2α in heifers. *J. Reprod. Fert.* **82**, 429–436.

Lamming, G.E. & Bulman, D.C. (1976) The use of milk progesterone radioimmunoassay in the diagnosis and treatment of subfertility in dairy cows. *Br. vet. J.* **132**, 507–517.

Shemesh, M., Ayalon, N., Marcus, S., Danielli, Y., Shore, L. & Lavi, S. (1981) Improvement of early pregnancy diagnosis based on milk progesterone by the use of progestin-impregnated vaginal sponges. *Theriogenology* **15**, 459–462.

Southee, J.A., Hunter, M.G. & Haresign, W. (1988a) Function of abnormal corpora lutea *in vivo* after GnRH-induced ovulation in the anoestrous ewe. *J. Reprod. Fert.* **84**, 131–137.

Southee, J.A., Hunter, M.G., Law, A.S. & Haresign, W. (1988b) Effect of hysterectomy on the short lifecycle corpus luteum produced after GnRH-induced ovulation in the anoestrous ewe. *J. Reprod. Fert.* **84**, 149–155.

Sreenan, J.M. & Diskin, M.G. (1985) The extent and timing of embryonic mortality in the cow. In *Embryonic Mortality in Farm Animals*, pp. 1–11. Eds J. M. Sreenan & M. G. Diskin. Martinus Nijhoff, Dordrecht.

Thatcher, W.W., Hansen, P.J., Gross, T.S., Helmer, S.D., Plante, C. & Bazer, F.W. (1989) Antiluteolytic effects of bovine trophoblast protein-1. *J. Reprod. Fert., Suppl.* **37**, 91–99.

Wiltbank, J.N., Hawk, H.W., Kidder, H.E., Ulberg, L.C. & Casida, L.E. (1956) Effect of progesterone therapy on embryo survival in cows of lowered fertility. *J. Dairy Sci.* **39**, 456–461.

J. Reprod. Fert., Suppl. **37** (1989), 253–260

Response to the antiprogestagen RU 486 (mifepristone) during early pregnancy and the menstrual cycle in women

I. M. Spitz*, Donna Shoupe†, Regine Sitruk-Ware‡§, and D. R. Mishell, Jr†

**Center for Biomedical Research, The Population Council, New York, NY 10021, U.S.A.;*
†*University of Southern California School of Medicine, Los Angeles, CA 90033, U.S.A.; and*
‡*Hopital Necker, Paris, France*

Summary. RU 486 has wide potential utility as an abortifacient drug when used within the first 6 weeks of pregnancy and has the ability to induce an abortion in about 80% of subjects. Administration of low doses of prostaglandins together with RU 486 increases the success rate. It is possible that alterations in metabolism of RU 486 may explain non-responsiveness to the drug in some women. Mid-luteal phase administration of RU 486 produces bleeding within 72 h and in one-third of subjects there was luteolysis with decrease in serum FSH, oestradiol and progesterone concentrations. Administration of RU 486 in the late luteal phase does not disturb menstrual cycle length, bleeding patterns, ovulation, or hormonal parameters in treatment or post-treatment cycles. However, the drug alone cannot be used as a 'menses regulator' or 'once monthly pill' since some pregnancies do continue. Possibly the efficacy of RU 486 may be enhanced when it is combined with prostaglandins or other agents. Administration of RU 486 in the follicular phase blocks ovulation, delays the LH surge, and is associated with low concentrations of oestradiol. This is presumably the result of gonadotrophin inhibition.

Keywords: RU 486; abortion; LH; FSH; oestradiol; progesterone

Introduction

RU 486 (17β-hydroxy-11β-[4-dimethylaminophenyl]-17α-1-[prop-1-ynyl]-oestra-4,9-dien-3-one), also known as mifepristone, is a 19-norsteroid derivative which was synthesized by Roussel UCLAF, Paris, France. This compound has been shown to have antiprogestational and antiglucocorticoid action in man and other animals (Philibert *et al.*, 1985, Baulieu *et al.*, 1987). It is estimated that throughout the world up to 55×10^6 pregnancies each year are terminated by abortion (Tietze, 1983). It has long been recognized that a major advance in contraceptive technology would be the development of an agent capable of inducing medical abortion. RU 486 has therefore aroused considerable interest because of its antiprogestagenic properties. In this review, we will evaluate the effect of RU 486 on abortion induction and also determine the effect of this antiprogestagen when administered at different phases of the menstrual cycle.

Abortion induction

In studies carried out by the Population Council on 125 women with amenorrhoea of less than 7 weeks, abortion was successfully induced in 76% of the subjects when RU 486 was administered in a dose of 100 mg daily for 7 days (Spitz *et al.*, 1988). Roussel UCLAF (France) have reported that,

§Present address: Medical Department, Ciba Geigy, Basel, Switzerland.

in 920 women with amenorrhoea of less than 6 weeks, the incidence of abortion was 79·5%. In these studies, RU 486 was given as a single dose (600 mg). Similar success rates were observed by Roussel UCLAF with single doses of 200–800 mg (unpublished observations). This is not unexpected since circulating RU 486 concentrations determined by radioimmunoassay in non-pregnant women during the luteal phase were similar with single doses ranging from 200 to 800 mg (Shoupe *et al.*, 1987a). With the Population Council regimen of 100 mg daily for 7 days, bleeding usually began on the 2nd or 3rd day of RU 486 administration and lasted for up to 14 days (Shoupe *et al.*, 1986a; Mishell *et al.*, 1987). Bleeding begins earlier and lasts longer in those subjects who abort. In the series reported by Shoupe *et al.* (1986a), in 47 subjects who received 100 mg/day for 7 days, 59% of subjects reported heavy bleeding. The reduction in haemoglobin was < 1 g/100 ml in 31 subjects and in 12 it ranged from 1 to 3 g/100 ml. In only 4 subjects did haemoglobin fall more than 3 g/100 ml. No subject required blood transfusion and, in all, haemoglobin returned to pretreatment levels by Day 21. Side-effects reported in this series included nausea and vomiting (40%), uterine cramps (42%), and headaches (9%). Weakness and tiredness have also been described. It is often difficult to dissociate these symptoms from those occurring in normal pregnancy.

RU 486 has also been shown to display antiglucocorticoid activity and doses ranging from 5 to 20 mg/kg/day have resulted in amelioration of the clinical and biochemical manifestations of Cushing's Syndrome (Nieman *et al.*, 1985). These doses are higher than those required for antiprogestagenic activity. While single doses of 200–800 mg do produce a dose-dependent transient rise in plasma cortisol, these concentrations usually remain within or just above the normal range and return to baseline within a few days (Shoupe *et al.*, 1986a, 1987a; Mishell *et al.*, 1987). No clinical manifestations of glucocorticoid deficiency have been reported during RU 486 administration for pregnancy interruption.

Attempts have been made to ascertain whether any index could predict which women will respond with successful termination of pregnancy. The most reliable factor appears to be the steady reduction in serum hCG-β values in the responders (Mishell *et al.*, 1987). In contrast, in those subjects who fail to abort, hCG-β concentrations remain the same or show further elevation. Other factors appear less reliable. Although pretreatment serum concentrations of oestradiol, progesterone and hCG-β were usually lower in the responders than in the non-responders, in individual cases these measurements appear to have little predictive value unless hCG-β values are < 10 000 m.i.u./ml (Mishell *et al.*, 1987). A gestational sac on ultrasound of < 10 mm may also be of some diagnostic aid.

A critical factor determining the successful response to RU 486 would appear to be the duration of pregnancy. The incidence of successful termination is higher in pregnancies of < 6 weeks than in those exceeding 7 weeks (Baulieu *et al.*, 1987). In pregnancies of > 8 weeks, only 3 out of 9 subjects aborted (Vervest & Haspels, 1985). Other factors involved in the non-responsiveness could be inadequate prostaglandin activation by RU 486. Studies with cultured decidual and endometrial tissue have shown that RU 486 increases prostaglandin secretion into the medium (Kelly *et al.*, 1985; Smith & Kelly, 1987). Bygdeman & Swahn (1985) have suggested that inadequate prostaglandin activation could account for the non-responsiveness to RU 486 and have shown that the addition of low doses of prostaglandin increase the success rate.

Finally, non-responsiveness could also be related to variations in absorption or metabolism of RU 486. In studies in mongrel dogs, we have observed that some animals respond with increases in ACTH and cortisol after RU 486 administration whereas others do not respond in this way. Repeated administration of RU 486 elicits the identical response in the same animals. On the other hand, all dogs respond uniformly to other stimuli for ACTH and cortisol secretion (Spitz *et al.*, 1985). The disappearance of circulating RU 486 and its metabolites is retarded in dogs that respond with increases in ACTH and cortisol after administration of RU 486. Since these were mongrel dogs, this implies some alteration in metabolism of RU 486 in different strains of the same species. In unpublished studies we have shown that dogs of the same strain uniformly respond with increases in ACTH and cortisol following the same dose schedules of RU 486. A similar phenomenon could possibly occur in women and may explain the non-responsiveness.

Administration of RU 486 in the mid-luteal phase

Administration of RU 486 in doses of 50–800 mg on Days 6–8 of the luteal phase induced bleeding within 72 h (Shoupe *et al.*, 1987a). The bleeding episode occurred despite high circulating concentrations of oestradiol and progesterone and is presumably due to a direct effect on the endometrium. In 36% of the subjects this represented the only bleeding episode and was associated with reduction in serum FSH, oestradiol and progesterone concentrations and a shortened cycle length (Fig. 1). In the remaining 74% of subjects, there were no changes in hormonal values (Fig. 1) and after some days there was further bleeding associated with spontaneous corpus luteum

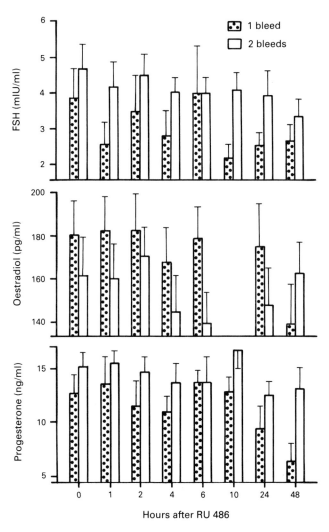

Fig. 1. Mean ± s.e.m. serum concentrations of FSH, oestradiol and progesterone in response to a single dose administration of RU 486 (50–800 mg) in normal women. RU 486 was administered on Days 6–8 of the luteal phase. Groups of 4 subjects received RU 486 doses of 50, 100, 200 and 400 mg; 5 subjects received 600 mg and 800 mg RU 486. In those subjects who had only one bleeding episode, analysis of variance showed a significant decline in FSH, oestradiol and progesterone concentrations (□); there was no decline in these hormones in those subjects who had 2 bleeding episodes (□).

256   *I. M. Spitz* et al.

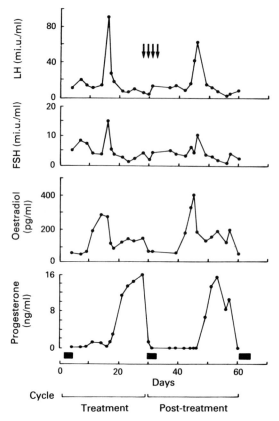

Fig. 2. Serum LH, FSH, oestradiol and progesterone response in the treatment and post-treatment cycle in a woman treated with RU 486 (indicated by the arrows) on Days 23–27 of the first cycle. Hormonal profiles are normal in both cycles.

regression. In these latter subjects, the cycle length was prolonged (Shoupe *et al.*, 1987a). These two distinct patterns were not related to the dose of the antiprogestagen or circulating RU 486 concentrations. There was a dose-dependent transient rise in serum prolactin concentrations which was independent of the bleeding patterns or steroid values (Shoupe *et al.*, 1987a).

Administration of RU 486 in the late luteal phase

When given in the late luteal phase in a dose of 100 mg/day for 4 days immediately before menstrual bleeding, RU 486 did not alter the serum concentrations of oestradiol, progesterone, LH or FSH in the post-treatment cycle (Fig. 2) or the length of the cycle (Croxatto *et al.*, 1987). Furthermore, there were no disturbances in menstrual cyclicity, bleeding patterns or hormonal profile when this same dose was given in identical fashion for 3 successive cycles. The elevation of urinary pregnanediol during the 3 treatment cycles was similar to that observed in two pre-treatment and two post-treatment placebo-treated cycles (Fig. 3). This indicates the presence of ovulation and corpus luteum function. Bleeding patterns were also not disturbed by RU 486 administration provided the drug was given late in the luteal phase (Croxatto *et al.*, 1987). Several workers have attempted to utilize this strategy and develop RU 486 as a 'menses regulator' or 'once-a-month pill'. RU 486 administered as a single dose of 400 mg or in divided doses over 4 days at the expected

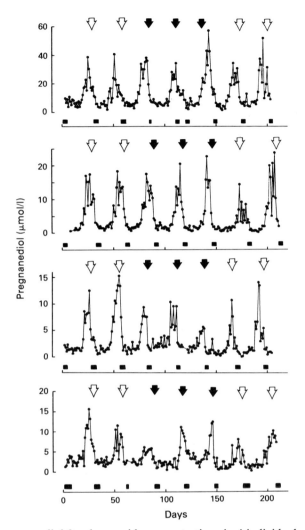

Fig. 3. Urinary pregnanediol 3α-glucuronide concentrations in 4 individual subjects during 7 successive cycles. These comprised 2 placebo, 3 RU 486 treatment and a further 2 placebo cycles. RU 486 administration (100 mg daily for 4 days) is indicated by closed arrows; placebo by open arrows. The elevation of urinary pregnanediol glucuronide is indicative of ovulation and corpus luteum function. Bleeding patterns are indicated by the solid bars. A disruption of the normal bleeding pattern occurred only in the first subject since RU 486 was administered too early in the 2nd and 3rd treatment cycles.

time of menses to unprotected women who have had sexual relations during that cycle have shown that some pregnancies can continue (van Santen & Haspels, 1987). A similar effect is seen with single doses of 600 mg (unpublished observations).

Administration of RU 486 in the follicular phase

When RU 486 was given in a dose of 100 mg from Days 10 to 17 of the cycle, the LH and FSH surges were attenuated and preovulatory oestradiol values were reduced (Shoupe *et al.*, 1987b). There was no rise in progesterone. This regimen resulted in demise of the dominant follicle (Liu *et*

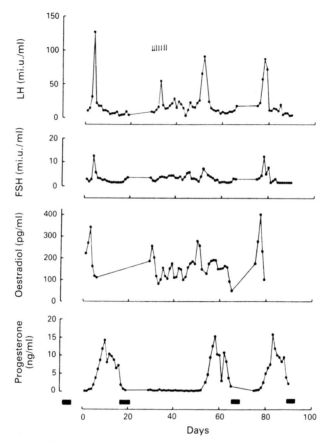

Fig. 4. Serum LH, FSH, oestradiol and progesterone concentrations in a woman during a control (pre-treatment), treatment and post-treatment cycle when RU 486 (arrows) was administered on Days 10–17. Solid bars indicate the bleeding pattern. Note the attenuated LH surge during RU 486 administration. Serum oestradiol concentrations are low compared to the pre-treatment and post-treatment cycles.

Table 1. Mean ± s.e.m. length (days) of the total cycle, as well as follicular and luteal phases in the pre-treatment, treatment and post-treatment cycles in 5 women treated with RU 486 from Days 10 to 17 of the treatment cycle

	Pre-treatment	Treatment	Post-treatment
Total cycle	28·8 ± 0·7	40·6 ± 2·6*	25·2 ± 0·9
Luteal phase	15·2 ± 0·8	13·8 ± 1·2	13·5 ± 4·0
Follicular phase	14·6 ± 1·3	28·0 ± 2·3*	13·5 ± 1·9

*$P < 0.05$ compared to pre-treatment and post-treatment cycles.

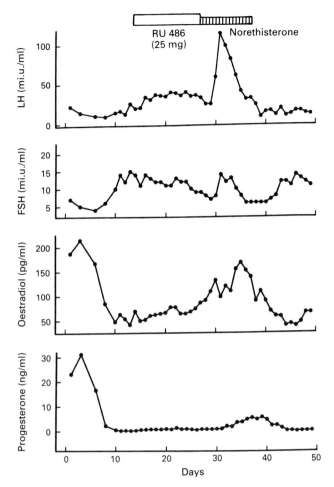

Fig. 5. LH, FSH, oestradiol and progesterone profiles in a woman treated with RU 486 from Days 5 to 15 of the cycle in a dose of 25 mg daily. This was followed by a 7-day course of norethisterone (5 mg/day).

al., 1987). Further follicular recruitment occurred and 14 days later there was an LH surge followed by a rise in progesterone (Fig. 4). This pharmacological manipulation produced a prolongation of the follicular phase of the treatment cycle when compared to the pre-treatment and post-treatment cycles (Table 1).

In further studies, RU 486 was given in a daily dose of 25 or 100 mg from Days 5 to 15 of the cycle. This was followed by norethisterone (5 mg/day) for 7 days. During RU 486 administration there was no LH or FSH surge and oestradiol values were low. After cessation of RU 486 treatment and during administration of the progestagen, there was a rise in oestradiol values and LH and FSH surges (Fig. 5). These results suggest that RU 486 may have an inhibitory effect on gonadotrophin secretion. Indeed, frequent blood sampling in the luteal phase has shown that there is a decrease in amplitude of LH pulses during RU 486 administration (Shoupe *et al.*, 1986b; Garzo *et al.*, 1988). However, no modification in the LH secretory pattern was observed when RU 486 was administered in the follicular phase (Liu *et al.*, 1987). It is also possible that RU 486 may directly affect the ovary and in-vitro studies with cultured granulosa cells have shown that RU 486 decreases progesterone but not oestradiol secretion (Dimattina *et al.*, 1986, 1987).

The RU 486 used in this study was kindly supplied by Roussel UCLAF, Paris, France. The study was supported by grants from the Ford and Mellon Foundations.

References

Baulieu, E.E., Ulmann, A. & Philibert, D. (1987) Contragestion by antiprogestin RU 486: A novel approach to human fertility control. In *Fertility Regulation Today and Tomorrow* (Serono Symp.) pp. 55–73. Eds E. Diczfalusy & M. Bygdeman. Raven Press, New York.

Bygdeman, M. & Swahn, M-L. (1985) Progesterone receptor blockage: effect on uterine contractility and early pregnancy. *Contraception* 32, 45–57.

Croxatto, H.B., Salvatierra, A.M., Romero, C. & Spitz, I.M. (1987) Late luteal phase administration of RU 486 for three successive cycles does not disrupt bleeding patterns or ovulation. *J. clin. Endocr. Metab.* 65, 1272–1277.

Dimattina, M., Albertson, B., Seyler, D.E., Loriaux, D.L. & Falk, R.J. (1986) Effect of the antiprogestagin RU 486 on progesterone production by cultured human granulosa cells: inhibition of the ovarian 3β-hydroxysteroid dehydrogenase. *Contraception* 34, 199–206.

Dimattina, M., Albertson, B.D., Tyson, V., Loriaux, D.L. & Falk, R.J. (1987) Effect of the antiprogestin RU 486 on human ovarian steroidogenesis. *Fert. Steril.* 48, 229–233.

Garzo, G.V., Liu, J., Ulmann, A., Baulieu, E. & Yen, S.S.C. (1988) Effects of the antiprogesterone (RU 486) on the hypothalamic-hypophyseal-ovarian-endometrial axis during the luteal phase of the menstrual cycle. *J. clin. Endocr. Metab.* 66, 508–517.

Kelly, R.W., Healy, D.L., Cameron, M.J., Cameron, I.T. & Baird, D.T. (1985) RU 486 stimulation of $PGF_2\alpha$ production in isolated endometrial cells in short term culture. In *The Antiprogestin Steroid RU 486 and Human Fertility Control*, pp. 259–262. Eds E. E. Baulieu & S. J. Segal. Plenum Press, New York.

Liu, J.H., Garzo, G., Morris, S., Stuenkel, C., Ulmann, A. & Yen, S.S.C. (1987) Disruption of follicular maturation and delay of ovulation after administration of the antiprogesterone RU 486. *J. clin. Endocr. Metab.* 65, 1135–1140.

Mishell, D.R., Shoupe, D., Brenner, P.F., Lacarra, M., Horenstein, P.J., Lahteenmaki, P. & Spitz, I.M. (1987) Termination of early gestation wth the antiprogestin RU486, medium versus low dosage. *Contraception* 35, 307–321.

Nieman, L.K., Chrousos, G.P., Kellner, C., Spitz, I.M., Nisula, B.C., Cutler, G.B., Jr, Merriam, G.R., Bardin, C.W. & Loriaux, D.L. (1985) Successful treatment of Cushing's syndrome with the glucocorticoid anatagonist RU 486. *J. clin. Endocr. Metab.* 61, 536–540.

Philibert, D., Moguilewsky, M., Mary, I., Lecaque, D., Tournemine, C., Secchi, J. & Deraedt, R. (1985) Pharmacological profile of RU 486 in animals. In *The Antiprogestin Steroid RU 486 and Human Fertility Control*, pp. 49–68. Eds E. E. Baulieu & S. J. Segal. Plenum Press, New York.

Shoupe, D., Mishell, D.R., Brenner, P.F. & Spitz, I.M. (1986a) Pregnancy termination with a high and medium dosage regimen of RU 486. *Contraception* 33, 455–461.

Shoupe, D., Spitz, I., Osborn, C., Page, M., Mishell, D. & Lobo, R. (1986b) Effects of progesterone antagonism on gonadotropin at midcycle and during the luteal phase. *Proc. 33rd Annual Meeting of Society for Gynecologic Investigation, Toronto, Ontario, Canada*, Abstract 20.

Shoupe, D., Mishell, D.R., Jr, Lahteenmaki, P., Heikinheimo, O., Birgerson, L., Madkour, H. & Spitz, I.M. (1987a) Effects of the antiprogesterone RU 486 in normal women. I. Single dose administration in the mid-luteal phase. *Am. J. Obstet. Gynecol.* 157, 1415–1420.

Shoupe, D., Mishell, D.R., Jr, Page, M.A., Madkour, H., Spitz, I.M. & Lobo, R.A. (1987b) Effects of antiprogesterone RU 486 in normal women. II. Administration in the late follicular phase. *Am. J. Obstet. Gynecol.* 157, 1421–1428.

Smith, S.K. & Kelly, R.W. (1987) The effect of the antiprogestins RU 486 and ZK 98734 on the synthesis and metabolism of prostaglandins $F_{2\alpha}$ and E_2 in separated cells from early human decidua. *J. clin. Endocr. Metab.* 65, 527–534.

Spitz, I.M., Wade, C.E., Krieger, D.T., Lahteenmaki, P. & Bardin, C.W. (1985) Effect of RU486 in the dog. In *The Antiprogestin Steroid RU 486 and Human Fertility Control*, pp. 315–329. Eds E. E. Baulieu & S. J. Segal. Plenum Press, New York.

Spitz, I.M., Sitruk-Ware, R., Shoupe, D., Croxatto, H., Lahteenmaki, P., Birgerson, L., Mishell, D., Johansson, E. & Bardin, C.W. (1988) Clinical effects of RU486. *Proc. Int. Symp. Fertil. Reg. Res. (Beijing)*.

Tietze, C. (1983) Induced abortion: a world review, 1983. In *A Population Council Fact Book*, 5th edn. The Population Council, New York.

van Santen, M.R. & Haspels, A.A. (1987) Interception IV: Failure of mifepristone (RU 486) as a monthly contragestive, 'Lunarette'. *Contraception* 35, 433–438.

Vervest, H.A.M. & Haspels, A.A. (1985) Preliminary results with the antiprogestational compound RU-486 (mifepristone) for interruption of early pregnancy. *Fert. Steril.* 44, 627–632.

J. Reprod. Fert., Suppl. **37** (1989), 261–267

Prostaglandin secretion by the blastocyst

G. S. Lewis

United States Department of Agriculture, Agricultural Research Service, Beltsville Agricultural Research Center, Livestock and Poultry Sciences Institute, Reproduction Laboratory, Building 200, Beltsville, Maryland 20705, U.S.A.

Summary. Conceptuses from some mammals synthesized prostaglandins (PG) *in vitro*. Blastocysts from cattle produced primarily PGF-2α; those from sheep produced mainly 6-keto-PGF-1α and PGF-2α; and those from pigs produced mostly PGE-2. Rabbits have not been shown to produce a predominant PG and mice and rats have not been shown to produce detectable amounts of PG. Other species do not appear to have been studied. Prostaglandins of conceptus origin appear to be involved directly in: intrauterine migration of embryos; blastocyst hatching from the zona pellucida; ion transport across trophectoderm; fluid accumulation in the blastocoele; increased endometrial capillary permeability; blastocystic glucose metabolism.

Keywords: blastocyst; trophoblast; prostaglandins; livestock; early pregnancy

Introduction

Before attaching to endometrium, conceptus membranes, mainly trophoblast, seem to be the physiological guardian of the embryo. Much as liver functions after birth, conceptus membranes probably process to some extent virtually all nutrients passing from the uterine lumen into the conceptus. Conceptus membranes use these nutrients to synthesize a variety of biochemicals, which are surely essential for embryonic survival and continuance of pregnancy. This review summarizes synthesis of one class of biochemicals, prostaglandins (PGs), and suggests some physiological functions for PG of conceptus origin.

Prostaglandin synthesis

Cattle

Radioimmunoassays (RIA) have indicated that blastocysts collected on Days 13, 15 or 16 of pregnancy released PGF (antibody crossreacted significantly with PGF-2α and PGF-1α) and PGE-2 *in vitro* (Shemesh *et al.*, 1979). Day-16 and -19 blastocysts incubated with [³H]arachidonic acid synthesized and released tritiated PGF-2α, PGE-2, 13,14-dihydro-15-keto-PGF-2α (PGFM; a major metabolite of PGF-2α) and several unidentified compounds (Lewis *et al.*, 1982). Blastocysts produced more PGF-2α than PGE-2 or PGFM and considerably more PGF-2α and PGE-2 than did endometrium, but the two tissues produced similar amounts of PGFM (Table 1; Shemesh *et al.*, 1979; Lewis *et al.*, 1982; Lewis & Waterman, 1983a).

Studies on control of PG synthesis indicated that endometrium co-incubated with blastocysts reduced (32% and 97%; Lewis & Waterman, 1983a; Lewis, 1986a, respectively) blastocystic production of PGF-2α. Factors in high-speed supernatants from early-pregnant endometrial homogenates reduced PG synthetase activity, and these factors may have reduced blastocystic production of PGF-2α *in vitro* (Wlodawer *et al.*, 1976; Basu & Kindahl, 1987; Gross *et al.*, 1987; G. S. Lewis, unpublished observations). In-vivo studies have not been conducted to determine whether endometrium secretes PG-inhibitory factors into the uterine lumen. Even though

G. S. Lewis

Table 1. Prostaglandins released by cattle blastocysts and endometrium incubated for 24 h *in vitro* (after Lewis *et al.*, 1982)

| | Quantity (ng)/mg tissue | | | |
| | Blastocyst | | Endometrium | |
Prostaglandin	Day 16	Day 19	Day 16	Day 19
PGF-2α	284 ± 76	111 ± 32	2 ± 0·4	2 ± 0·4
PGE-2	66 ± 37	18 ± 5	0·6 ± 0·1	1 ± 0·5
PGFM	3 ± 1	2 ± 1	3 ± 1	5 ± 1

Values are mean ± s.e.m. for 5 observations on Day 16 and 6 on Day 19. Blastocysts from both days of pregnancy released more ($P < 0.01$) PGF-2α than PGE-2 or PGFM and more ($P < 0.05$) PGE-2 than PGFM. Blastocysts released more ($P < 0.001$) PGF-2α and PGE-2 than did endometrium. Neither tissue nor day affected release of PGFM.

endogenous arachidonic acid will sustain maximal endometrial synthesis of PGF-2α for 24 h *in vitro*, that available for blastocystic PGF-2α synthesis appears to become limiting after 8 h, indicating that blastocysts *in utero* may need a continuous maternal supply of arachidonic acid to support PG-mediated developmental events (Lewis, 1986a).

Sheep

Day-12, -14, -15 and -16 blastocysts and Day-20 and -24 chorionic membranes incubated with radioactive arachidonic acid released radiolabelled 6-keto-PGF-1α (a major metabolite of PGI-2), PGF-2α, PGE-2, PGFM and several unidentified compounds (Marcus, 1981; Lewis & Waterman, 1985). Summarization of studies with conceptuses indicated that the relative amounts of PG produced *in vitro* were: 6-keto-PGF-1α ≥ PGF-2α > PGE-2 ≥ PGFM (Table 2; Marcus, 1981; Hyland *et al.*, 1982; Lacroix & Kann, 1982; Lewis & Waterman, 1985; Rawlings & Hyland, 1985).

Table 2. Prostaglandins (ng/mg tissue) released by sheep blastocysts and endometrium incubated for 24 h *in vitro* (after Lewis & Waterman, 1985)

	6-keto-PGF-1α	PGF-2α	PGE-2	PGFM
Blastocyst				
Day 14	41 ± 5[a]*	32 ± 18[a]†	12 ± 8[a]*	8 ± 6[a]
Day 16	16 ± 3[a]*	9 ± 4[a]†	1 ± 0·2[b]*	0·5 ± 0·1[b]
Endometrium				
Day 14	5 ± 0·4[a]*	0·6 ± 0·1[b]†	0·1 ± 0·04[b]*	3 ± 0·1[c]
Day 16	3 ± 0·2[a]*	0·4 ± 0·05[b]†	0·03 ± 0·01[b]*	3 ± 0·2[a]

Values are mean ± s.e.m. for 4 observations.
For incubation, average wet weights for Day-14 and -16 blastocysts were 32 and 184 mg, respectively, and were 502 mg for endometrium.
[a,b,c]Within rows, means with different superscript letters differed ($P < 0.05$).
*Means differed between tissue types ($P < 0.05$) and days ($P < 0.05$), but there was a tissue type-by-day interaction ($P < 0.05$).
†Means differed ($P < 0.05$) between tissue types.

Day-14 and -16 blastocysts produced (ng/mg tissue) more 6-keto-PGF-1α, PGF-2α and PGE-2 but not more PGFM than did endometrium (Table 2; Lewis & Waterman, 1985). Because sheep and cattle blastocysts had more PGF-2α as substrate for PGFM synthesis, and yet they did not produce more PGFM than did endometrium, we speculated that 15-hydroxy-PG dehydrogenase and 13,14-PG reductase activities were less in blastocysts than in endometrium (Lewis *et al.*, 1982; Lewis & Waterman, 1985; Lewis, 1986a). However, sheep blastocysts metabolized (per mg tissue) at least as much [^{3}H]PGF-2α as did endometrium (Table 3; Lewis, 1987). Blastocysts metabolized [^{3}H]PGF-2α primarily to material more polar than PGF-2α, while endometrium primarily produced material less polar than PGF-2α, which includes PGFM (Table 4; Lewis, 1987). The polar metabolites of PGF-2α have not yet been indentified.

Table 3. Metabolism of [^{3}H]PGF-2α by sheep blastocysts and endometrium incubated for 8 h *in vitro* (Lewis, 1987)

	Least-squares means [% ÷ tissue weight (mg)]*	
	Day 14 ($n = 5$)	Day 16 ($n = 6$)
Blastocyst	0·8	0·4
Endometrium	0·5	0·5

For incubation, average wet weights of Day-14 blastocysts were 38 mg and of Day-16 blastocysts and endometrium were 130 mg.
*Day × tissue interaction ($P < 0·05$). The standard error from the model used to analyse the data was 0·1.

Table 4. Production of ^{3}H-labelled material more polar than PGF-2α and [^{3}H]PGFM (13,14-dihydro-15-keto-PGF-2α) by sheep blastocysts and endometrium incubated with [^{3}H]PGF-2α for 8 h *in vitro* (Lewis, 1987)

	Least-squares means [(% of total d.p.m.) ÷ tissue weight (mg)]		
	Day 14 ($n = 5$)	Day 16 ($n = 6$)	Overall
	Material more polar than [^{3}H]PGF-2α*		
Blastocyst	0·5	0·3	0·4
Endometrium	0·05	0·06	0·06
			s.e. = 0·02†
	[^{3}H]PGFM		
Blastocyst	0·03	0·004	0·02‡
Endometrium	0·1	0·1	0·1
			s.e. = 0·01†

*Day × tissue interaction ($P < 0·01$).
†s.e. = standard error from the model used to analyse the data.
‡Tissue affected production of [^{3}H]PGFM ($P < 0·001$).

Studies of arachidonic acid utilization indicated that conceptuses rapidly take up arachidonic acid from incubation medium, incorporate it into less polar materials, including triglycerides, and then liberate arachidonic acid from the less polar materials and use it for PG synthesis (Waterman

& Lewis, 1983; Lewis & Waterman, 1985). This process seemed more active in Day-16 blastocysts than in Day-20 and -24 chorion (Lewis & Waterman, 1985). In Day-24 chorion incubated for 6 h with radioactive arachidonic acid, triglycerides contained about 3 times as much radio-labelled arachidonic acid as did phospholipids (3606 *vs* 1254 d.p.m./μg of each lipid class), and phospholipids contained about 4 times as much radiolabelled arachidonic acid as did cholesterol esters (310 d.p.m./μg), which is consistent with data on Day-12 and -15 blastocysts (Marcus, 1981; Waterman & Lewis, 1983; R. A. Waterman & G. S. Lewis, unpublished observations). These results indicate that triglycerides probably are an important source of arachidonic acid for conceptus synthesis of PG.

Table 5. Production (ng/g tissue) of PGF-2α and PGFM (13,14-dihydro-15-keto-PGF-2α) by pig conceptuses and endometrium incubated for 3 h *in vitro* (after Guthrie & Lewis, 1986)

Day after first mating (n)	Conceptus		Endometrium	
	PGF-2α	PGFM	PGF-2α	PGFM
13 (5)	777[a]	10[a]	70[a,b]	15[a]
16 (4)	788[a]	19[a]	96[b]	26[a]
19 (4)	248[a,b]	32[a]	110[b]	40[a]
25 (4)	26[b]	21[a]	32[a]	36[a]
Standard error*	141	4	10	6

[a,b]Within columns, means without any superscripts in common differed ($P < 0.05$).
*Standard error from the model used to analyse the data.

Pigs

Based upon RIA, Day-4, -13, -16, -19, -22 and -25 blastocysts or conceptus membranes released PGF-2α or PGE-2 *in vitro* (Watson & Patek, 1979; Guthrie & Lewis, 1986; Stone *et al.*, 1986). Day-16 blastocysts incubated with radioactive arachidonic acid synthesized and released radiolabelled PGF-2α, PGE-2, PGFM and several unidentified compounds (Lewis & Waterman, 1983b). In contrast to sheep, pig and cattle conceptuses did not produce detectable amounts of 6-keto-PGF-1α. Day-7, -8, -9, -10, -11 and -12 blastocysts contained PGF and PGE-A (the antibody crossreacted significantly with PGAs); numerically, content of both PGs increased with day of pregnancy (Davis *et al.*, 1983). Pig blastocysts produced at least twice as much E- as F- series PG, PGF-2α production declined after Day 16, and PGF-2α production on Days 13, 16 and 19 was greater than that of PGFM (Table 5; Davis *et al.*, 1983; Lewis & Waterman, 1983b; Guthrie & Lewis, 1986; Stone *et al.*, 1986). Conceptus and endometrium produced similar amounts of PGFM (Table 5) and, unlike sheep, metabolized similar percentages (about 52) of [^{3}H]PGF-2α to [^{3}H]PGFM (Guthrie & Lewis, 1986).

Laboratory animals

Based upon RIA, Day-4, -5, -6 and -7 rabbit blastocysts contained and released *in vitro* PGE and PGF (Dickmann & Spilman, 1975; Dey *et al.*, 1980; Harper *et al.*, 1983; Kasamo *et al.*, 1986). After lipid pools were loaded with [^{14}C]arachidonic acid and treatment with calcium ionophore *in vitro*, Day-6 rabbit blastocysts synthesized and released radiolabelled PGF-2α, PGE-2, PGD-2, PGA-2 (a major non-enzymic metabolite of PGE-2) and thromboxane B-2 (TXB-2; a non-enzymic hydrolysis product of TXA-2); PGA-2 predominated (Racowsky & Biggers, 1983). Whether the predominance of PGA-2 indicates that PGE-2 was the primary cyclooxygenase product is unclear, because Dey *et al.* (1980) found with RIA that Day-6 rabbit blastocysts produced more PGF than PGE–A–B.

Little is known about mechanisms controlling blastocystic synthesis of PG, but in rabbits catechol oestrogens were potent stimulators of blastocystic synthesis of PGF and PGE–A; oestradiol was less effective (Pakrasi & Dey, 1983). Although rabbit blastocysts have not been shown to produce catechol oestrogens, pig blastocysts can synthesize these compounds (Mondschein *et al.*, 1985).

Day-2, -3 and -4 mouse blastocysts incorporated radioactive arachidonic acid into neutral lipids and phospholipids, incorporation increased with day of pregnancy, calcium ionophore stimulated release of radioactive arachidonic acid from the lipid pools, but there was no biochemical evidence for PG synthesis (Racowsky & Biggers, 1983). Based upon RIA, Day-5 rat blastocysts did not produce detectable amounts of PGF or PGE *in vitro* (Kennedy & Armstrong, 1981).

Some possible functions of prostaglandins

Pig embryos migrate and become spaced in the uterus between Days 7 and 12 of pregnancy (Pope *et al.*, 1982). Local myometrial contractions seem to be involved in controlling migration, and blastocystic PG may stimulate these contractions (Pope *et al.*, 1982).

Inhibitors of PG synthesis and PG antagonists reduced the rate of hatching of mouse embryos from the zona pellucida (Biggers *et al.*, 1978; Baskar *et al.*, 1981; Hurst & MacFarlane, 1981, Chida *et al.*, 1986). Prostaglandin F-2α but not PGE-2 partly reversed the effects of indomethacin on hatching (Chida *et al.*, 1986). Because they hatch in serum-free medium without exogenous PG and because of the effect of PG inhibitors on hatching rate, circumstantial evidence indicates that mouse blastocysts synthesize PG. Biggers *et al.* (1978) proposed that PG inhibitors reduced hatching rate because they reduced blastocystic synthesis of PG, which interfered with PG-mediated ion transport across trophectoderm and accumulation of blastocoelic fluid; this interference with fluid dynamics prevented blastocystic expansion necessary for hatching. Later studies (Baskar *et al.*, 1981; Hurst & MacFarlane, 1981; Chida *et al.*, 1986) supported the hypothesis of Biggers *et al.* (1978).

Indomethacin reduced PG synthesis by and transport of ^{22}Na across Day-16 sheep trophoblast, and it prevented formation of trophoblastic vesicles (Lewis, 1986b). This in-vitro study indicated that PG may be involved in controlling fluid accumulation during the period of rapid blastocystic elongation.

Localized increases in endometrial capillary permeability precede implantation in many mammals (for reviews, see Hoos & Hoffman, 1983; Pakrasi *et al.*, 1985). Prostaglandins seem involved in initiating increases in capillary permeability in rabbits, rats and hamsters (Evans & Kennedy, 1978; Kennedy & Armstrong, 1981; Hoos & Hoffman, 1983; Jones *et al.*, 1986). In rabbits, blastocysts appear to be the source of PGs that initiate increases in capillary permeability, but this conclusion is somewhat controversial (Snabes & Harper, 1984; Pakrasi *et al.*, 1985; Jones *et al.*, 1986). Between Days 11 and 12 of pregnancy in pigs, endometrial capillaries adjacent to conceptus membranes became permeable to albumin-bound dye, blastocystic content of PGE-A doubled and content of PGF and PGE-2 in uterine flushings more than doubled; taken together these data indicate that PGs may be involved in increasing capillary permeability in pigs (Geisert *et al.*, 1982; Davis *et al.*, 1983; Keys *et al.*, 1986).

Prostaglandin E-2 reduced [^{14}C]glucose incorporation into acid-soluble glycogen in Day-4 mouse blastocysts, while PGE-2 and PGF-2α increased [^{14}C]glucose incorporation into non-glycogen macromolecules (Khurana & Wales, 1987). The amount of [^{14}C]glucose in Day-19 cattle blastocysts and concentration of PGE-2 in medium after a 24-h incubation were negatively correlated (McCarther *et al.*, 1985). These studies indicate that PGs, perhaps of blastocyst origin, influence energy metabolism in blastocysts.

Future studies with conceptuses should determine more precisely when during development genes controlling PG synthesis and metabolism are expressed, what regulates PG synthesis and the roles of PG during critical developmental events. Every effort should be made to conduct these studies *in vivo* and to use the data to improve reproductive performance of animals.

References

Baskar, J.F., Torchiana, D.F., Biggers, J.D., Corey, E.J. Andersen, N.H. & Subramanian, N. (1981) Inhibition of hatching of mouse blastocysts *in vitro* by various prostaglandin inhibitors. *J. Reprod. Fert.* **63**, 359–363.

Basu, S. & Kindahl, H. (1987) Prostaglandin biosynthesis and its regulation in the bovine endometrium: A comparison between nonpregnant and pregnant status. *Theriogenology* **28**, 175–193.

Biggers, J.D., Leonov, B.V., Baskar, J.F. & Fried, J. (1978) Inhibition of hatching of mouse blastocysts *in vitro* by prostaglandin antagonists. *Biol. Reprod.* **19**, 519–533.

Chida, S., Uehara, S., Hoshiai, H. & Yajima, A. (1986) Effects of indomethacin, prostaglandin E_2, prostaglandin $F_2\alpha$ and 6-keto-prostaglandin $F_1\alpha$ on hatching of mouse blastocysts. *Prostaglandins* **31**, 337–342.

Davis, D.L., Pakrasi, P.L. & Dey, S.K. (1983) Prostaglandins in swine blastocysts. *Biol. Reprod.* **28**, 1114–1118.

Dey, S.K., Chien, S.M., Cox, C.L. & Crist, R.D. (1980) Prostaglandin synthesis in the rabbit blastocyst. *Prostaglandins* **19**, 449–453.

Dickmann, Z. & Spilman, C.H. (1975) Prostaglandins in rabbit blastocysts. *Science, N.Y.* **190**, 997–998.

Evans, C.A. & Kennedy, T.G. (1978) The importance of prostaglandin synthesis for the initiation of blastocyst implantation in the hamster. *J. Reprod. Fert.* **54**, 255–261.

Geisert, R., Renegar, R.H., Thatcher, W.W., Roberts, R.M. & Bazer, F.W. (1982) Establishment of pregnancy in the pig. I. Interrelationships between preimplantation development of the pig blastocyst and uterine endometrial secretions. *Biol. Reprod.* **27**, 925–939.

Gross, T.S., Thatcher, W.W. & Hansen, P.J. (1987) Regulation of prostaglandin synthesis in cyclic and pregnant bovine endometrium. *J. Anim. Sci.* **65**, (Suppl. 1), 383, Abstr.

Guthrie, H.D. & Lewis, G.S. (1986) Production of prostaglandin $F_2\alpha$ and estrogen by embryonal membranes and endometrium and metabolism of prostaglandin $F_2\alpha$ by embryonal membranes, endometrium and lung from gilts. *Domestic Anim. Endocr.* **3**, 185–198.

Harper, M.J.K., Norris, C.J. & Rajkumar, K. (1983) Prostaglandin release by zygotes and endometria of pregnant rabbits. *Biol. Reprod.* **28**, 350–362.

Hoos, P.C. & Hoffman, L.H. (1983) Effect of histamine receptor antagonists and indomethacin on implantation in the rabbit. *Biol. Reprod.* **29**, 833–840.

Hurst, P.R. & MacFarlane, D.W. (1981) Further effects of nonsteroidal anti-inflammatory compounds on blastocyst hatching *in vitro* and implantation rates in the mouse. *Biol. Reprod.* **25**, 777–784.

Hyland, J.H., Manns, J.G. & Humphrey, W.D. (1982) Prostaglandin production by ovine embryos and endometrium *in vitro*. *J. Reprod. Fert.* **65**, 299–304.

Jones, M.A., Cao, Z.-d., Anderson, W., Norris, C & Harper, M.J.K. (1986) Capillary permeability changes in the uteri of recipient rabbits after transfer of blastocysts from indomethacin-treated donors. *J. Reprod. Fert.* **78**, 261–273.

Kasamo, M., Ishikawa, M., Yamashita, K., Sengoku, K. & Shimizu, T. (1986) Possible role of prostaglandin F in blastocyst implantation. *Prostaglandins* **31**, 321–336.

Kennedy, T.G. & Armstrong, D.T. (1981) The role of prostaglandins in endometrial vascular changes at implantation. In *Cellular and Molecular Aspects of Implantation*, pp. 349–358. Ed S. R. Glasser & D. W. Bullock. Plenum Press, New York.

Keys, J.L., King, G.J. & Kennedy, T.G. (1986) Increased uterine vascular permeability at the time of embryonic attachment in the pig. *Biol. Reprod.* **34**, 405–411.

Khurana, N.K. & Wales, R.G. (1987) Effects of prostaglandins E-2 and F-2α on the metabolism of [U-^{14}C]glucose by mouse morulae-early blastocysts *in vitro*. *J. Reprod. Fert.* **79**, 275–280

Lacroix, M.C. & Kann, G. (1982) Comparative studies of prostaglandins $F_2\alpha$ and E_2 in late cyclic and early early pregnant sheep: *In vitro* synthesis by endometrium and conceptus; effects of *in vivo* indomethacin treatment on establishment of pregnancy. *Prostaglandins* **23**, 507–526.

Lewis, G.S. (1986a) Effects of superovulation, arachidonic acid or endometrium on release of prostaglandins and synthesis of proteins by bovine trophoblast. *Prostaglandins* **32**, 275–290.

Lewis, G.S. (1986b) Indomethacin inhibits the uptake of ^{22}sodium by ovine trophoblastic tissue *in vitro*. *Prostaglandins* **31**, 111–122.

Lewis, G.S. (1987) Metabolism of prostaglandin $F_2\alpha$ by ovine trophoblast and endometrium. *J. Anim. Sci.* **65** (Suppl. 1), 383–384, Abstr.

Lewis, G.S. & Waterman, R.A. (1983a) Effects of endometrium on metabolism of arachidonic acid by bovine blastocysts *in vitro*. *Prostaglandins* **25**, 881–889.

Lewis, G.S. & Waterman, R.A. (1983b) Metabolism of arachidonic acid *in vitro* by porcine blastocysts and endometrium. *Prostaglandins* **25**, 871–880.

Lewis, G.S. & Waterman, R.A. (1985) Metabolism of arachidonic acid *in vitro* by ovine conceptuses recovered during early pregnancy. *Prostaglandins* **30**, 263–283.

Lewis, G.S. Thatcher, W.W., Bazer, F.W. & Curl, J.S. (1982) Metabolism of arachidonic acid *in vitro* by bovine blastocysts and endometrium. *Biol. Reprod.* **27**, 431–439.

Marcus, G.J. (1981) Prostaglandin formation by the sheep embryo and endometrium as an indication of maternal recognition of pregnancy. *Biol. Reprod.* **25**, 56–64.

McCarther, C.E., Williams, W.F., Lewis, G.S. & Gross, T.S. (1985) The effect of Banamine (flunixin meglumide) on *in vitro* arachidonic acid and glucose metabolism by bovine 19 day blastocysts. *J. Anim. Sci.* **61** (Suppl. 1), 362, Abstr.

Mondschein, J.S., Hersey, R.M., Dey, S.K., Davis, D.L. & Weisz, J. (1985) Catechol estrogen formation by pig blastocysts during the preimplantation period: Biochemical characterization of estrogen-2/4-hydrolase and correlation with aromatase activity. *Endocrinology* **117**, 2339–2346.

Pakrasi, P.L. & Dey, S.K. (1983) Catechol estrogens stimulate synthesis of prostaglandins in the preimplantation rabbit blastocyst and endometrium. *Biol. Reprod.* **29**, 347–354.

Pakrasi, P.L., Becka, R. & Dey, S.K. (1985) Cyclooxygenase and lipoxygenase pathways in the preimplantation rabbit uterus and blastocyst. *Prostaglandins* **29**, 481–495.

Pope, W.F., Maurer, R.R. & Stormshak, F. (1982) Intrauterine migration of the porcine embryo-Interaction of embryo, uterine flushings and indomethacin

on myometrial function *in vitro*. *J. Anim. Sci.* **55**, 1169–1178.

Racowsky, C. & Biggers, J.D. (1983) Are blastocyst prostaglandins produced endogenously? *Biol. Reprod.* **29**, 379–388.

Rawlings, N.C. & Hyland, J.H. (1985) Prostaglandin F and E levels in the conceptus, uterus and plasma during early pregnancy in the ewe. *Prostaglandins* **29**, 933–951.

Shemesh, M., Milaguir, F., Ayalon, N. & Hansel, W. (1979) Steroidogenesis and prostaglandin synthesis by cultured bovine blastocysts. *J. Reprod. Fert.* **56**, 181–185.

Snabes, M.C. & Harper, M.J.K. (1984) Site of action of indomethacin on implantation in the rabbit. *J. Reprod. Fert.* **71**, 559–565.

Stone B.A., Seamark, R.F., Kelly, R.W. & Deam, S. (1986) Production of steroids and release of prostaglandins by spherical pig blastocysts *in vitro*. *Aust. J. Biol. Sci.* **39**, 283–293.

Waterman, R.A. & Lewis, G.S. (1983) Arachidonic acid incorporation into sheep conceptus lipids at 24 days after insemination. *J. Anim. Sci.* **57** (Suppl. 1), 379, Abstr.

Watson, J. & Patek, C.E. (1979) Steroid and prostaglandin secretion by the corpus luteum, endometrium and embryos of cyclic and pregnant pigs. *J. Endocr.* **82**, 425–428.

Wlodawer, P., Kindahl, H. & Hamberg, M. (1976) Biosynthesis of prostaglandin $F_2\alpha$ from arachidonic acid and prostaglandin endoperoxides in the uterus. *Biochim. Biophys. Acta* **431**, 603–614.

J. Reprod. Fert., Suppl. **37** (1989), 269–276

Printed in Great Britain
© 1989 Journals of Reproduction & Fertility Ltd

Regulation of prostaglandin synthesis during early pregnancy in the cow

H. Kindahl, S. Basu, S. Aiumlamai, K. Odensvik and G. Stabenfeldt

*Department of Obstetrics and Gynaecology, Swedish University of Agricultural Sciences,
S-750 07 Uppsala, Sweden*

Keywords: PG biosynthesis; PG metabolites; luteolysis; early pregnancy; flunixin meglumine; cow

Introduction

After liberation from cell membrane phospholipids, arachidonic acid, a polyunsaturated fatty acid is metabolized via the cyclo-oxygenase pathway to several biologically active metabolites (Fig. 1) (Samuelsson *et al.*, 1975, 1978). Prostaglandin (PG) F-2α, a product of arachidonic acid metabolism, is synthesized and released from the endometrium and causes regression of the corpus luteum at the end of the oestrous cycle (see reviews, Horton & Poyser, 1976; Kindahl *et al.*, 1984; Basu, 1985). The formation of PGF-2α is therefore due to the action of phospholipase, cyclo-oxygenase, prostaglandin–endoperoxide reductase and several co-factors. In addition, intracellular transport of substrate and product is involved in the release of PGF-2α. When proper conception occurs, the synthesis of PGF-2α in the endometrium is decreased and the release pattern is altered (Kindahl *et al.*, 1976a, 1981; Poyser, 1981; Thatcher *et al.*, 1984; Basu & Kindahl, 1987a; Basu *et al.*, 1988). It is obvious that some biochemical mechanism should exist in the endometrium to regulate the synthesis and release of PGF-2α in a very accurate manner during different stages of the oestrous cycle and early pregnancy. In this article, some of the major studies which have been performed at our laboratory are reviewed.

Synthesis and release of prostaglandin F-2α *in vivo*

To follow the synthesis and release of F-2α *in vivo*, the major initial plasma metabolite of PGF-2α, 15-ketodihydro-PGF-2α is a reliable parameter (Granström & Kindahl, 1982). To depict a true picture of the PG release the samples must be collected frequently. In non-pregnant animals samples have been collected at 3- or 1-h intervals and it was found that PGF-2α was released during the 2–3 days of luteolysis (Kindahl *et al.*, 1976a, b). The duration of the peaks was 1–5 h. The rapid increase of the PG metabolite in each peak as well as the rapid decrease indicate that the PGF-2α synthesis and release are like an on–off mechanism. In one animal the 15-ketodihydro metabolite was monitored during early pregnancy and it was found that no significant increase in the metabolite level occurred when plasma progesterone levels remained constant (Kindahl *et al.*, 1976a). Similar findings have been seen in early pregnant cows, although the samples have been collected less frequently (Kindahl *et al.*, 1982; Madej *et al.*, 1986).

In a detailed study of PGF-2α release, blood was collected continuously before luteolysis (Days 15–17), during luteolysis (Days 16–22) and early pregnancy (Days 16–21) (Basu & Kindahl, 1987a). A double-lumen catheter made of tubing of two different diameters was used for blood collection. The inner tubing delivered an anticoagulant (heparin–saline), and the outer tubing was used to collect blood. Approximately 7000 blood samples were collected continuously from 4 heifers

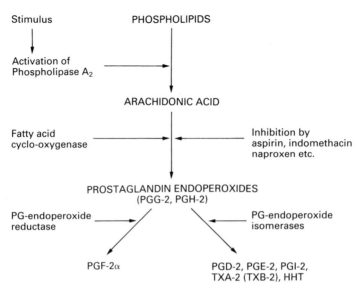

Fig. 1. Biosynthesis of prostaglandins and thromboxanes from arachidonic acid through the cyclo-oxygenase pathway. Arachidonic acid is liberated from phospholipids through an activation of phospholipase A_2 and undergoes oxygenation through cyclo-oxygenase to endoperoxides PGG-2 and PGH-2. They convert to different prostaglandins and thromboxanes through several isomerases and a reductase.

(2 cyclic, 2 pregnant) at intervals of 3·7 min. All samples were analysed for 15-ketodihydro-PGF-2α and every twentieth sample for its progesterone content by radioimmunoassay. Heifer 1 showed no significant peak in its 15-ketodihydro metabolite level during Days 15–17 of the oestrous cycle when plasma progesterone concentrations remained constant. In Heifer 2, 7 large peaks of 15-ketodihydro-PGF-2α were seen during Days 17–21 (Fig. 2) concomitant with luteolysis when plasma progesterone concentrations started to decline on Day 19. Each of these peaks developed and diminished by successive increments and decrements of the metabolite. The mean ($\pm$s.d.) duration of each peak was 4·1 $\pm$ 1·0 h. Therefore, about 65 samples were included in each peak. The maximum levels of the prostaglandin metabolite were seen about 20 min after onset. This indicates a very rapid triggering of PG biosynthesis since it takes about 20 min after onset of exogenous PGF-2α infusion to obtain maximal constant levels (Kindahl et al., 1976a). Similarly, the PG metabolite levels in each luteolytic peak diminished rapidly with a half-life close to that seen after intravenous infusion of PGF-2α. These results strongly indicate that the biosynthesis and release of PGF-2α really are like an on–off mechanism. There were no significant peaks of 15-ketodihydro-PGF-2α in the 2 pregnant heifers, Nos 3 and 4 (Days 16–21), but the basal values were slightly higher than those of the 2 non-pregnant ones (basal levels, non-pregnant: 137 $\pm$ 29·3 and 149 $\pm$ 24·5 pmol/l; pregnant: 183 $\pm$ 29·7 and 192 $\pm$ 32·4 pmol/l). Progesterone concentrations remained very high in both of these heifers during Days 16–21. Figure 3 shows the peripheral plasma concentration of 15-ketodihydro-PGF-2α during early pregnancy in Heifer 4.

An alternative method to follow PG release in the cow is to monitor 11-ketotetranor PGF metabolites, the more degraded metabolites of PGF-2α, in the urine (Granström & Kindahl, 1976; Basu et al., 1987). During corpus luteum regression, 11-ketotetranor PGF metabolites were much increased for 2–3 days in urine. When these metabolites were measured in urinary samples from early pregnant cows, the increase of 11-ketotetranor PGF metabolites as seen during luteolysis did not occur (Fig. 4). However, there was a trend to a slight increase in 11-ketotetranor PGF metabolites after Day 20 (Harvey et al., 1984).

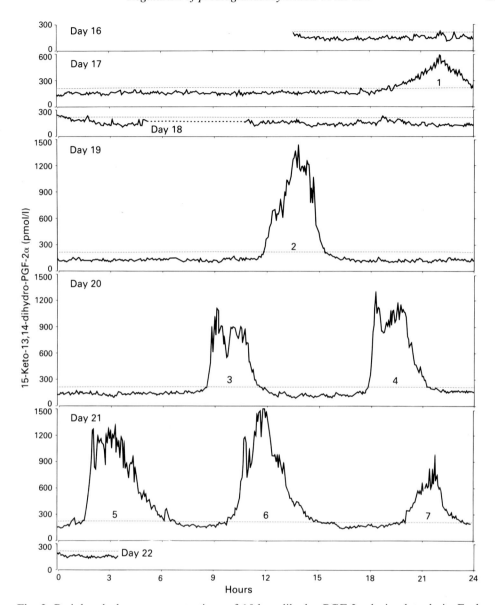

Fig. 2. Peripheral plasma concentrations of 15-ketodihydro-PGF-2α during luteolysis. Each panel represents the pattern of the metabolite over 1 whole day. Line of lowest skewness is drawn by dotted line. During Day 18 blood samples are missing for a period of 5 h. (From Basu & Kindahl, 1987a.)

Biosynthesis of PGs from arachidonic acid by bovine endometrium *in vitro*

In in-vitro studies, the conversion of $[1-^{14}C]$arachidonic acid by different endometrial preparations of cows have been performed to investigate their ability to synthesize PGs (Basu & Kindahl, 1987b). The endometrial preparations were from different days of the oestrous cycle and early pregnancy. Among homogenates, particle-free high-speed supernatant (cytosol) and microsomal

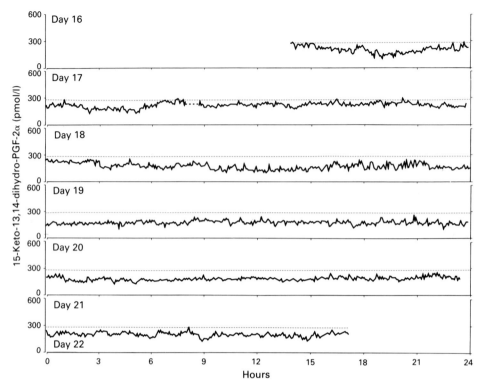

Fig. 3. Peripheral plasma concentrations of 15-ketodihydro-PGF-2α during early pregnancy in a heifer. Each panel represents the pattern of the metabolite over 1 whole day. Line of lowest skewness is drawn by dotted line. (From Basu & Kindahl, 1987a.)

fractions of endometrial tissue, the highest fatty acid cyclo-oxygenase activity was found in the microsomal fractions. However, the enzymic conversion of labelled arachidonic acid was of low order, as observed for endometrial preparations of guinea-pigs and cows (Wlodawer *et al.*, 1976). By increasing the amount of microsomes the formation of total PGs was increased in a dose-dependent manner only up to a certain level. These results indicate the presence of an endogenous inhibiting factor in the endometrial preparations. Endometrium from four different stages of the oestrous cycle (Days 1, 4, 14 and 17) was studied and an increase in total PG formation is seen towards the end of the oestrous cycle (Day 17). This increase in PG synthesis *in vitro* from arachidonic acid parallels the increase seen when PGF-2α metabolites were measured in both plasma and urine (see above).

Endometrium from seven different days (Days 16–20, 25 and 31) of early pregnancy was studied for its ability to convert [1-^{14}C]arachidonic acid to various PGs. Formation of total PGs was very low until Day 19 of pregnancy. A slight increase in PG synthetic capacity is seen from Day 20. The lowest capacity of endometrial microsomes to convert labelled arachidonic acid to PGs was on Day 18 out of the tested days. Day-17 pregnant endometrium had about 50% lower ability to form PGs than had the non-pregnant Day 17 endometrium. The biosynthesis of PGs therefore varies during different stages of oestrous cycle and early pregnancy due to different levels of potency of the endometrial cyclo-oxygenase at that time. These changes in the conversion of arachidonic acid to PGs depend on various factors. One of the major factors is the involvement of endogenous inhibitors of PG synthesis in the endometrium which is discussed below.

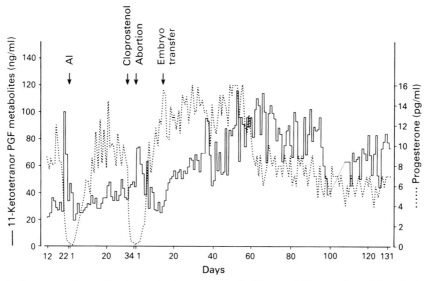

Fig. 4. Concentrations of urinary 11-ketotetranor PGF metabolites and peripheral plasma values of progesterone during the oestrous cycle and early pregnancy, after induced abortion and after embryo transfer at Day 14. Urinary metabolites were not corrected for variations in glomerular filtration rate. (After Basu *et al.*, 1987.)

Inhibition of prostaglandin synthesis by bovine endometrial preparations

Sheep seminal vesicular gland microsomes (SVGM) were used as a source of PG cyclo-oxygenase. In a validated test system, these microsomes efficiently converted arachidonic acid to various PGs ($81 \cdot 6 \pm 3 \cdot 0\%$) including PGF-2α (Fig. 5) (Basu & Kindahl, 1987b). All endometrial preparations (homogenates, cytosolic fractions and microsomes) had the ability to inhibit the PG synthesizing system of the highly efficient SVGM. Inhibitory ability was of different degrees. Highest inhibitory activity was as follows: microsomes > cytosolic fractions > homogenates as calculated by the content of proteins in these preparations. The presence of an inhibitor was first described by Wlodawer *et al.* (1976) but its variation in potency during oestrous cyclicity and early pregnancy is not known.

In a comparative study, both cytosolic and microsomal fractions of different days of oestrous cycle (Days 1, 4, 14 and 17) and early pregnancy (Days 16–20, 25 and 31) were checked for their ability to inhibit PG formation from labelled arachidonic acid by SVGM. Inhibition was highest on Day 14 and lowest on Day 17 out of Days 1, 4, 14 and 17 of the oestrous cycle by both cytosolic and microsomal fractions. A representative radiochromatogram shows the conversion of labelled arachidonic acid by SVGM alone (Fig. 5a) and in the presence of endometrial cytosolic fractions of non-pregnant Day-17 animal (Fig. 5b).

The presence of different cytosolic and microsomal fractions from pregnant endometrium (Days 16–20, 25 and 31) resulted in a higher inhibition of PG formation from labelled arachidonic acid. The percentage of inhibition was highest on Day 18 and lowest on Day 25 for cytosolic fractions. Similarly, the percentage of inhibition was highest on Day 17 and lowest on Day 31 for microsomes. A representative radiochromatogram shows the conversion of labelled arachidonic acid by SVGM in the presence of endometrial cytosolic fractions of Day-17 pregnant animal (Fig. 5c). When comparing the inhibitory potency of this endometrial inhibitory factor, as calculated by IC_{50} values (inhibitory concentration resulting in 50% inhibition), the potency

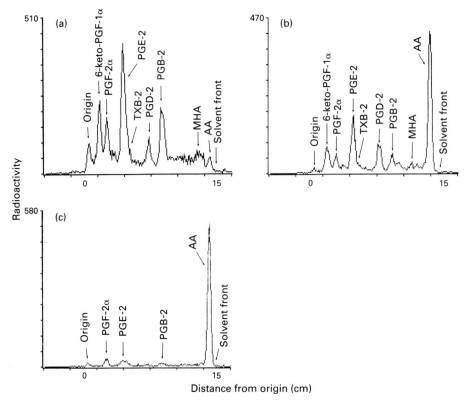

Fig. 5. Radiochromatograms representing the conversion of ^{14}C-labelled arachidonic acid by sheep seminal vesicular gland microsomes alone (a), in the presence of cytosolic fractions of non-pregnant Day-17 endometrium (b) and pregnant Day-17 endometrium (c). (After Basu & Kindahl, 1987b.)

was about 8 times higher for Day-17 pregnant than Day-17 non-pregnant endometrial cytosolic fractions.

In conclusion, the endometrium of non-pregnant and pregnant cows comprises a PG synthetase system and a potent inhibitor(s) that controls prostaglandin biosynthesis in this tissue. This inhibitor blocks arachidonic acid metabolism by acting on fatty acid cyclo-oxygenase. During luteolysis, the inhibitory potency falls and a higher synthesis of PGs including PGF-2α occurs and the corpus luteum regresses. During early pregnancy, presumably by an unknown signal from the conceptus, the inhibitory capacity of the endometrium is much increased and thus possibly blocks PG biosynthesis. This results in maintenance of the corpus luteum during early pregnancy in the cow.

Use of flunixin meglumine to control prostaglandin biosynthesis

Flunixin meglumine (Essex, Stockholm, Sweden) is an anti-inflammatory drug used, e.g. for treatment of endotoxaemia. The effect of the drug is believed to be an inhibition of the PG cyclo-oxygenase and thus causes decreased formation of PGs and related substances. To clarify the potency of the drug to inhibit the cyclo-oxygenase, studies were conducted with the above-mentioned sheep vesicular gland microsome system and different known cyclo-oxygenase inhibitors were tested (Odensvik *et al.*, 1988). It was found that flunixin meglumine was about 10 times less potent than indomethacin when calculated as IC_{50} values. However, flunixin meglumine was about 200 times more potent than acetylsalicylic acid. Since flunixin meglumine is a water-soluble substance and so easy to administer, it can be used in studies in which decreased synthesis of prostaglandins is required.

Since many of our studies *in vivo* are aimed at studying PG metabolites as indicators of PG production and release it is also important to know whether flunixin meglumine has any effect on the metabolizing enzymes, e.g. on the 15-hydroxy prostanoate dehydrogenase and Δ^{13}-reductase. In a study in pigs, it was shown that flunixin meglumine in therapeutic concentrations had no effect on the metabolizing enzymes (Odensvik *et al.*, 1988). It can therefore be concluded that an observed effect on PG metabolite levels in plasma after flunixin treatment is due to a decreased synthesis of primary PGs and not due to inhibited formation of the metabolites.

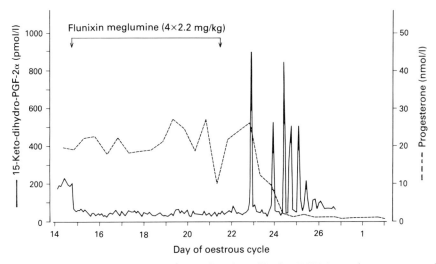

Fig. 6. Peripheral plasma concentrations of 15-ketodihydro-PGF-2α and progesterone in a heifer treated with flunixin meglumine 4 times daily from Day 15 of the oestrous cycle.

In a preliminary study 2 cows received flunixin meglumine intravenously in a dose of 2·2 mg/kg body weight. Blood cannulae were inserted to collect continuous samples according to the procedure described by Basu & Kindahl (1987a). Blood samples were collected before and after flunixin injection and basal plasma concentrations of 15-ketodihydro-PGF-2α were analysed. A rapid decrease in the concentrations was seen after flunixin meglumine and then values were slowly increased again. A clear effect on the metabolite levels was seen for about 6 h. It can therefore be recommended that flunixin meglumine should be injected at least 4 times daily to obtain a full effect on PG synthesis.

Three heifers were used in a study to mimic a situation of decreased PG output. Flunixin meglumine was administered 4 times daily from Day 15 of the oestrous cycle and plasma concentrations of 15-ketodihydro-PGF-2α and progesterone were measured. The drug was administered during 7 days. The basal levels decreased after treatments and the expected pulsatile release was delayed (Fig. 6). Normal release resumed about 1 day after cessation of treatment and luteolysis then occurred.

It is therefore possible to use an efficient PG cyclo-oxygenase inhibitor like flunixin meglumine to control primary PG production and delay normal luteolysis. The effect of flunixin meglumine thus resembles the effect of the endogenous cyclo-oxygenase inhibitor described above. It is not excluded that also other mechanisms act in the control of primary prostaglandin synthesis but one of the key events is inhibition of PG cyclo-oxygenase in early pregnancy.

We thank the Swedish Council for Forestry and Agricultural Research for financial support.

References

Basu, S. (1985) Maternal recognition of pregnancy. *Nord. VetMed.* **37**, 57–79.

Basu, S. & Kindahl, H. (1987a) Development of a continuous blood collection technique and a detailed study of prostaglandin $F_{2\alpha}$ release during luteolysis and early pregnancy in heifers. *J. vet. Med. A.* **34**, 487–500.

Basu, S. & Kindahl, H. (1987b) Prostaglandin biosynthesis and its regulation in the bovine endometrium: a comparison between nonpregnant and pregnant status. *Theriogenology* **28**, 175–193.

Basu, S., Kindahl, H., Harvey, D. & Betteridge, K.J. (1987) Metabolites of $PGF_{2\alpha}$ in blood plasma and urine as parameters of $PGF_{2\alpha}$ release in cattle. *Acta vet. scand.* **28**, 409–420.

Basu, S., Albihn, A. & Kindahl, H. (1988) Studies on endogenous inhibitors of prostaglandin biosynthesis in bovine endometrial tissues collected by biopsy. *J. vet. Med. A.* **35**, 141–151.

Granström, E. & Kindahl, H. (1976) Radioimmunoassay for urinary metabolites for prostaglandin $F_{2\alpha}$. *Prostaglandins* **12**, 759–783.

Granström, E. & Kindahl, H. (1982) Species differences in circulating prostaglandin metabolites: Relevance for the assay of prostaglandin release. *Biochim. Biophys. Acta* **713**, 555–569.

Harvey, D., Basu, S., Betteridge, K.J., Goff, A.K. & Kindahl, H. (1984) The influence of pregnancy on $PGF_{2\alpha}$ secretion in cattle. II. Urinary levels of 11-ketotetranor PGF metabolites and plasma progesterone concentrations during the oestrous cycle and early pregnancy. *Anim. Reprod. Sci.* **7**, 217–234.

Horton, E.W. & Poyser, N.L. (1976) Uterine luteolytic hormone: A physiological role for prostaglandin $F_{2\alpha}$. *Physiol. Rev.* **56**, 595–651.

Kindahl, H., Edqvist, L.-E., Bane, A. & Granström, E. (1976a) Blood levels of progesterone and 15-keto-13,14-dihydro-prostaglandin $F_{2\alpha}$ during the normal oestrous cycle and early pregnancy in heifers. *Acta endocr., Copenh.* **82**, 134–149.

Kindahl, H., Edqvist, L.-E., Granström, E. & Bane, A. (1976b) The release of prostaglandin $F_{2\alpha}$ as reflected by 15-keto-13,14-dihydro-prostaglandin $F_{2\alpha}$ in the peripheral circulation during normal luteolysis in heifers. *Prostaglandins* **11**, 871–878.

Kindahl, H., Lindell, J.-O. & Edqvist, L.-E. (1981) Release of prostaglandin $F_2\alpha$ during the oestrous cycle. *Acta vet. scand., Suppl.* **77**, 143–158.

Kindahl, H., Edqvist, L.-E., Larsson, K. & Malmqvist, Å. (1982) Influence of prostaglandins on ovarian function post partum. *Curr. Topics vet. Med. Anim. Sci.* **20**, 173–196.

Kindahl, H., Basu, S., Fredriksson, G., Goff, A., Kunavongkrit, A. & Edqvist, L.-E. (1984) Levels of prostaglandin $F_{2\alpha}$ metabolites in blood and urine during early pregnancy. *Anim. Reprod. Sci.* **7**, 133–148.

Madej, A., Kindahl, H., Larsson, K. & Edqvist, L.-E. (1986) Sequential hormonal changes in the postpartum dairy cow. *Acta vet. scand.* **27**, 280–295.

Odensvik, K., Cort, N., Basu, S. & Kindahl, H. (1988) Effect of flunixin meglumine on prostaglandin $F_{2\alpha}$ synthesis and metabolism. In *Proc. 4th Eur. Assoc. Vet. Pharmacol. & Toxicol.,* Budapest, p. 25.

Poyser, N.L. (1981) Uterine prostaglandins in luteolysis and menstruation. In *Prostaglandins in Reproduction,* pp. 83–131. Ed. N. L. Poyser. Research Studies Press, Chichester.

Samuelsson, B., Granström, E., Gréen, K., Hamberg, M. & Hammarström, S. (1975) Prostaglandins. *Ann. Rev. Biochem.* **44**, 669–695.

Samuelsson, B., Goldyne, M., Granström, E., Hamberg, M., Hammarström, S. & Malmsten, C. (1978) Prostaglandins and Thromboxanes. *Ann. Rev. Biochem.* **47**, 997–1029.

Thatcher, W.W., Wolfenson, D., Curl, J.S., Rico, L.-E., Knickerbocker, J.J., Bazer, F.W. & Drost, M. (1984) Prostaglandin dynamics associated with development of the bovine conceptus. *Anim. Reprod. Sci.* **7**, 149–176.

Wlodawer, P., Kindahl, H. & Hamberg, M. (1976) Biosynthesis of prostaglandin $F_{2\alpha}$ from arachidonic acid and prostaglandin endoperoxides in the uterus. *Biochim. Biophys. Acta* **431**, 603–614.

J. Reprod. Fert., Suppl. **37** (1989), 277–286

Sequences of pituitary, ovarian and uterine hormone secretion during the first 5 weeks of pregnancy in dairy cattle

E. Schallenberger, D. Schams and H. H. D. Meyer

Lehrstuhl für Physiologie der Fortpflanzung und Laktation, Technische Universität München, 8050 Freising-Weihenstephan, Federal Republic of Germany

Summary. Blood samples were collected frequently from permanent catheters placed in the aorta and caudal vena cava of 36 heifers in order to monitor the release pattern of LH, FSH, progesterone, oestradiol-17β, oxytocin, PGF-2α, PGE-2 and PGI-2 (determined as its 6-keto-PGF-1α metabolite). The frequency of secretory bursts of both gonadotrophins and progesterone was similar in early pregnant and cyclic animals, whereas the amplitude of LH and progesterone increased between 2 and 4 weeks of gestation. Concentrations of circulating oestradiol-17β and oxytocin were already lower at Days 4–7 in pregnant than in cyclic animals. Oestradiol-17β originated after Day 14 from the uterus rather than the ovary. A sustained release of oxytocin most probably from the posterior pituitary gland and a concomitant decrease of progesterone occurred in about two-thirds of pregnant animals during Days 19–23. Insemination could induce releases of PGF-2α lasting up to 2 h. In addition, basal concentrations of PGF-2α during the first 6 days after oestrus were ~2-fold higher in inseminated than in non-inseminated cyclic heifers. A parallel increase of PGF-2α and PGI-2 occurred between Days 30 and 33 of gestation. Early embryonic mortality resulted, at least up to Day 35, in 4–7 concomitant secretory bursts of PGF-2α and luteal oxytocin. There was a delay of 20–26 h between the first and second release. The present results from in-vivo experiments point towards major endocrine changes in cattle within a few days after conception, resulting in an early inhibition of follicular oestradiol-17β and luteal oxytocin facilitating the suppression of luteolytic releases of PGF-2α.

Keywords: gonadotrophins; ovarian hormones; prostaglandins; pregnancy; cattle

Introduction

The period from 14 to 30 days after conception is considered very important for the recognition and maintenance of early pregnancy in cattle. Initially binuclear and later on multiple-nucleated cells of the trophoblast, first described by Wimsatt (1951), facilitate the local exchange of substances between embryo and dam in ruminants. The continuation of pregnancy may involve the specific recognition of gestational signals by the mother and the early suppression of luteolysis. Between Days 14 and 25, the trophoblast produces specific proteins of 22 000–25 000 molecular weight (bovine trophoblast proteins) which are secreted only into the lumen of the uterus and do not appear in the peripheral circulation. These substances possess some luteotrophic but primarily anti-luteolytic abilities (Knickerbocker *et al.*, 1986). The aim of our experiments was to characterize during the first 5 weeks of pregnancy in-vivo changes of the relative concentrations and sequences of secretion of both gonadotrophins, ovarian hormones as well as uterine prostaglandins.

Materials and Methods

Experimental animals. The study is based upon data from 36 heifers (aged 22–26 months) of the local Brown Swiss breed. Blood samples were collected from 5 heifers during a complete control oestrous cycle or starting before spontaneous oestrus ($N = 19$) or before luteolysis induced with an analogue of prostaglandin F-2α (500 µg Estrumate; Coopers, Burgwedel, FRG) ($N = 17$) as described earlier (Schallenberger *et al.*, 1984). Artificial insemination (AI) was carried out twice within 12 h: 24 heifers conceived after the initial double insemination (duration of gestation 279–302 days) and 12 heifers returned to oestrus after 19–36 days.

Blood sampling. Indwelling Silastic (Dow Corning, Midland, MI, U.S.A.) or vinyl (Dural Plastics, Dural, N.S.W., Australia) catheters were placed via the tail vessels in the caudal vena cava as described by Walters *et al.* (1984). A similar approach was used to cannulate the aorta abdominalis. Blood samples (5 ml) were obtained simultaneously from both vessels every 2–12 h. In addition, series of intensive bleedings (every 15 min for 6 h) were carried out at intervals of 2–4 days. The tip of the catheter was placed in the vena cava either proximal or just distal to the inflow of the common utero-ovarian vessels in order to obtain a sample of the uterine as well as the ovarian drainage or selectively only part of the uterine ouflow. Comparing estimations of the parallel samples enabled the establishment of arterio-venous differences. Only this approach allowed the differentiation of short-term hormone releases arising from the uterus, the ovary or from sources outside of the reproductive tract.

The samples were collected in tubes containing 6 mM-EDTA and 0·2% sodium salicylic acid. They were immediately chilled in an ice-water bath and centrifuged within 5–10 min at 4°C and 2500 g for 15 min. The separated plasma fraction was stored at $-20°C$ until hormone assays were carried out.

Hormone determinations. All evaluations were done by specific and earlier validated RIAs: LH (Schams & Karg, 1969), FSH (Schams & Schallenberger, 1976), oestradiol-17β (Schallenberger *et al.*, 1985), progesterone (Hoffmann *et al.*, 1973), oxytocin (Schams, 1983), prostaglandins (PG) F-2α and E-2 and the metabolite of PGI-2, 6-keto-PGF-1α (Meyer *et al.*, 1988).

Results

Gonadotrophins

Frequency of release of gonadotrophins was similar in cyclic and pregnant animals. Pulses of LH occurred regularly at about the same time as the luteal phase progressed in pregnant heifers (Fig. 1). Basal concentrations decreased slightly, whereas amplitudes increased in general between 2 and 4 weeks. Secretion of FSH was much more frequent (up to 5 secretory bursts/6 h) than that of LH (1–2 releases/6 h). Average concentrations, frequency and amplitude of secretion of FSH remained about constant throughout the first 5 weeks of gestation (Fig. 1).

Ovarian hormones

Short-term changes of progesterone occurred similar to the oestrous cycle concomitantly with FSH (Fig. 1). Parallel releases of progesterone and luteal oxytocin were present only in the early luteal phase. Thereafter, oxytocin was secreted in a rather constant fashion and levels in the vena cava were only slightly higher than in the aorta (Figs 1 & 2). A temporal relationship between releases of LH and oestradiol-17β was obvious only up to Day 9 of the luteal phase (Fig. 1). The release of oestradiol from ovarian follicles during the early luteal phase was highly variable in pregnant animals, in general much lower than in the cyclic controls and was already missing in some 5 pregnant individuals. Concentrations of oestradiol-17β in the vena cava were slightly higher than in the artery after 2 weeks of gestation independently of the position of the catheter tip (Fig. 3) proximal or distal to the inflow of the ovarian vessels, indicating a secretion out of the pregnant uterus. A nadir of oestradiol-17β was reached after about 3 weeks (Fig. 2) when progesterone secretion decreased also in about two thirds of the heifers for several days (Fig. 2). However, oxytocin increased between Days 19 and 23 in those animals exhibiting the progesterone decrease, and values in the aorta exceeded those in the vena cava (Figs 2 & 4), indicating a non-luteal, most probably neurohypophysial, site of secretion.

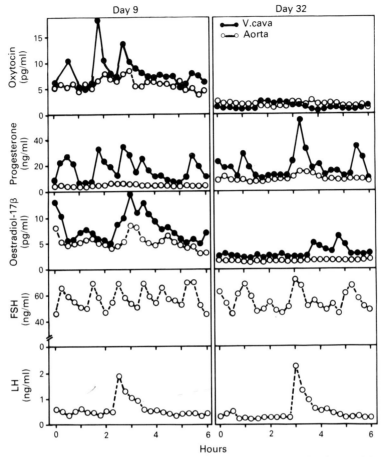

Fig. 1. Secretory pattern of gonadotrophins and ovarian hormones in the caudal vena cava
(●—●) and aorta (○—○) at Days 9 and 32 of gestation. Blood samples were collected
simultaneously from both vessels every 15 min for 6 h from 08:00 to 14:00 h.

Prostaglandins

Out of 8 heifers examined 4 revealed an increase of PGF-2α within 10 min after the start of
manipulation during artificial insemination, but there was no difference in the conception rate of
cattle exhibiting or not exhibiting releases of PGF-2α. Concentrations remained higher for about 6
days in the inseminated than in the cyclic animals (Fig. 5) but were not dependent upon the success
of AI. From Days 7 to 30 only basal concentrations (< 200 fmol/ml) of PGF-2α as well as PGE-2
were found. Secretion of PGF-2α and PGI-2 from the pregnant uterus increased concomitantly up
to 10-fold between Days 31 and 33 (Fig. 6). Concentrations of PGI-2 were slightly higher in the vein
than in the artery, but, unlike at the start of luteolysis, values of both prostaglandins remained
continuously high for several days.

Luteolysis after early pregnancy

Twelve heifers returned to oestrus after AI, 5 of them between Days 22 and 34. Luteolysis was
characterized by 4–7 episodes of massive releases of PGF-2α interrupted by several hours of basal
concentrations (Fig. 7). There was a delay of 20–26 h between the first and second release, but
progesterone had already started to decrease after the first output of PGF-2α. Only the first 3 (–4)

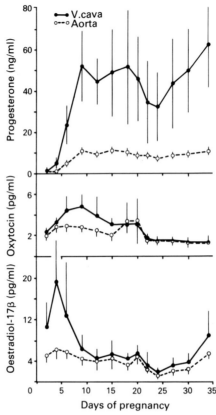

Fig. 2. Ovarian hormones in the caudal vena cava and aorta of a heifer during the first 35 days of pregnancy. Values are the means ($\pm$ s.d.) of a series of frequent samplings performed every 2–4 days.

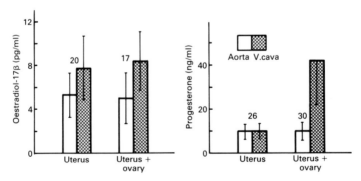

Fig. 3. Comparison of average concentrations of oestradiol-17β and progesterone in the caudal vena cava and aorta between Days 15 and 18 of pregnancy. Values are from animals in which either only the venous drainage of the uterus (left panel) or in which the common uterine and ovarian drainage (right panel) was monitored. The numbers of paired samples involved are indicated.

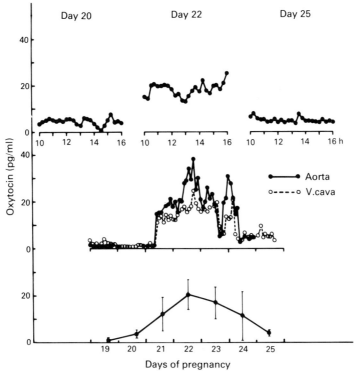

Fig. 4. Concentrations of oxytocin in the caudal vena cava (○—○) or aorta (●—●) of a heifer between Days 19 and 25 of early pregnancy. Samples were collected every 2 h (middle panel) and, in addition, every 15 min for 6 h at Days 20, 22 and 25 (top panel). The average daily concentrations (± s.d.) are given for comparison in the lower panel.

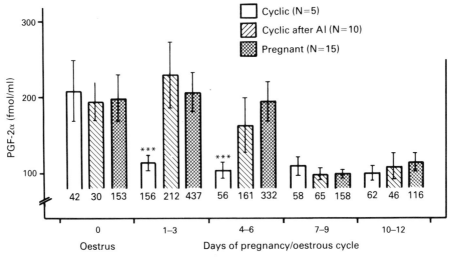

Fig. 5. Basal secretion (mean ± s.d.) of PGF-2α in the vena cava of heifers at the day of oestrus and during the first 12 days of oestrous cycles or early pregnancy. The numbers of animals and samples evaluated are indicated. ***$P < 0.001$ compared with the other two values.

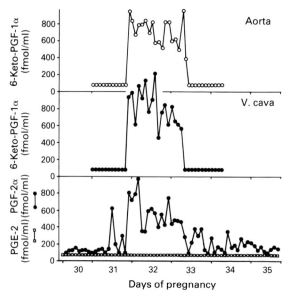

Fig. 6. Concentrations of prostaglandins of a heifer between Days 30 and 35 of early pregnancy. Samples were collected every 2 h synchronously from the vena cava and aorta.

episodes of PGF-2α were accompanied by secretory bursts of luteal oxytocin (Figs 7 & 8). Massive releases of PGF-2α and oxytocin were preceded by slightly rising basal concentrations of both hormones as well as of progesterone (Fig. 8).

Discussion

The maintenance of early pregnancy depends on the transformation of the corpus luteum of the oestrous cycle into one of pregnancy ('Rescue of the CL': Knobil, 1973). The continuous secretion of progesterone prolongs the secretory phase of the endometrium and inhibits the spontaneous motility of the uterine myometrium. At least locally acting links have to be established between embryo and dam until Day 16 (Heap *et al.*, 1973). It is possible only up to this stage of luteal development to inhibit luteolysis by the transfer of embryos into the ipsilateral but not the contralateral horn of the uterus in ruminants (Moor & Rowson, 1966). Various groups have described proteins which are secreted by the early embryo or its membranes into the uterus starting around Day 15 (Roberts & Parker, 1974; Laster, 1977; Bazer *et al.*, 1985; Knickerbocker *et al.*, 1986). One of the induced effects is the suppression of the oestrogen-mediated release of PGF-2α, and so direct luteotrophic properties of these conceptus proteins are less probable. Our own in-vivo experiments strongly support this hypothesis.

Only low basal concentrations of PGF-2α and PGE-2 are detectable until Day 31 after a certain initial increase of basal PGF-2α during the first days after AI (Fig. 5). The low levels of oestradiol-17β at least after the first week of gestation (Figs 2 & 3) might contribute to this relative inhibition of PGF-2α. As tertiary follicles are present at the ovary at all stages of early pregnancy (Rüsse, 1971), as during the oestrous cycle in cattle, we have to postulate an inhibition of synthesis and release of oestrogens within a few days after conception. This effect can be reversed again very soon after early embryonic mortality (Fig. 7).

Luteotrophic signals from the embryo or uterus may reach the ovary by countercurrent transport (Mapletoft *et al.*, 1976), by local transfer by diffusion through tissue (Krzymowski *et al.*, 1982) or by the lymphatic drainage (Magness & Ford, 1982). The secretion of progesterone by the

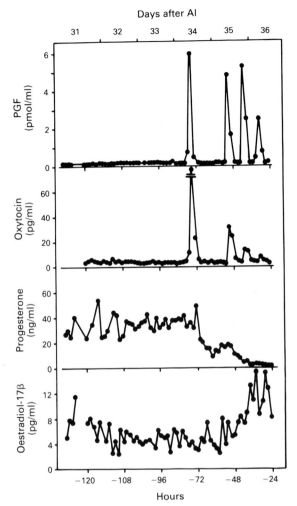

Fig. 7. Spontaneous luteolysis of a previously pregnant heifer during the 5th week after AI. Samples were collected from the vena cava every 2 h.

corpus luteum of pregnancy (Fig. 2) is faster and reaches higher plateau concentrations than during the oestrous cycle (Godkin *et al.*, 1978; Lukaszweska & Hansel 1980). This is not necessarily due to the direct luteotrophic action of embryonic signals upon the corpus luteum. This could also be influenced by the low concentrations of circulating oestradiol-17β leading to a less expressed negative feed-back action of ovarian steroids upon synthesis and release of LH, but not FSH, from the pituitary gland. This might result in the presence of an unchanged frequency of release with slightly increased amplitudes of LH (Fig. 1; Schallenberger *et al.*, 1986). This might secondarily result in higher pulsatile releases of progesterone (see Fig. 1), contributing to somewhat higher average concentrations. Concentrations of oestradiol-17β are higher than basal during Days 4–7 of the oestrous cycle (Glencross *et al.*, 1973; Schallenberger *et al.*, 1985). This occurs still in some pregnant animals (Fig. 2), but average concentrations are already lower than in the cyclic controls and decrease further until reaching a nadir around Day 21 after AI. Nevertheless, the early embryo also seems to secrete *in vivo* some amounts of oestradiol-17β (Fig. 3) after about 2 weeks of pregnancy. This confirms earlier in-vitro data of Shemesh *et al.* (1979). This weak local increase of oestradiol-17β, which does not lead to a striking increase of peripheral concentrations (Fig. 3), may

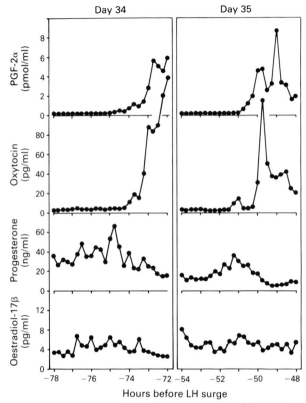

Fig. 8. Release of ovarian hormones and PGF-2α during series of frequent bleedings (from the vena cava every 15 min for 6 h) at Days 34 and 35 after AI during spontaneous luteolysis (same heifer as in Fig. 7).

have a functional role in increasing the local blood flow to the pregnant horn of the uterus and from there to the ovary (Fabian, 1981; Ford *et al.*, 1981). Changes in the secretory pattern of oestradiol-17β may therefore have multiple actions to contribute to the inhibition of luteolysis and to the regulation of blood flow.

We have not yet been able to report a direct effect of luteal oxytocin initiating luteolysis in cattle (Schams *et al.*, 1985). Walters *et al.* (1984) demonstrated considerably higher releases of oxytocin during the luteal phase of cyclic cattle than during early pregnancy (Figs 1 & 2), when the secretion of oxytocin from the ovary is inhibited within a few days after conception. As for oestradiol-17β, this effect can be overridden after embryonic mortality (Figs 7 & 8). Basal secretion of PGF-2α might originate during early gestation from the endometrium (Thatcher *et al.*, 1984) as well as the early preimplantation trophoblast (Shemesh *et al.*, 1979). The sequences leading to the spiking releases inducing luteolysis are inhibited as long as pregnancy is maintained, and also during the period of continuously enhanced concentrations of PGF-2α around placentation (Fig. 6) when maximal values do not exceed 1–2 pmol/ml (Fig. 6), whereas luteolytic spikes at about the same time after AI exceed these values 3–5 times (Figs 7 & 8).

The continuously high concentrations of oxytocin, most probably from the posterior pituitary gland around Day 21 of gestation (Figs 2 & 4), cannot stimulate releases of PGF-2α. They occur in about two-thirds of pregnant animals when progesterone secretion is somewhat reduced at the same time (Fig. 2) (see also Bulman & Lamming, 1978; Karg *et al.*, 1980). We cannot give reasons for the increase of oxytocin in pregnant cattle 3 weeks after AI, but there might be functional links to the stages of apposition and adhesion (Leiser, 1975) which the embryo just passes. Blood flow is considerably increased in the pregnant horn after Day 28 of gestation (Ford *et al.*, 1981) when the trophoblast is increasingly secreting oestrogens (Fig. 2). The synchronous release of PGF-2α and PGI-2 after this period might reflect a local tissue reaction to the invasion of microvilli of the chorion into the surface of the endometrium (Leiser, 1975; King *et al.*, 1980). The secretion of PGI-2 causes vasodilatation in addition to the already increased blood flow facilitating maximal exchange of fluids through the membranes. The inhibition of secretion of oestradiol-17β from ovarian follicles, of oxytocin from the corpus luteum and of PGF-2α from the endometrium is terminated within a few hours after embryonic mortality. Luteolysis before or after this is initiated by a first pulse of PGF-2α, causing immediately a considerable decrease of progesterone. The second pulse is delayed up to 26 h, and subsequent pulses follow within a few hours (Fig. 7). The parallel release of oxytocin is most probably due to secretion from storage pools in the luteal cells because the corpus luteum is exhausted after about 3 bursts.

We conclude that cattle have acquired an alternative method of maintenance of early pregnancy initially not depending upon the action of specific luteotrophic factors from the early embryo. The mechanisms leading within few days after AI to the functional very important inhibition of oestradiol and oxytocin are yet not elucidated. They might involve active recognition of pregnancy by the dam but it is also possible that this pregnancy-type release is the 'normal' pattern and that non-pregnant cyclic animals have to induce luteolysis by additional mechanisms.

This project was generously supported by the Deutsche Forschungsgemeinschaft.

References

Bazer, F.W., Roberts, R.M., Thatcher, W.W. & Sharp, D.C. (1985) Mechanism related to establishment of pregnancy. In *Early Pregnancy Factors*, pp. 13–24. Eds F. Ellendorff & E. Koch. Perinatology Press, Ithaca.

Bulman, D.C. & Lamming, G.E. (1978) Milk progesterone levels in relation to conception, repeat breeding and factors influencing acyclicity in dairy cows. *J. Reprod. Fert.* **54**, 447–458.

Fabian, G. (1981) The cyclical changes in the uterine lymphatics of the pig. Investigations on the perimetrium. *Lymphology* **14**, 17–23.

Ford, S.P., Chenault, J.R., Christenson, R.K., Echternkamp, S.E. & Ford, J.J. (1981) Effects of preimplantation bovine and porcine conceptuses on blood flow and steroid content of the uterus. In *Cellular and Molecular Aspects of Implantation*, pp. 436–438. Eds S. R. Glasser & D. W. Bullock. Plenum Press, New York.

Glencross, R.G., Monro, I.B., Senior, B.E. & Pope, G.S. (1973) Concentrations of oestradiol-17β, oestrone and progesterone in jugular venous plasma of cows during the oestrous cycle and in early pregnancy. *Acta endocr., Copenh.* **73**, 374–384.

Godkin, J.D., Cote, C. & Duby, R.T. (1978) Embryonic stimulation of ovine and bovine corpora lutea. *J. Reprod. Fert.* **54**, 375–378.

Heap, R.B., Perry, J.S. & Challis, J.R.G. (1973) Hormonal maintenance of pregnancy. In *Handbook of Physiology*, Section 7, Endocrinology, Part II, pp. 217–260. Eds American Physiological Society, Washington, D.C.

Hoffmann, B., Kyrein, H.J. & Ender, M.L. (1973) An efficient procedure for the determination of progesterone by radioimmunoassay applied to bovine peripheral plasma. *Hormone Res.* **4**, 302–310.

Karg, H., Claus, R., Günzler, O., Rattenberger, E., Hahn, R. & Hocke, P. (1980) Milk progesterone assay for assessing cyclicity and ovarian dysfunction in cattle. *Proc. 9th Int. Congr. Anim. Reprod. & AI, Madrid* II, 119–124.

King, G.J., Atkinson, B.A. & Robertson, H.A. (1980) Development of the bovine placentome from Days 20 to 29 of gestation. *J. Reprod. Fert.* **59**, 95–100.

Knickerbocker, J.J., Thatcher, W.W., Bazer, F.W., Barron, D.H. & Roberts, R.M. (1986) Inhibition of uterine prostaglandin-F2α production by bovine conceptus secretory proteins. *Prostaglandins* **31**, 777–793.

Knobil, E. (1973) On the regulation of the primate corpus luteum. *Biol. Reprod.* **8**, 246–258.

Krzymowski, T., Kotwica, J., Stefanczyk, S., Czarnocki, J. & Debek, J. (1982) A subovarian exchange mechanism for the countercurrent transfer of ovarian steroid hormones in the pig. *J. Reprod. Fert.* **65**, 457–465.

Laster, D.B. (1977) A pregnancy-specific protein in the bovine uterus. *Biol. Reprod.* **11**, 566–577.

Leiser, R. (1975) Kontaktaufnahme zwischen Trophoblast und Uterusepithel während der frühen Implantation beim Rind. *Anat. Histol. Embryol.* **4**, 63–86.

Lukaszewska, J. & Hansel, W. (1980) Corpus luteum maintenance during early pregnancy in the cow. *J. Reprod. Fert.* **59**, 485–493.

Magness, R.R. & Ford, S.P. (1982) Steroid concentrations in uterine lymph and uterine arterial plasma of gilts during the estrous cycle and early pregnancy. *Biol. Reprod.* **27**, 871–877.

Mapletoft, R.J., Lapin, D.R. & Ginther, O.J. (1976) The ovarian artery as the final component of the local luteotropic pathway between a gravid uterine horn and ovary in ewes. *Biol. Reprod.* **15**, 414–421.

Meyer, H.H.D., Enzenhöfer, G. & Feck, H. (1988) Improvement of radioimmunoassays for prostaglandins in bovine blood plasma and their application to monitor reproductive functions. *Theriogenology* (in press).

Moor, R.M. & Rowson, L.E.A. (1966) Local maintenance of the corpus luteum in sheep with embryos transferred to various isolated portions of the uterus. *J. Reprod. Fert.* **12**, 539–550.

Roberts, G.P. & Parker, J.M. (1974) Macromolecular components of the luminal fluid from the bovine uterus. *J. Reprod. Fert.* **40**, 291–303.

Rüsse, I. (1971) Größe des Corpus luteum und Follikelanbildung während der Gravidität bei Rind und Schaf. *Zuchthygiene* **6**, 126–134.

Schallenberger, E., Schams, D., Bullermann, B. & Walters, D. L. (1984) Pulsatile secretion of gonadotrophins, ovarian steroids and ovarian oxytocin during prostaglandin-induced regression of the corpus luteum in the cow. *J. Reprod. Fert.* **71**, 493–501.

Schallenberger, E., Schöndorfer, A.M. & Walters, D. L. (1985) Gonadotrophins and ovarian steroids in cattle. I. Pulsatile changes of concentrations in the jugular vein throughout the oestrous cycle. *Acta endocr., Copenh.* **108**, 312–321.

Schallenberger, E., Meyer, H.H.D., Schams, D., & Karg, H. (1986) Alternative hormonale Mechanismen zur Erhaltung der Frühgravidität beim Rind. In *Fortschritte in der Fertilitätsforschung* 13, pp. 16–23. Ed. C. Schirren. Grosse Verlag, Berlin.

Schams, D. (1983) Oxytocin determination by radioimmunoassay—III. Improvement to subpicogram sensitivity and application to blood levels in cyclic cattle. *Acta endocr., Copenh.* **103**, 180–183.

Schams, D. & Karg, H. (1969) Radioimmunologische LH-Bestimmung im Blutserum vom Rind unter besonderer Berücksichtigung des Brunstzyklus. *Acta endocr., Copenh.* **61**, 96–103.

Schams, D. & Schallenberger, E. (1976) Heterologous radioimmunoassay for bovine follicle-stimulating hormone and its application during the oestrous cycle in cattle. *Acta endocr., Copenh.* **81**, 461–473.

Schams, D., Schallenberger, E., Meyer, H.H.D., Bullermann, B., Breitinger, H.-J., Enzenhöfer, G., Koll, R., Kruip, T.A.M., Walters, D.L. & Karg, H. (1985) Ovarian oxytocin during the estrous cycle in cattle. In *Oxytocin, Clinical and Laboratory Studies*, pp. 317–334. Eds J. A. Amico & A. G. Robinson. Excerpta Medica, Amsterdam.

Shemesh, M., Milaguir, F., Ayalon, N. & Hansel, W. (1979) Steroidogenesis and prostaglandin synthesis by cultured bovine blastocysts. *J. Reprod. Fert.* **56**, 181–185.

Thatcher, W.W., Wolfenson, D., Curl, J.S., Rico, L.E., Knickerbocker, J.J., Bazer, F.W. & Drost, M. (1984) Prostaglandin dynamics associated with development of the bovine conceptus. *Anim. Reprod. Sci.* **7**, 149–176.

Walters, D.L., Schams, D. & Schallenberger, E. (1984) Pulsatile secretion of gonadotrophins, ovarian steroids and ovarian oxytocin during the luteal phase of the oestrous cycle in the cow. *J. Reprod. Fert.* **71**, 479–491.

Wimsatt, W.A. (1951) Observation on the morphogenesis, cytochemistry, and significance of the binucleate giant cells of the placenta of ruminants. *Am. J. Anat.* **89**, 233–282.

INTRACELLULAR SIGNALLING

Chairmen

H. Behrman
Y. Solomon

J. Reprod. Fert., Suppl. **37** (1989), 287–293

Inositol lipids and LHRH action in the rat ovary

P. C. K. Leung and J. Wang

Department of Obstetrics and Gynaecology, University of British Columbia, Grace Hospital, Vancouver, Canada V6H 3V5

Keywords: LHRH; calcium; protein kinase C; ovary; steroid hormones

Introduction

In the past few years, there has been increasing evidence that the initial action of luteinizing hormone-releasing hormone (LHRH) may involve a rapid alteration in the metabolism of cellular inositol lipids in the ovary. Specifically, ^{32}P labelling studies with rat ovarian cells have demonstrated that LHRH induces a rapid turnover of phosphatidylinositol (Naor & Yavin, 1982; Leung *et al.*, 1983; Leung, 1985; Minegishi & Leung, 1985a) and, more recently, in polyphosphoinositides. LHRH causes a rapid decrease in the level of radiolabel found in phosphatidylinositol 4-phosphate and phosphatidylinositol 4,5-bisphosphate, while increasing the level of phosphatidylinositol and phosphatidic acid (Leung *et al.*, 1986). These findings are consistent with the concept of a role of inositol lipid breakdown in early signal transduction. At the level of the ovarian cell, therefore, it is postulated that the hydrolysis of phosphatidylinositol 4,5-bisphosphate (by phospholipase C) may immediately follow LHRH receptor occupancy, and lead to rapid generation of inositol triphosphate (IP_3) and 1,2-diacylglycerol. In support of this hypothesis, it has been shown that LHRH markedly stimulates the accumulation of inositol phosphates (i.e. inositol 1-phosphate, inositol diphosphate and IP_3) in radiolabelled ovarian cells, concomitant with the alterations in cellular levels of phospholipids (Fig. 1) (Ma & Leung, 1985; Leung *et al.*, 1986; Davis *et al.*, 1986). The stimulatory effect of LHRH on inositol phosphate accumulation could be blocked completely by the presence of a potent LHRH antagonist. IP_3 has been suggested to function as a second messenger for mobilizing intracellular calcium (Burgess *et al.*, 1984) and it is known that Ca^{2+} is required in the action of LHRH at the level of the ovarian cell (Ranta *et al.*, 1983; Dorflinger *et al.*, 1984). On the other hand, it is now well established that 1,2-diacylglycerol activates protein kinase C in various tissues (Nishizuka *et al.*, 1984). Indeed, it has been proposed that protein kinase C may also be involved in the action of LHRH in ovarian cells (Davis & Clark, 1983; Noland & Dimino, 1986; Veldhuis & Demers, 1986). Thus these results implicate the involvement of a calcium-dependent as well as a protein kinase C-mediated pathway in the mechanism of LHRH action, which may well be correlated with the well-known inhibitory effect of LHRH on the steroidogenic response of rat ovarian cells to gonadotrophins (Hsueh & Jones, 1981; Leung, 1985).

Effect of LHRH on ovarian progesterone production

Numerous studies have shown that LHRH and its synthetic agonists can directly affect steroid hormone production in the ovary. These extrapituitary, intraovarian actions are either stimulatory or inhibitory, depending on the duration of LHRH treatment as well as the simultaneous presence of other ovarian cell regulators (such as gonadotrophins) during the culture period (Hsueh & Jones, 1981). In the presence of FSH, LHRH is predominantly inhibitory to progesterone production in cultured granulosa cells (Fig. 2). LHRH agonists progressively inhibit adenylate cyclase and stimulate phosphodiesterase activities in cultured granulosa cells, indicating that blockade of FSH action is attributable in part to the combined effects of decreased production and increased

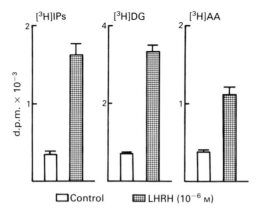

Fig. 1. Effect of LHRH (5 min) on the liberation of radiolabelled inositol phosphates (IPs), diacylglycerol (DG) and unesterified arachidonic acid (AA) in rat granulosa cells. Values are the means ± s.e.m. of quadruplicate determinations. Similar results were observed in at least 2 separate experiments. (From Wang & Leung, 1988.)

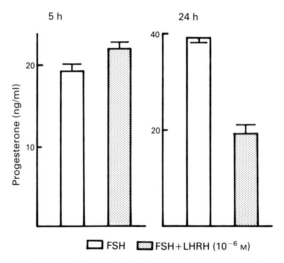

Fig. 2. Effect of LHRH for 5 or 24 h on FSH-induced progesterone production in rat granulosa cells. Values are mean ± s.e.m. of quadruplicate determinations. Similar results were observed in at least 2 separate experiments.

degradation of cyclic AMP (Knecht & Catt, 1981). Direct inhibition of steroidogenic enzymes by LHRH in ovarian cells has also been reported (Hsueh & Jones, 1981).

Role of calcium and protein kinase C in LHRH action

In the ovary, the precise relationship between Ca^{2+} mobilization and steroidogenesis is not understood. It has been reported that LHRH and its agonists rapidly increase cytosolic free Ca^{2+} levels, as measured by Quin 2 fluorescence (Davis *et al.*, 1986). Although the addition of A 23187 by

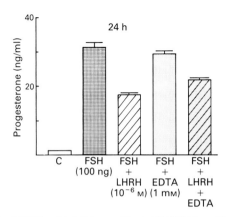

Fig. 3. Partial reversal by EDTA of inhibitory effect of LHRH on FSH-induced progesterone production in rat granulosa cells. Values are mean $\pm$ s.e.m. for quadruplicate determinations. Similar results were obtained in at least 2 separate experiments.

itself slightly enhances basal progesterone production in granulosa cells, the calcium ionophore markedly antagonizes the stimulation of progesterone by gonadotrophins or cholera toxin or cAMP derivatives (Leung *et al.*, 1988). Further, calcium is required for the inhibitory action of LHRH on cAMP and steroid production during long-term incubation of ovarian cells (Ranta *et al.*, 1983; Dorflinger *et al.*, 1984; Fig. 3). It has therefore been proposed that LHRH action in ovarian cells is partly mediated by intracellular Ca^{2+}. Activation of protein kinase C stimulates basal progesterone production in rat granulosa cells but inhibits the progesterone response to stimulation by gonadotrophins or cAMP derivatives (Welsh *et al.*, 1984; Kawai & Clark, 1985; Shinohara *et al.*, 1986; Leung *et al.*, 1988). The steroidogenic effect of LHRH can be partly blocked by a potent inhibitor of protein kinase C (Wang & Leung, 1987). Protein kinase C activity has been characterized in ovarian tissues (Davis & Clark, 1983; Noland & Dimino, 1986; Veldhuis & Demers, 1986). The highest specific activities are found in the cytosol, followed by microsomes and mitochondria (Noland & Dimino, 1986). At the level of the ovarian cell, therefore, the hydrolysis of inositol lipids may immediately follow LHRH receptor occupancy and lead to the rapid generation of IP_3 and diacylglycerol. The resultant changes in calcium mobilization and/or protein kinase C activity may well be correlated with the modulatory effects of LHRH on ovarian steroidogenesis. This hypothesis is clearly supported by several studies (Welsh *et al.*, 1984; Kawai & Clark, 1985; Shinohara *et al.*, 1986; Leung *et al.*, 1988), in which a calcium ionophore as well as a protein kinase C activator mimic the inhibitory effect of LHRH on gonadotrophin-stimulated progesterone production in granulosa cells.

Effects of calcium ionophore and/or protein kinase C activators

Treatment with 12-0-tetradecanoyl phorbol-13-acetate (TPA) or A 23187 suppresses the steroidogenic response of rat granulosa cells to FSH stimulation. The effects of both TPA and A 23187 can be seen as early as 5 h after drug addition (Fig. 4). However, at 5 h, the FSH-stimulated progesterone production is attenuated only 30–45% by 10^{-7} M-TPA or 10^{-7} M-A 23187, suggesting that the inhibitory actions at this time are relatively weak. By comparison, during a 24-h incubation of granulosa cells (Fig. 5), 50% suppression of FSH-stimulated progesterone production is caused by $\sim 10^{-10}$ M and $\sim 10^{-8}$ M for TPA and A 23187, respectively. The effect of TPA is probably due to activation of protein kinase C, since other phorbol derivatives which are not potent

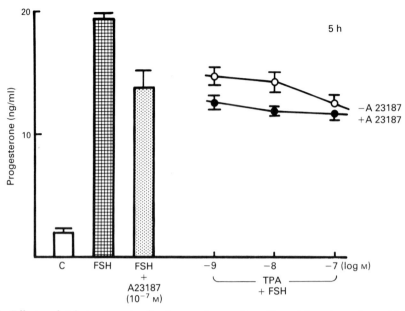

Fig. 4. Effects of 5-h treatment of rat granulosa cells with calcium ionophore (A 23187) and/or protein kinase C activator (TPA) on FSH-induced progesterone production. Values are mean ± s.e.m. for quadruplicate determinations. Similar results were obtained in at least 2 separate experiments.

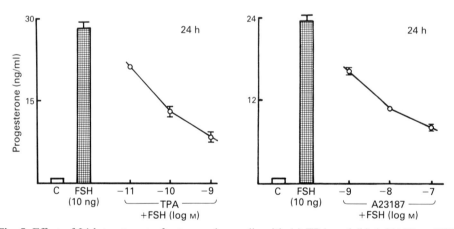

Fig. 5. Effect of 24-h treatment of rat granulosa cells with (a) TPA and (b) A 23187 on FSH-induced progesterone production. Values are mean ± s.e.m. for quadruplicate determinations. Similar results were obtained in at least 2 separate experiments.

protein kinase C activators are ineffective. Likewise, Shinohara *et al.* (1986) have reported that TPA does not affect the elevated progesterone production in granulosa cells incubated for 2 h in the presence of hCG, cholera toxin or forskolin. On the other hand, Kawai & Clark (1985) have shown that TPA significantly decreases the progesterone response of granulosa cells to LH during a 5-h incubation period. The inhibition of gonadotrophin-stimulated progesterone production is more

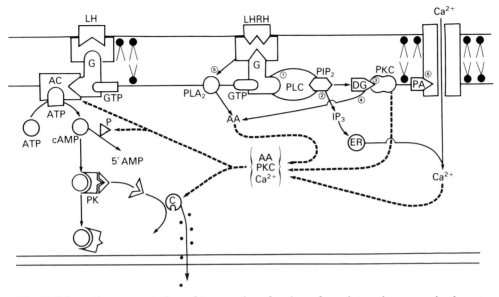

Fig. 6. Schematic representation of two modes of action of regulatory hormones in the rat ovarian cell. First, the binding of LH to a receptor located on the plasma membrane stimulates adenylate cyclase (AC) activity via a GTP-binding protein (G). Changes in intracellular cAMP levels then modulate cAMP-dependent protein kinase (PK) activity and subsequently lead to enhanced cholesterol (C) side-chain cleavage and progesterone production. On the other hand, LHRH may act via an alternative mechanism involving alterations in inositol phospholipid metabolism: (1) pre-existing polyphosphoinositides such as PIP_2 may be hydrolysed by a specific phospholipase C (PLC); (2) inositol triphosphate (IP_3) may be released into the cytoplasm to function as a second messenger for mobilizing intracellular Ca^{2+}; (3) diacylglycerol (DG) may activate protein kinase C (PKC); (4) arachidonic acid (AA) may be liberated from phospholipids via a DG lipase, or (5) by the action of a phospholipase A_2 (PLA_2); (6) phosphatic acid (PA) may also serve as a Ca^{2+} ionophore. Thus, the subsequent mobilization of Ca^{2+}, activation of PKC, and liberation of AA or its metabolites may all mediate the action of LHRH in the ovarian cell.

pronounced when granulosa cells are treated with TPA for 2 days (Welsh *et al.*, 1984). Our observation that the inhibitory effects of A 23187 or TPA could be seen even in the presence of a phosphodiesterase inhibitor also suggests that the suppression of the progesterone response to FSH is exerted, in part at least, at step(s) beyond cAMP generation and degradation (Leung *et al.*, 1988). Likewise, in rat luteal cells, it has been shown that A 23187 or TPA inhibits progesterone production by the cAMP analogues (8-bromo-cAMP or dibutyryl-cAMP), implicating an inhibition not only on adenylate cyclase but also on the steroidogenic enzymes (Baum & Rosberg, 1987). A synergistic role of calcium and protein kinase C pathways for eliciting full cellular responses has already been proposed in many different systems (Nishizuka *et al.*, 1984). However, our results fail to demonstrate a synergistic action of A 23187 and TPA in affecting the steroidogenic capacity of the ovary (Fig. 4). In this regard, while A 23187 has been shown to enhance acutely the TPA-induced production of prostaglandin F-2α in pig granulosa cells (Veldhuis & Demers, 1987), a report on the inhibitory effects of the phorbol ester and calcium ionophore on LH-induced progesterone production in rat luteal cells has not described this potential amplifying mechanism (Baum & Rosberg, 1987).

Treatment of granulosa cells with LHRH for 5 h fails to affect FSH-induced progesterone production, whereas FSH-stimulated progesterone concentrations are markedly attenuated by LHRH during a 24-h treatment (Fig. 2). On the assumption that calcium and protein kinase C

P. C. K. Leung and J. Wang

pathways indeed partly mediate LHRH action in the ovarian cell, it could be postulated that their potential inhibitory effects at 5 h might have been blocked or antagonized by some other LHRH-induced intracellular messenger(s). Possibly one such candidate is arachidonic acid, which is released rapidly from cellular phospholipid pools after LHRH addition to granulosa cells (Minegishi & Leung, 1985b; Minegishi *et al.*, 1987) (Fig. 1). There is increasing evidence that arachidonic acid and/or its metabolites might play an important role in hormone signal transduction (Lapetina *et al.*, 1981; Kolesnick *et al.*, 1984; Reich *et al.*, 1985; Lin, 1985; Milvae *et al.*, 1986; Chang *et al.*, 1986; Abou-Samra *et al.*, 1986). Moreover, arachidonic acid has been reported to activate protein kinase C in some systems (McPhail *et al.*, 1984; Murakami & Routtenberg, 1985). In the absence of FSH, treatment of granulosa cells with arachidonic acid and TPA for 5 h synergically stimulates progesterone production (Wang & Leung, 1988). The potential interaction between arachidonic acid (or its metabolites), calcium and protein kinase C on gonadotrophin-stimulated progesterone production in ovarian cells is depicted in Fig. 6.

Conclusion

It is becoming clear that remarkable similarities exist between LHRH actions in the pituitary and gonads. Identical receptors for LHRH are presumably present in both tissues. Enhanced inositol lipid metabolism has been reported following the exposure of gonadotrophes or ovarian cells to LHRH. Calcium ionophores and activators of protein kinase C have now been shown to mimic the biological actions of LHRH in the pituitary (stimulation of LH release) and the ovary (inhibition of progesterone response to gonadotrophins). Taken together, these findings strongly support the hypothesis that stimulation of polyphosphoinositide metabolism is intimately involved in the mechanism of LHRH action at the pituitary and ovarian levels.

This research has been supported by the Medical Research Council of Canada.

References

Abou-Samra, A.B., Catt, K.J. & Aguilera, G. (1986) Role of arachidonic acid in the regulation of adrenocorticotropin release from rat anterior pituitary cell cultures. *Endocrinology* 119, 1427–1431.

Baum, M.S. & Rosberg, S. (1987) A phorbol ester, phorbol 12-myristate 13-acetate, and a calcium ionophore, A23187, can mimic the luteolytic effect of prostaglandin $F_{2\alpha}$ in isolated rate luteal cells. *Endocrinology* 120, 1019–1026.

Burgess, G.M., Godfrey, P.P., McKinney, J.S., Berridge, M.J., Irvine, R.F. & Putney, J.W., Jr (1984) The second messenger linking receptor activation to internal Ca release in liver. *Nature, Lond.* 309, 63–66.

Chang, J.P., Graeter, J. & Catt, K.J. (1986) Coordinate actions of arachidonic acid and protein kinase C in gonadotropin-releasing hormone-stimulated secretion of luteinizing hormone. *Biochem. Biophys. Res. Commun.* 134, 134–139.

Davis, J.S. & Clark, M.R. (1983) Activation of protein kinase C in the bovine corpus luteum by phospholipids and Ca^{2+}. *Biochem. J.* 214, 569–574.

Davis, J.S., West, L.A. & Farese, R.V. (1986) Gonadotropin-releasing hormone (GnRH) rapidly stimulates the formation of inositol phosphates and diacylglycerol in rat granulosa cells: further evidence for the involvement of Ca^{2+} and protein kinase C in the action of GnRH. *Endocrinology* 118, 2561–2571.

Dorflinger, L.J., Albert, P.J., Williams, A.T. & Behrman, H.R. (1984) Calcium is an inhibitor of luteinizing hormone-sensitive adenylate cyclase in the luteal cells. *Endocrinology* 114, 1208–1215.

Hsueh, A.J.W. & Jones, P.B.C. (1981) Extrapituitary actions of gonadotropin-releasing hormone. *Endocrine Rev.* 2, 437–461.

Kawai, Y. & Clark, M.R. (1985) Phorbol ester regulation of rat granulosa cell prostaglandin and progesterone accumulation. *Endocrinology* 116, 2320–2326.

Knecht, M. & Catt, K.J. (1981) Gonadotropin-releasing hormone: regulation of adenosine-3',5'-monophosphate in ovarian granulosa cells. *Science, N.Y.* 214, 1346–1348.

Kolesnick, R.N., Musacchio, I., Thaw, C. & Gershengorn, M.C. (1984) Arachidonic acid mobilizes calcium and stimulates prolactin secretion from GH_3 cells. *Am. J. Physiol.* 246, E458–E462.

Lapetina, E.G., Billah, M.M. & Cuatrecasas, P. (1981) The phosphatidylinositol cycle and the regulation of arachidonic acid production. *Nature, Lond.* 292, 367–369.

Leung, P.C.K. (1985) Mechanisms of gonadotropin-releasing hormone and prostaglandin action on luteal cells. *Can. J. Physiol. Pharmacol.* 63, 249–256.

Leung, P.C.K., Raymond, V. & Labrie, F. (1983) Stimulation of phosphatidic acid and phosphatidylinositol labeling in luteal cells by luteinizing hormone-releasing hormone. *Endocrinology* **112**, 1138–1140.

Leung, P.C.K., Minegishi, T., Ma, F., Zhou, F.Z. & Ho Yuen, B. (1986) Induction of polyphosphoinositide breakdown in rat corpus luteum by prostaglandin $F_{2\alpha}$. *Endocrinology* **119**, 12–18.

Leung, P.C.K., Minegishi, T. & Wang, J. (1988) Inhibition of FSH and cyclic adenosine-3′,5′-monophosphate induced progesterone production by calcium and protein kinase C in the rat ovary. *Am. J. Obstet. Gynecol.* **158**, 350–356.

Lin, T. (1985) Mechanism of action of gonadotropin-releasing hormone-stimulated Leydig cell steroidogenesis. III. The role of arachidonic acid and calcium/phospholipid dependent protein kinase. *Life Sci.* **36**, 1255–1264.

Ma, F. & Leung, P.C.K. (1985) Luteinizing hormone-releasing hormone enhances polyphosphoinositide breakdown in rat granulosa cells. *Biochem. Biophys. Res. Commun.* **130**, 1201–1208.

McPhail, L.C., Clayton, C.C. & Snyderman, R. (1984) A potential second messenger role for unsaturated fatty acids: actions of Ca^{2+}-dependent protein kinase. *Science, N.Y.* **224**, 622–625.

Milvae, R.A., Alila, H.W. & Hansel, W. (1986) Involvement of lipoxygenase products of arachidonic acid metabolism in bovine luteal cells. *Biol. Reprod.* **35**, 1210–1215.

Minegishi, T. & Leung, P.C.K. (1985a) Effects of prostaglandins and LHRH on phosphatidic acid-phosphatidylinositol labeling in rat granulosa cells. *Can. J. Physiol. Pharmacol.* **63**, 320–324.

Minegishi, T. & Leung, P.C.K. (1985b) Luteinizing hormone-releasing hormone stimulates arachidonic acid release in rat granulosa cells. *Endocrinology* **117**, 2001–2007.

Minegishi, T., Wang, J. & Leung, P.C.K. (1987) Luteinizing hormone-releasing hormone (LHRH)-induced arachidonic acid release in rat granulosa cells: role of calcium and protein kinase C. *FEBS Lett.* **214**, 139–142.

Murakami, K. & Routtenberg, A. (1985) Direct activation of purified protein kinase C by unsaturated fatty acids (oleate and arachidonate) in the absence of phospholipids and Ca^{2+}. *FEBS Lett.* **192**, 189–193.

Naor, Z. & Yavin, E. (1982) Gonadotropin releasing hormone stimulates phospholipid labeling in cultured granulosa cells. *Endocrinology* **111**, 1615–1619.

Nishizuka, Y., Takai, Y., Kishimoto, A., Kikkawa, U. & Kaibuchi, K. (1984) Phospholipid turnover in hormone action. *Recent Prog. Horm. Res.* **40**, 301–341.

Noland, T.A. & Dimino, M.J. (1987) Characterization and distribution of protein kinase C in ovarian tissue. *Biol. Reprod.* **35**, 863–872.

Ranta, T., Knecht, M., Darbon, J.-M., Baukal, A.J. & Catt, K.J. (1983) Calcium dependence of the inhibitory effect of gonadotropin-releasing hormone on luteinizing hormone-induced cyclic AMP production in rat granulosa cells. *Endocrinology* **113**, 427–429.

Reich, R., Kohen, F., Slager, R. & Tsafriri, A. (1985) Ovarian lipoxygenase activity and its regulation by gonadotropin in the rat. *Prostaglandins* **30**, 581–590.

Shinohara, O., Knecht, M., Feng, P. & Catt, K.J. (1986) Activation of protein kinase C potentiates cyclic AMP production and stimulates steroidogenesis in differentiated ovarian granulosa cells. *J. Steroid Biochem.* **24**, 161–168.

Veldhuis, J.D. & Demers, L.M. (1986) An inhibitory role for the protein kinase C pathway in ovarian steroidogenesis: studies with cultured swine granulosa cells. *Biochem. J.* **239**, 505–511.

Veldhuis, J.D. & Demers, L.M. (1987) Activation of protein kinase C is coupled to prostaglandin $F_{2\alpha}$ synthesis in the ovary: studies in cultured swine granulosa cells. *Molec. cell. Endocrin.* **49**, 249–254.

Wang, J. & Leung, P.C.K. (1987) Role of protein kinase C in luteinizing hormone-releasing hormone (LHRH)-stimulated progesterone production in rat granulosa cells. *Biochem. Biophys. Res. Commun.* **146**, 939–944.

Wang, J. & Leung, P.C.K. (1988) Role of arachidonic acid in luteinizing hormone-releasing hormone action: stimulation of progesterone production in rat granulosa cells. *Endocrinology* **122**, 906–911.

Welsh, T.H., Jr, Jones, P.B.C. & Hsueh, A.J.W. (1984) Phorbol ester of ovarian and testicular steroidogenesis in vitro. *Cancer Res.* **44**, 885–892.

J. Reprod. Fert., Suppl. **37** (1989), 295–300

Mechanism of action of gonadotrophin-releasing hormone on pituitary gonadotrophin secretion

Z. Naor, H. Dan-Cohen, J. Hermon* and R. Limor†

*Department of Biochemistry, The George S. Wise Faculty of Life Sciences, Tel Aviv University, Ramat Aviv 69978, Israel; *Department of Hormone Research, The Weizmann Institute of Science, Rehovot 76100, Israel; and †Timsit Institute of Reproductive Endocrinology, Sackler School of Medicine, Tel Aviv University, Ramat Aviv 69978, Israel*

Keywords: GnRH; pituitary; gonadotrophins; Ca^{2+}; protein kinase C

Introduction

Gonadotrophin-releasing hormone (GnRH) binds to and preferentially activates the pituitary gonadotrophs to stimulate gonadotrophin secretion and biosynthesis (Naor & Childs, 1986). Peptide hormones, neurotransmitters, growth factors and antigens operate via formation of second messengers. The messenger molecules can activate a respective protein kinase which phosphorylates key proteins and enzymes participating in the physiological response. Since cAMP, cGMP and prostaglandins have been ruled out as mediators of GnRH-induced gonadotrophin secretion (Naor & Childs, 1986), we investigated the role of phosphoinositide turnover, Ca^{2+} mobilization and protein kinase C activation in the neuropeptide action.

Effect of GnRH on phosphoinositide turnover

Ca^{2+}-mobilizing receptors operate via GTP-binding proteins (Gp), analogous to Gs and Gi of the adenylate cyclase system (Cockcroft, 1987). Activation of Gp is now thought to enhance phospholipase C activity. The activated enzyme hydrolyses phosphatidylinositol-4,5-bis phosphate (PIP_2) to 1,2-diacylglycerol and *myo*-inositol-1,4,5-trisphosphate (IP_3). The two products are regarded as 'second messengers' since diacylglycerol activates the Ca^{2+}/phospholipid-dependent protein kinase (C-kinase; Nishizuka, 1984, 1986) and IP_3 mobilizes intracellular Ca^{2+} (Berridge & Irvine, 1984). Diacylglycerol is then phosphorylated to phosphatidic acid and IP_3 is converted to inositol. Other inositol polyphosphates such as IP_4, IP_5, IP_6 and cyclic inositol phosphates were also described, but their biological significance awaits further investigation (Majerus *et al.*, 1986; Irvine & Moor, 1986; Putney, 1986; Vallejo *et al.*, 1987). The activated diacylglycerol and inositol will produce phosphatidylinositol (PI) and phosphorylation of PI will result in the formation of phosphatidylinositol-4-phosphate (PIP) and PIP_2. It has been suggested that, while IP_3 is formed from PIP_2, most of the diacylglycerol is produced from direct hydrolysis of PI rather than PIP_2 (Majerus *et al.*, 1986). The importance of the cycle is therefore the production of the second messengers diacylglycerol and IP_3 which are involved in signal transduction mechanisms (Michell, 1975).

Rapid hydrolysis of pituitary PIP_2 by GnRH has been demonstrated (Schrey, 1985; Naor *et al.*, 1986; Morgan *et al.*, 1987). We found that addition of GnRH to pituitary cells prelabelled with *myo*-[2-³H]inositol stimulated the appearance of labelled IP_3 (~ 10 sec) in the presence of Li^+ in the medium (Naor *et al.*, 1986; Fig. 1). Activation of phospholipase C by GnRH does not require elevation of cytosolic free Ca^{2+} levels ($[Ca^{2+}]_i$) and therefore might represent an early process induced by GnRH in order to mobilize cellular Ca^{2+} pools. The stimulatory effect of GnRH on inositol phosphate production is not inhibited by pertussis toxin, suggesting that the GTP-binding protein involved in GnRH action is not Gi (Naor *et al.*, 1986). We therefore suggest that one of the earliest effects induced by GnRH in pituitary gonadotrophs is a rapid Ca^{2+}-independent phosphodiesteric hydrolysis of phosphoinositides to generate the second messengers IP_3 and diacylglycerol required for further processing of the receptor-evoked signal.

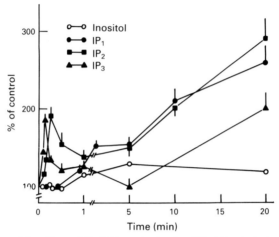

Fig. 1. Time course of the effect of GnRH on the levels of [^{3}H]inositol phosphate formation in cultured rat pituitary cells. Values are mean $\pm$ s.e.m. for 3 observations at each point. (From Naor *et al.*, 1986.)

Effect of GnRH on $[Ca^{2+}]_i$

Many investigators have documented that extracellular Ca^{2+} is required for GnRH stimulation of gonadotrophin secretion (Conn *et al.*, 1981). Nevertheless, detailed studies on changes in $[Ca^{2+}]_i$ in pituitary cells stimulated by GnRH have only recently been performed (Chang *et al.*, 1986; Limor *et al.*, 1987). Such measurements are now possible with fluorescent probes such as Quin 2 (Tsien *et al.*, 1982), and enriched fractions of rat pituitary gonadotrophs separated by centrifugal elutriation (Hyde *et al.*, 1982; Limor *et al.*, 1987). GnRH induced a rapid transient (~ 10 sec) increase in gonadotroph $[Ca^{2+}]_i$ followed by a prolonged decay phase of elevated $[Ca^{2+}]_i$ which lasted several minutes (Fig. 2). The first peak is composed of an ionomycin-sensitive intracellular Ca^{2+} pool and a second component of Ca^{2+} entry via voltage-dependent Ca^{2+} channels (Naor *et al.*, 1988; Davidson *et al.*, 1988). The second phase involves Ca^{2+} influx via voltage-sensitive and insensitive channels. The cellular Ca^{2+} pool is most probably mediated via IP_3 formation since addition of IP_3 to permeabilized pituitary cells resulted in a transient increase of Ca^{2+} which was released from a nonmitochondrial pool capable of maintaining ambient free Ca^{2+} concentrations around 170 nM in an ATP-dependent mechanism. The intracellular Ca^{2+} pool mobilized rapidly by GnRH accounts for 55% of the peak $[Ca^{2+}]_i$ induced by GnRH and might be responsible for the first burst phase of the LH exocytotic response (Smith *et al.*, 1987; Davidson *et al.*, 1988). Since ionomycin mobilizes the cellular Ca^{2+} pool but also induces Ca^{2+} influx, it is an ideal tool to investigate the role of Ca^{2+} in exocytosis. Indeed, elevation of gonadotroph $[Ca^{2+}]_i$ by ionomycin to levels equivalent to those induced by GnRH resulted in LH release amounting to only 45% of the response to GnRH (Naor *et al.*, 1988). Others have reported that extracellular Ca^{2+} pools are necessary and

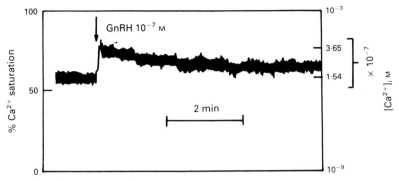

Fig. 2. Effect of GnRH on $[Ca^{2+}]_i$ in cultured rat gonadotrophs. The enriched cells were prepared by centrifugal elutriation as described by Limor *et al.* (1987). Traces of Quin-2 fluorescence are shown. Note the early 'spike phase' of GnRH action which is followed by a sustained phase of elevated $[Ca^{2+}]_i$.

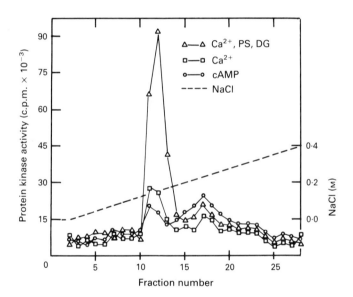

Fig. 3. DEAE-cellulose (DE-52) chromatography of pituitary protein kinase C. PS, phosphatidylserine; DG, diacylglycerol. (Data from Naor *et al.*, 1985b; Hermon *et al.*, 1986.)

sufficient for mediating the full exocytotic response of GnRH (Conn, 1986). However, we have suggested that Ca^{2+} mobilization, first from cellular sources followed by influx via nifedipine-sensitive and -insensitive channels, is involved in mediating part of the LH response of pituitary gonadotrophs to a GnRH challenge (Naor *et al.*, 1988).

Role of protein kinase C

Since its discovery (Nishizuka, 1984, 1986) the Ca^{2+} and phospholipid-dependent protein kinase (C-kinase) gained recognition as a key element in the regulatory network of cellular processes. C-kinase is thought to be involved in synaptic transmission, neuronal development, axonal regeneration, exocytosis, growth, differentiation, learning and tumour promotion. Among others

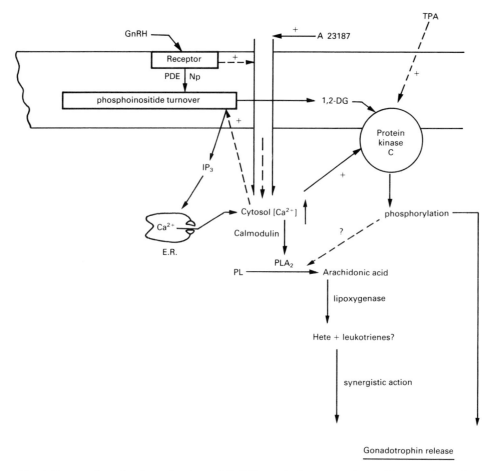

Fig. 4. Proposed mechanism of action of GnRH on pituitary gonadotrophin secretion. PDE, phosphodiesterase; Np or Gp is a GTP-binding protein; E.R., endoplasmic reticulum; PL, phospholipids; Hete, hydroxyeicosatetraenoic acid; DG, diacylglycerol.

C-kinase mediates the pleiotropic actions of the tumour-promoting phorbol esters such as 12-0-tetradecanoyl phorbol-13-acetate (TPA). Although it was previously regarded as a single mono-meric entity, analysis of cDNA clones of the enzyme revealed a multiple gene family encoding at least 4 subspecies (Parker *et al.*, 1986; Coussens *et al.*, 1986; Kikkawa *et al.*, 1988).

C-kinase is activated by association with membrane phospholipids, in particular phosphatidyl-serine, in the presence of elevated Ca^{2+}. Unsaturated diacylglycerol increases the apparent affinity of C-kinase for phosphatidylserine and decreases the Ca^{2+} concentration needed for maximal enzyme activity (Nishizuka, 1984, 1986).

Since diacylglycerol is generated during enhanced phosphoinositide turnover, C-kinase is most probably involved in signal transduction mechanisms of Ca^{2+}-mobilizing receptors. The presence of C-kinase in the pituitary has been reported (Turgeon *et al.*, 1984; Hirota *et al.*, 1985; Naor *et al.*, 1985b; Hermon *et al.*, 1986). Pituitary C-kinase is mostly soluble (70%) and partly particulate (30%, Fig. 3). However, while the soluble form is recovered in an inactive state, the particulate form is found in a cofactor-insensitive state. Therefore, the soluble form of the enzyme can also be detected in a crude cytosolic preparation, while the particulate enzyme is detectable only after solubilization and anion exchange chromatography (Naor *et al.*, 1985b; Hermon *et al.*, 1986).

Pituitary C-kinase is redistributed from the cytosol to the membrane upon GnRH or TRH challenge (Hirota *et al.*, 1985; Naor *et al.*, 1985b; Drust & Martin, 1985; Fearon & Tashjian, 1985). Translocation of C-kinase to the membrane by GnRH or TRH following increased PI turnover will expose the inactive enzyme to diacylglycerol and phosphatidylserine present in the membrane and permit activation even in the face of submicromolar concentrations of Ca^{2+}.

Fearon & Tashjian (1987) have demonstrated that the cellular Ca^{2+} pool mobilized by TRH in GH_3 cells and the newly formed diacylglycerol are most probably responsible for C-kinase translocation. Therefore it seems that the IP_3-mobilized cellular Ca^{2+} pool might have a dual function: redistribution of C-kinase and mediation of the first phase of exocytosis.

Studies with cultured cells demonstrated that the simultaneous presence of the Ca^{2+} ionophore A 23187 and the C-kinase activator TPA produced a synergistic response that mimicked the exocytotic response of GnRH (Naor & Eli, 1985; Naor *et al.*, 1987). We therefore suggest that the simultaneous activation of the bifurcating Ca^{2+} messenger system, namely elevation of $[Ca^{2+}]_i$ and C-kinase activation, is necessary for full expression of GnRH stimulation of gonadotrophin secretion (Fig. 4). The C-kinase subspecies present in the pituitary and their possible role in GnRH action await further investigation (Kikkawa *et al.*, 1988).

Arachidonic acid and its lipoxygenase or epoxygenase metabolites have also been implicated in GnRH action (Naor & Catt, 1981; Naor *et al.*, 1985a; Snyder *et al.*, 1983; Hulting *et al.*, 1985). Two possible sites of action are considered. The first is that arachidonic acid is formed early in the process from diacylglycerol by diacylglycerol-lipase and might participate in cellular Ca^{2+} mobilization, C-kinase activation and the first phase of exocytosis. The second possibility is that activation of phospholipase A_2 is the result of the combined action of Ca^{2+} and C-kinase via phosphorylation of a regulatory protein. In this case it is likely that arachidonic acid and/or its metabolites will participate with C-kinase in eliciting the second phase of GnRH-induced gonadotrophin secretion. The well-documented biphasic response of pituitary gonadotrophs to GnRH challenge might be mediated by a complex interaction of different Ca^{2+} pools, activated C-kinase subspecies and arachidonic acid and its metabolites.

This work was supported by the United States–Israel Binational Science Foundation. We thank Dr K. Catt, Dr G. Childs, Dr A. Capponi and Dr Y. Nishizuka for active collaboration; and A. Azrad, Y. Eli and T. Hannoch for technical assistance.

References

Berridge, M.J. & Irvine, R.F. (1984) Inositol trisphosphate a novel second messenger in cellular signal transduction. *Nature, Lond.* **312**, 315–321.

Chang, J.P., McCoy, E.E., Graeter, J., Tasaka, K. & Catt, K.J. (1986) Participation of voltage-dependent calcium channels in the action of gonadotroph releasing hormone. *J. biol. Chem.* **261**, 9105–9108.

Cockcroft, S. (1987) Polyphosphoinositide phosphodiesterase: regulation by a novel guanine nucleotide binding protein, Gp. *Trends Biochem. Sci.* **12**, 75–78.

Conn, P.M. (1986) The molecular basis of gonadotrophin releasing hormone action. *Endocr. Rev.* **7**, 3–10.

Conn, P.M., Marian, J., McMillan, M., Stern, J., Rogers, D., Hamby, M., Penna, A. & Grant, E. (1981) Gonadotropin releasing hormone action in the pituitary: a three step mechanism. *Endocr. Rev.* **2**, 174–185.

Coussens, L., Parker, P.J., Rhee, L., Yang-Feng, T.L., Chen, E, Waterfield, M.D., Francke, U. & Ullrich, A. (1986) Multiple, distinct forms of bovine and human protein kinase C suggest diversity in cellular signalling pathways. *Science, N.Y.* **233**, 859–866.

Davidson, J.S., Wakefield, I.K., King, J.A., Mulligan, G.P. & Millar, P. (1988) Dual pathways of calcium entry in spike and plateau phase of luteinizing hormone release from chicken pituitary cells: sequential activation of receptor-operated and voltage-sensitive calcium channels by gonadotropin-releasing hormone. *Molec. Endocr.* **2**, 382–390.

Drust, D.S. & Martin, T.F.J. (1985) Protein kinase C translocates from cytosol to membrane upon hormone activation: Effects of thyrotropin-releasing hormone in GH_3 cells. *Biochem. Biophys. Res. Commun.* **128**, 531–537.

Fearon, C.W. & Tashjian, A.H., Jr (1985) Thyrotropin-releasing hormone induces redistribution of protein-kinase C in GH_4C_1 rat pituitary cells. *J. biol. Chem.* **260**, 8366–8371.

Fearon, C.W. & Tashjian, A.H., Jr (1987) Ionomycin inhibits thyrotropin-releasing hormone induced translocation of protein kinase C in GH_4C_1 pituitary cells. *J. biol. Chem.* **262**, 9515–9520.

Hermon, J., Reiss, N. & Naor, Z. (1986) Phospholipid-dependent Ca^{2+} activated protein kinase (C-kinase) in the pituitary: further characterization and endogenous redistribution. *Molec. cell. Endocrinol.* **47**, 201–208.

Hirota, K., Hirota, T., Aquileria, G. & Catt, K.J. (1985) Hormone induced redistribution of calcium activated phospholipid dependent protein kinase in pituitary gonadotrophs. *J. biol. Chem.* **260**, 3243–3246.

Hulting, A.L., Lindgren, J.A., Hokfelt, T., Eneroth, P., Werner, S., Patrono, C. & Samuelsson, B. (1985) Leukotriene C_4 as a mediator of luteinizing hormone release from rat anterior pituitary cells. *Proc. natn. Acad. Sci. U.S.A.* **82**, 3834–3838.

Hyde, C.L., Childs (Moriarty), G., Wahl, L.M., Naor, Z. & Catt, K.J. (1982) Preparation of gonadotroph enriched cell population from adult rat anterior pituitary cells by centrifugal elutriation. *Endocrinology* **111**, 1421–1423.

Irvine, R.F. & Moor, R.M. (1986) Micro-injection of inositol 1,3,4,5-tetrakisphosphate activates sea urchin eggs by a mechanism dependent on external Ca^{2+}. *Biochem. J.* **240**, 917–920.

Kikkawa, U., Ogita, K., Shearman, M.S., Ase, K., Sekiguchi, K., Naor, Z., Ido, M., Nishizuka, Y., Saito, N., Tanaka, C., Ono, Y., Fujii, T. & Igarashi, K. (1988) The heterogeneity and differential expression of protein kinase C in nervous tissues. *Phil. Trans. Roy. Soc. Lond.* (In Press).

Limor, R., Ayalon, D., Capponi, A.M., Childs, G.V. & Naor, Z. (1987) Cytosolic free calcium levels in cultured pituitary cells separated by centrifugal elutriation: effect of gonadotropin releasing hormone. *Endocrinology* **120**, 497–503.

Majerus, P.W., Connolly, T.M., Deckmyn, H., Ross, T.S., Bross, T.E., Ishii, H., Bansal, K.S. & Wilson, D.B. (1986) The metabolism of phosphoinositide derived messenger molecules. *Science, N.Y.* **234**, 1519–1526.

Michell, R.H. (1975) Inositol phospholipids and cell surface receptor function. *Biochim. Biophys. Acta* **415**, 81–147.

Morgan, R.O., Chang, J.P. & Catt, K.J. (1987) Novel aspects of gonadotropin releasing hormone action on inositol polyphosphate metabolism in cultured pituitary gonadotrophs. *J. biol. Chem.* **262**, 1166–1171.

Naor, Z. & Catt, K.J. (1981) Mechanism of action of gonadotropin releasing hormone: involvement of phospholipid turnover in luteinizing hormone release. *J. biol. Chem.* **256**, 2226–2229.

Naor, Z. & Childs, G.V. (1986) Binding and activation of gonadotropin releasing hormone receptors in pituitary and gonadal cells. *Int. Rev. Cytol.* **103**, 147–187.

Naor, Z. & Eli, Y. (1985) Synergistic stimulation of luteinizing hormone release by protein kinase C activators and Ca^{2+} ionophore. *Biochem. Biophys. Res. Commun.* **130**, 848–853.

Naor, Z., Kiesel, L., Vanderhoek, J.Y. & Catt, K.J. (1985a) Mechanism of action of gonadotropin releasing hormone: role of lipoxygenase products of arachidonic acid in luteinizing hormone release. *J. Steroid Biochem.* **23**, 711–717.

Naor, Z., Zer, J., Zakut, H. & Hermon, J. (1985b) Characterization of pituitary calcium activated phospholipid dependent protein kinase: redistribution by gonadotropin releasing hormone. *Proc. natn. Acad. Sci. U.S.A.* **82**, 8203–8207.

Naor, Z., Azrad, A., Limor, R., Zakut, H. & Lotan, M. (1986) Gonadotropin releasing hormone activates a rapid Ca^{2+}-independent phosphodiester hydrolysis of polyphosphoinositides in pituitary gonadotrophs. *J. biol. Chem.* **261**, 12506–12512.

Naor, Z., Schvartz, I., Hazum, E., Azrad, A. & Hermon, J. (1987) Effect of phorbol ester on stimulus-secretion coupling mechanisms in gonadotropin releasing hormone stimulated pituitary gonadotrophs. *Biochem. Biophys. Res. Commun.* **148**, 1312–1322.

Naor, Z., Capponi, A.M., Rossier, M.F., Ayalon, D. & Limor, R. (1988) Gonadotropin releasing hormone-induced rise in cytosolic free Ca^{2+} levels: mobilization of cellular and extracellular Ca^{2+} pools and relationship to gonadotropin secretion. *Molec. Endocr.* **2**, 512–520.

Nishizuka, Y. (1984) The role of protein kinase C in cell surface signal transduction and tumor promotion. *Nature, Lond.* **308**, 693–698.

Nishizuka, Y. (1986) Studies and perspectives of protein kinase C. *Science, N.Y.* **233**, 305–312.

Parker, P.J., Coussens, L., Totty, N., Rhee, L., Young, S., Chen, E., Stabel, S., Waterfield, M.D. & Ullrich, A. (1986) The complete primary structure of protein kinase C—the major phorbol ester receptor. *Science, N.Y.* **233**, 853–859.

Putney, J.W., Jr (1986) A model for receptor-regulated calcium entry. *Cell Calcium* **7**, 1–12.

Schrey, M.P. (1985) Gonadotroph releasing hormone stimulates the formation of inositol phosphates in rat anterior pituitary tissue. *Biochem. J.* **226**, 563–569.

Smith, C.E., Wakefield, I., King, J.A., Naor, Z., Millar, R.P. & Davidson, J.S. (1987) The initial phase of GnRH-stimulated LH release from pituitary cells is independent of calcium entry through voltage-gated channels. *FEBS Lett.* **225**, 247–250.

Snyder, G.D., Capdevila, J., Chacos, N., Manna, S. & Falck, J.R. (1983) Action of luteinizing hormone releasing hormone: involvement of novel arachidonic acid metabolites. *Proc. natn. Acad. Sci. U.S.A.* **80**, 3504–3507.

Tsien, R.Y., Pozzan, T. & Rink, T.J. (1982) Calcium homeostasis in intact lymphocytes: cytoplasmic free calcium monitored with a new intracellularly trapped fluorescent indicator. *J. Cell Biol.* **94**, 325–334.

Turgeon, J.L., Ashcroft, S.J.H., Waring, D.W., Milewski, M.A. & Walsh, D.A. (1984) Characteristics of adenohypophyseal Ca^{2+}-phospholipid dependent protein kinase. *Molec. cell. Endocrinol.* **34**, 107–112.

Vallejo, M., Jackson, T., Lightmans, S. & Hanley, M.R. (1987) Occurrence and extracellular actions of inositol pentakis- and hexakis phosphate in mammalian brain. *Nature, Lond.* **330**, 656–658.

J. Reprod. Fert., Suppl. **37** (1989), 301–309

Printed in Great Britain
© 1989 Journals of Reproduction & Fertility Ltd

Role of phosphoinositol metabolism and phospholipases C and A_2/A_1 in signal transduction in isolated rat adrenal cells

D. Schulster*, A. D. Smith† and I. M. Bird*†

*Department of Endocrinology, National Institute for Biological Standards & Control, South Mimms, Potters Bar, Hertfordshire EN6 3QG, U.K. and †Department of Chemical Pathology, U.C. & Middlesex Medical School, Mortimer Street, London W1P 7PN, U.K.

Summary. Isolated rat adrenal glomerulosa cells were prelabelled with [^{3}H]inositol and stimulated with 25 nM-angiotensin II in the presence of Li$^+$. The resulting inositol monophosphates were separated using h.p.l.c. and 2 major peaks of radioactivity were detected. These showed the same characteristics as inositol 4-phosphate and inositol 1-phosphate and stimulation with angiotensin II increased activity 4–5-fold and 7–8-fold respectively. A minor peak with the characteristics of inositol 1:2 cyclic phosphate increased 1·5-fold after stimulation. No material corresponding to inositol 2-phosphate or inositol 5-phosphate was detected. The results establish the identity of the main inositol phosphate products in angiotensin II-stimulated rat glomerulosa cells.

Analysis by h.p.l.c. has been similarly used to assess the inositol phosphates produced after $ACTH_{1-39}$-stimulation of isolated rat adrenal fasiculata–reticularis cells. A low dose of $ACTH_{1-39}$ (10^{-12} M) stimulated production of small but significant amounts of both glycerophosphoinositol and inositol monophosphate. Using superfused isolated fasiculata–reticularis cells it was also found that $ACTH_{1-39}$ (10^{-9} M and 10^{-12} M) rapidly increased efflux of $^{45}Ca^{2+}$ from $^{45}Ca^{2+}$-prelabelled cells.

It is concluded that although the results are consistent with a role for phospholipase C in the action of angiotensin II on adrenal glomerulosa cells, in the action of ACTH on adrenal fasciculata–reticularis cells a role for phospholipase A_2/A_1 is implicated.

Keywords: adrenal; angiotensin II; ACTH; phosphoinositides; phosphoinositols; rat

Introduction

The hormonal activation of phospholipase C with consequent enhanced turnover of the polyphosphoinositides is a well recognized signal transduction mechanism for Ca^{2+}-mobilizing hormones (Berridge & Irvine, 1984). Such a mechanism is involved when rat adrenal glomerulosa cells are stimulated by the Ca^{2+}-mobilizing hormone, angiotensin II. Rapid degradation of phosphatidylinositol 4-phosphate and phosphatidyl-inositol 4,5-bisphosphate and correspondingly rapid synthesis of inositol trisphosphate and inositol bisphosphate has been demonstrated (Enyedi *et al.*, 1985). The observations of Farese *et al.* (1984) and Enyedi *et al.* (1985), invoking a role for polyphosphoinositide metabolism in the angiotensin II effect, have been confirmed and extended by Balla *et al.* (1986). These workers established that the inositol trisphosphate isomer that accumulates seconds after angiotensin II stimulation is inositol 1,4,5-trisphosphate which has Ca^{2+}-mobilizing capability (see Berridge & Irvine, 1984, for review) and that the isomer accumulating in a sustained manner, in the presence of Li$^+$, is inositol 1,3,4-trisphosphate. They suggested, moreover, that the inositol monophosphate isomers accumulating were inositol 1-phosphate and inositol 4-phosphate, although their identification was uncertain and the accumulation of inositol

2-phosphate and inositol 5-phosphate by the glomerulosa cell was not rigorously excluded. We have therefore developed an h.p.l.c. system utilizing a shallow salt gradient (Bird *et al.*, 1987), to re-examine the angiotensin II-stimulated glomerulosa cell and further extend the results of Balla *et al.* (1986).

The mechanism of the steroidogenic response of the adrenal fasciculata cell to ACTH stimulation, on the other hand, has long been held to involve the classical cyclic AMP second messenger system (Schimmer, 1980), although not all of the evidence is fully consistent with this concept (Ramachandran *et al.*, 1980). For some ACTH analogues (e.g. $ACTH_{5-24}$ and the *o*-nitrophenyl-sulphenyl derivative of sheep $ACTH_{1-39}$) there is stimulation of corticosteroidogenesis without the evident production of cyclic AMP (Seelig & Sayers, 1973; Moyle *et al.*, 1973; Schulster & Salmon 1984). Several studies have therefore been undertaken into possible alternative or additional second messenger systems for the ACTH mechanism. Farese *et al.* (1983) have shown, using a crude adrenal preparation, that $ACTH_{1-24}$, at low doses which are steroidogenic but not cyclic AMP stimulatory, promoted ^{32}P incorporation into phosphoinositides. At high doses, ACTH did not have this effect. Similar observations were made by Whitley *et al.* (1984). In more recent work, Farese *et al.* (1986), using a crude, whole, rat adrenal cell preparation prelabelled with [^3H]inositol, demonstrated stimulation of phosphoinositol formation by $ACTH_{1-24}$. This occurred over the same low dose-range as that previously reported to stimulate ^{32}P incorporation into phospho-inositides.

In the studies reported here we have used h.p.l.c. analysis to assess the inositol phosphates produced from phosphoinositides after ACTH stimulation of rat adrenal fasciculata–reticularis cells. In contrast to earlier studies, the present study used $ACTH_{1-39}$, the physiological hormone which has been shown to have different characteristics from synthetic $ACTH_{1-24}$ (see Storring *et al.*, 1984).

Materials and Methods

Materials. The preparation and stimulation of isolated glomerulosa cells were as described by Bird *et al.* (1987), using the method of Hanning *et al.* (1970). $ACTH_{1-39}$ was World Health Organisation International Working Standard (Bangham *et al.*, 1962). (Asp^1, Ile^5)angiotensin II and (Asp^1, Val^5)angiotensin II were World Health Organisation Standards (code nos 70/302 and 64/15) obtained from NIBSC. For steroidogenesis assay, polypropylene tubes for cell incubations were obtained from Sarstedt (Beaumont Leys, Leicester, U.K.), sulphuric acid (BDH, Poole, Dorset, U.K.) was purchased as Aristar grade while dichloromethane (BDH) was purchased as FDPC grade. [2-^3H]*Myo*-inositol (sp. act. 15 Ci/mmol, 1 mCi/ml in water) and $^{45}Ca^{2+}$ (as $^{45}CaCl_2$ 10–40 mCi/mg) were from Amersham plc, Amersham, Bucks, U.K. Sephadex G10 was obtained from Pharmacia (Hounslow, U.K.) and swollen in 1 M-HCl before use. Radioactive standards were prepared as described by Bird *et al.* (1987).

Cell preparation and incubation. Adrenal glands were excised from female Sprague–Dawley rats (180–200 g) and the zona glomerulosa cells were isolated by incubating adrenal capsules for 60 min with Krebs–Ringer–bicarbonate buffer (pH 7·4)/11 mM-glucose/0·5% (w/v) human serum albumin (KRBGA) containing 2 mg collagenase/ml. The details of their preparation, their 3-h preincubation with 50 μCi [^3H]inositol and subsequent incubation with angio-tensin II were as described by Bird *et al.* (1987). Stimulation with angiotensin II was terminated after 30 min by extraction with 1·8 ml chloroform/methanol/X (100:200:1 by vol.) where X is concentrated HCl for acid extraction or water for neutral extraction. Phase separation was as described by Bird *et al.* (1987).

Cells of the zona fasciculata–reticularis were prepared by digestion of the decapsulated adrenal bisects for 45 min in KRBGA medium containing 1 mg collagenase/ml modified from the method of Richardson & Schulster (1972). These cells were labelled by preincubation in KRBGA with [^3H]inositol (160 μCi for 2 h at 37°C). Cells were then washed and resuspended in KRBGA containing 20 mM-LiCl and 10 mM-*myo*-inositol. Stimulation with ACTH was terminated after 30 min, as described above for acid extraction.

Statistical significance of the data was assessed using Student's *t* test.

Dowex-column chromatography and subsequent h.p.l.c. analysis. After solvent extraction, the aqueous phase was made 1 mM with respect to EDTA and applied to a 1-ml Dowex column (Cl$^-$ form). The column was then washed with 2·5 ml water and a 20-ml linear gradient of 0–400 mM-LiCl was applied.

Freeze-dried fractions eluted from the Dowex column were desalted using ethanol and subjected to h.p.l.c. on a 15 cm × 0·5 cm column of Partisil SAX-10 preceded by a 5 cm × 0·5 cm guard column of this material. Flow-rate was 1·3 ml/min and the h.p.l.c. procedure was as described by Bird *et al.* (1987) unless otherwise specified.

$^{45}Ca^{2+}$*-efflux after* $ACTH_{1-39}$ *stimulation of superfused cells of the zona fasciculata–reticularis.* The superfusion column and methodology was as described by Schulster *et al.* (1984) except that the internal diameter of the column was reduced to 6 mm and screw-fitting ends were used at both top and bottom to facilitate loading and unloading. Three such Teflon columns were used in parallel and packed with Sephadex G10 to retain the cells. Labelling with $^{45}Ca^{2+}$ and subsequent superfusion of cells was performed as described by Williams *et al.* (1981). Adrenal fasciculata–reticularis cells, prepared as above, were preincubated with 10 µCi $^{45}CaCl_2$ in 1·5 ml KRBGA buffer for 90 min in a shaking water-bath (37°C; 95% O_2/5% CO_2 atmosphere). Cells were then drawn onto the columns and washed for 30 min with KRBGA to remove free, extracellular $^{45}Ca^{2+}$, cell debris and the smaller cells (such as erythrocytes, glomerulosa and the bulk of the reticularis cells), leaving a highly purified population of zona fasciculata cells on the columns. Infusions of $ACTH_{1-39}$ were then made for 10 min, after which time KRBGA infusions were resumed for a further 30 min. Flow-rate was maintained at 0·5 ml/min throughout. At the end of superfusion the total remaining intracellular $^{45}Ca^{2+}$ in each column was determined by assessing the $^{45}Ca^{2+}$ released by acid lysis (see legend Fig. 4). Then 1-ml fractions were collected and the steroid content of half of each fraction was assayed as described (see Schulster *et al.*, 1984). Radioactivity in the other half was assessed as a percentage of radioactivity remaining in the system at the beginning of the collection of that fraction.

$$\text{Thus the percentage fractional release} = \frac{R_N}{\sum_N^{35} R + A} \times 100\%$$

where: 35 = total number of fractions and N = any fraction number, R_N = radioactivity in fraction N, $\sum_N^{35} R$ = total radioactivity in fractions N to 35, and A = total radioactivity in acid wash at end of experiment.

Abbreviations. PtdIns = phosphatidylinositol; PtdIns4P = phosphatidylinositol 4-phosphate; PtdIns(4,5)P_2 = phosphatidylinositol 4,5-bisphosphate; GroPIns = glycerophosphoinositol; GroPInsP = glycerophosphoinositol phosphate; Ins1P = inositol 1-phosphate; Ins2P = inositol 2-phosphate; Ins4P = inositol 4-phosphate; Ins5P = inositol 5-phosphate; Ins[1:2(cyc)]P = inositol 1:2-cyclic phosphate; Ins(1,4)P_2 = inositol 1,4-bisphosphate; Ins(1,4,5)P_3 = inositol 1,4,5-trisphosphate; Ins(1,3,4)P_3 = inositol 1,3,4-trisphosphate.

Results

[^{3}H]Inositol-prelabelled glomerulosa cells were stimulated with 25 nM of (Asp^1, Ile^5)angiotensin II or (Asp^1, Val^5)angiotensin II for 30 min in the presence of 10 mM-Li$^+$ to allow accumulation of products. The extracted phosphoinositols were purified by h.p.l.c. on Partisil SAX-10 as described in the 'Methods'. The quantitatively major, radiolabelled products formed in response to both analogues of angiotensin II are shown in Table 1. The time-course of the accumulation of these phosphoinositols both in the presence and absence of (Asp^1, Val^5)angiotensin II was determined using h.p.l.c. on Partisil SAX-10 (see 'Methods'). Results were obtained at zero time, 15 sec, 1 min, 15 min and 30 min. Figure 1 shows that rapid (within 15 sec) labelling of Ins(1,3,4)P_3 and Ins(1,4)P_2 was observed while labelling of InsP increased slowly (between 1 and 15 min). No change in GroPIns labelling was observed in response to agonist at any time (data not shown). When total phosphoinositide radioactivity was monitored, a significant decrease was observed within 1 min followed by a subsequent decrease of over 50% (Fig. 1). Similar results to those shown in Fig. 1 were also obtained with (Asp^1, Ile^5)angiotensin II (data not shown).

The inositol monophosphates produced after incubation for 30 min using the above procedures were subjected to closer examination. They were extracted using acidic or neutral procedures as described in 'Methods' and then separated from the other phosphoinositols by elution from Cl$^-$ Dowex with a LiCl gradient, as described by Bird *et al.* (1987). The material eluted by 50–100 mM-LiCl, co-migrated with [^{14}C]Ins1P standard, was desalted and then subjected to h.p.l.c. on Partisil SAX-10 (Fig. 2). This shows that the major inositol monophosphate products accumulating in the presence of Li$^+$, after stimulation with angiotensin II are Ins1P and Ins4P with significant increases in each of these monophosphates ($P < 0.0005$). In addition, a significant ($P < 0.001$) angiotensin II-stimulated accumulation of Ins[1:2(cyc)]P was observed under neutral extraction conditions. The identification of this material was supported by its absence under acidic extraction conditions (Fig. 3). Angiotensin II did not significantly stimulate the production of GroPIns in samples extracted from these glomerulosa cells under either acidic or neutral extraction procedures (Fig. 3).

Adrenal fasciculata cells were prelabelled with [^{3}H]inositol and incubated for 0, 1, 15 or 30 min in the presence or absence of 10^{-12} M-ACTH. After the incubation, radiolabelled phosphoinositols,

Table 1. Direct comparison of the phosphoinositide response (% of control) of adrenal glomerulosa cells stimulated by 25 nM-(Asp¹Ile⁵)angiotensin II or 25 nM-(Asp¹Val⁵)angiotensin II

	Angiotensin II analogue	
	(Asp^1Ile^5)	(Asp^1Val^5)
Total phosphoinositides	45 ± 1	45 ± 1
Ins1P	881 ± 12	764 ± 43
Ins4P	323 ± 13	320 ± 35
$Ins(1,4)P_2$	2208 ± 61	1953 ± 82
$Ins(1,3,4)P_3$	450 ± 11	415 ± 5

The radioactive phosphoinositols were assessed by h.p.l.c. on Partisil SAX-10 by a combination of the methods described by Irvine *et al.* (1985) and Bird *et al.* (1987) using a 24-min linear gradient of 0–300 nM-ammonium formate pH 5·0 followed by a linear gradient of 0–1 M-ammonium formate (buffered to pH 3·7 with orthophosphoric acid).

Results are expressed as % increase over the control which is taken as 100% and represent the mean ± s.e.m. from 3 incubations. All the values are significantly different from the control ($P < 0.0005$, Student's *t* test).

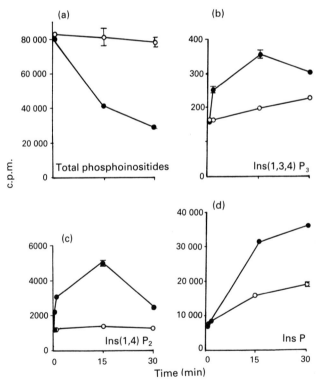

Fig. 1. Time-course of the angiotensin II-stimulated phosphoinositide and phosphoinositol response in zona glomerulosa cells. Zona glomerulosa cells prelabelled with [³H]inositol were resuspended in media containing 10 mM-Li⁺ and 10 mM-inositol and incubated with (●) and without (○) 25 nM-(Asp¹ Val⁵) angiotensin II. Values are mean ± s.e.m. of data from 3 incubations.

glycerophosphoinositols and phosphoinositides were extracted as described in 'Methods'. Phosphoinositols and glycerophosphoinositols were then assessed and identified after h.p.l.c. analysis on Partisil SAX-10 with 0·1 M-ammonium formate, pH 3·7, using radioactive standards (see 'Methods') chromatographed under identical conditions. The results given in Table 2 show that, in the presence of 10^{-12} M-ACTH, a significant ($P < 0.01$) transient increase in glycerophosphoinositol was evident after 15 min. After 1 min the increase in this product was not statistically significant. A similar small increase (significant at $P < 0.05$) in inositol monophosphate was observed after incubation for 15 min in the presence of 10^{-12} M-ACTH. However, no statistically significant changes in Ins(1,4)P$_2$, Ins(1,3,4)P$_3$ and GroPInsP were observed in response to ACTH (data not shown).

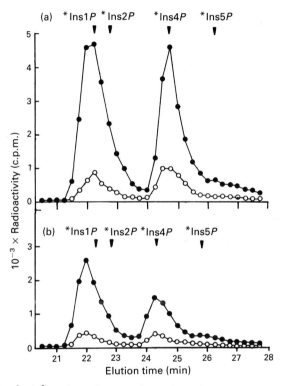

Fig. 2. Effect of (Asp^1, Ile^5)angiotensin II on formation of Ins1P and Ins4P in zona glomerulosa cells. [^{3}H]Phosphoinositol products were recovered from angiotensin II-stimulated (●) and unstimulated (○) incubations of zona glomerulosa cells by using acid (a) or neutral (b) extraction procedures. After h.p.l.c. on Partisil SAX-10 with a linear gradient of 0–300 nM-ammonium formate, the elution times of the ^{14}C-labelled radioactive (*) standards were as indicated (▼). The data are representative of those from 2 separate experiments each performed in triplicate. (From Bird *et al.*, 1987.)

Adrenal fasciculata cells were also examined in a superfusion system, for the effect of ACTH$_{1-39}$ on ^{45}Ca^{2+}-efflux (Fig. 4). Cells were preloaded with ^{45}Ca^{2+}, loaded onto superfusion columns and washed for 30 min. Media containing 10^{-12} M or 10^{-9} M ACTH$_{1-39}$ or saline, pH 4 (control), were perfused through each column for 10 min. Fractions (2 min) were collected and analysed for corticosteroid and ^{45}Ca^{2+} content. The lag-time of the system was also determined using dextran (Fig. 4b). ACTH$_{1-39}$ at both doses rapidly increased the ^{45}Ca^{2+} efflux expressed as a percentage of the fractional release. This stimulation of ^{45}Ca^{2+}-efflux by 10^{-9} M-ACTH$_{1-39}$

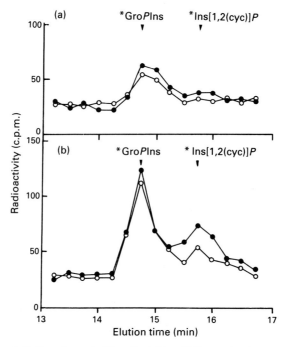

Fig. 3. Effect of (Asp¹, Ile⁵)angiotensin II on Ins1,2(cyc)P formation in zona glomerulosa cells. [³H]Phosphoinositol products were recovered from (Asp¹, Ile⁵)angiotensin II-stimulated (●) and unstimulated (○) incubations of cells by using acid (a) or neutral (b) extraction procedures. The data are representative of 2 separate experiments, each performed in triplicate. (From Bird *et al.*, 1987.)

Table 2. Time-course of the $ACTH_{1-39}$-stimulated phosphoinositide, glycerophosphoinositol and phosphoinositol response of zona fasciculata–reticularis cells

Time (min)	Presence or absence of 10^{-12} M-ACTH	Total phosphoinositides (c.p.m.)	GroPIns (c.p.m.)	InsP (c.p.m.)
0	−	58 948 ± 622	2303 ± 146	4443 ± 141
	+	60 321 ± 956	2034 ± 190	4081 ± 201
1	−	60 568 ± 980	2223 ± 86	4731 ± 221
	+	58 415 ± 1535	2492 ± 318	4637 ± 377
15	−	61 549 ± 1256	2163 ± 109	4465 ± 342
	+	61 812 ± 1228	2547 ± 192**	5156 ± 300*
30	−	64 585 ± 1769	2267 ± 188	4081 ± 418
	+	63 037 ± 930	2141 ± 97	4735 ± 621

[³H]Inositol-prelabelled cells were washed and resuspended in fresh media containing 20 mM-Li⁺ and 10 mM-inositol. Glycerophosphoinositols and phosphoinositols were separated by h.p.l.c. on Partisil SAX-10 using 0–1 M-ammonium formate pH 3·7.

Results are the mean ± s.e.m. of radioactivity in the peaks identified using radio-labelled standards run under identical h.p.l.c. conditions. Three experiments were performed in duplicate and 1 in triplicate; therefore data are from 9 separate incubations.

*$P < 0.05$; **$P < 0.01$ compared with unstimulated controls.

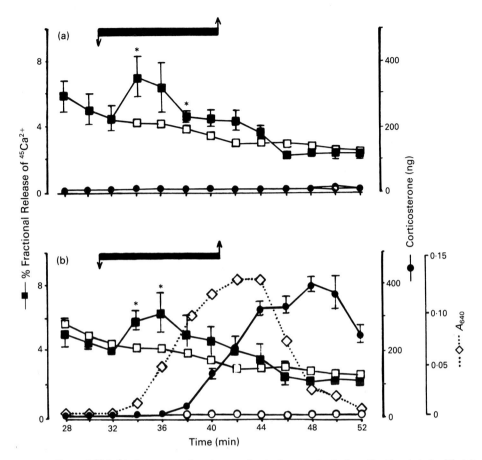

Fig. 4. Efflux of $^{45}Ca^{2+}$ from superfused zona fasciculata–reticularis cells stimulated with (a) 10^{-12} M- or (b) 10^{-9} M-ACTH$_{1-39}$ ($\bullet$,$\blacksquare$) Adrenal cells were prelabelled with $^{45}Ca^{2+}$, loaded onto superfusion columns and washed for 30 min (see 'Methods'). The perfusion time is shown as a solid bar. After a further 30 min $^{45}Ca^{2+}$ remaining in the cells was released by lysis with perchloric acid (10 ml, 1 M) followed by 15 ml water: 2-min fractions were collected and steroid content (circles) and $^{45}Ca^{2+}$ content (squares) were determined. On another column, dextran solution was infused for 10 min through each column in a manner identical to the ACTH$_{1-39}$ infusion. The dextran content ($\cdot \diamond \cdot$) of each fraction was measured by absorbance at 640 nm. For comparison, these results are shown superimposed on the steroid and $^{45}Ca^{2+}$-efflux data of panel (b). All results are the mean $\pm$ s.e.m. of the data from 3 completely separate experiments. *$P < 0.05$ (Student's t test) compared with control.

was observed within 3 min of infusing the ACTH and about 4 min before the stimulation of corticosteroid was evident.

Discussion

These studies attempt to clarify the relative roles of polyphosphoinositide metabolism in angiotensin II-stimulated glomerulosa cells and ACTH-stimulated fasciculata–reticularis cells.

The results using angiotensin II-stimulated glomerulosa cells indicate that there are substantial increases in the inositol mono-, bis- and tris-phosphates regardless of the angiotensin II analogue that is used. Previous workers in this field have used (Asp[1], Ile[5])angiotensin II (e.g. Enyedi *et al.*, 1985), although this is not the endogenous rat angiotensin II and it differs in amino acid composition at position 5. However, the responses to (Asp[1], Val[5])angiotensin II, the analogue present in the rat, and to (Asp[1], Ile[5])angiotensin II were identical (Table 1).

In the presence of Li^+ there are substantial increases in Ins1P as well as in Ins4P. After acidic or neutral extraction, increases in (Asp[1], Ile[5])angiotensin II-stimulated cells (compared with the control cells) were about 8-fold for Ins1P and 5-fold for Ins4P (see Fig. 2). This confirms the proposal of Balla *et al.* (1986) that Ins1P and Ins4P are the major inositol monophosphate products after stimulation of glomerulosa cells with angiotensin II. The large accumulation of Ins4P indicates that substantial degradation of PtdIns4P and PtdIns(4,5)$_2$ occurs after stimulation with angiotensin II.

No measurable quantities of Ins2P or Ins5P were detected after acidic or neutral extraction, indicating that Ins1P and Ins4P were the only major inositol monophosphate products. However, there were small increases (of ~ 1.5-fold over control values) seen in Ins[1:2(cyc)]P extracted under neutral conditions and accumulating in the cells stimulated with (Asp[1], Ile[5])angiotensin II. The identification of this material as Ins[1:2(cyc)]P is supported by its absence under acidic extraction conditions (see Figs 3a and 3b).

The presence of Ins[1:2(cyc)]P suggests the possible formation of cyclic derivatives of Ins(1,4,5)P$_3$ and Ins(1,4)P$_2$ by hormone-sensitive phospholipase C, and their subsequent dephosphorylation to Ins[1:2(cyc)]P (Conolly *et al.*, 1986). Alternatively, the direct breakdown of PtdIns in response to angiotensin II stimulation may have occurred, as discussed by Dixon & Hokin (1985). Regardless of the actual pathway in glomerulosa, however, it is clear that the quantity of Ins[1:2(cyc)]P formed is extremely small. These pathways are therefore not major alternative routes of phosphatidyl- inositol metabolism in the rat adrenal glomerulosa cell.

The adrenal fasciculata cell was also examined for its response to ACTH$_{1-39}$ both in terms of changes with time in the total phosphoinositides and in the h.p.l.c.-purified inositol phosphates and GroPIns. Only in the presence of 10^{-12} M-ACTH$_{1-39}$ (a low dose which was barely, if at all, steroidogenic (Richardson & Schulster 1972; Rafferty *et al.* 1983)) were statistically significant increases in some of these intermediates observed. Increases were found in GroPIns (117% of control; $P < 0.01$) and InsP (117% of control; $P < 0.05$) after 15 min incubation with hormone (see Table 1). The small magnitude of this response to ACTH$_{1-39}$ was consistent with the ^{32}P-labelling of the phosphoinositides seen in the response to ACTH$_{1-24}$ (Farese *et al.*, 1983; Whitley *et al.*, 1984).

The ACTH-stimulated increase in the labelling of GroPIns, as well as that of InsP, indicates possible phosphoinositide degradation by a phospholipase A$_2$/A$_1$, rather than (or additional to) the previously proposed phospholipase C (Farese *et al.*, 1986). Involvement of such a phospholipase A would be expected to be Ca^{2+}-dependent, whereas hormone-sensitive phospholipase C would be expected to be Ca^{2+}-independent. The use of Ca^{2+}-free medium to examine the ACTH response is not possible, since ACTH requires Ca^{2+} to bind its receptor (Cheitlin *et al.* 1985). The involvement of Ca^{2+} was, however, indirectly shown by examining the ACTH-stimulated efflux of $^{45}Ca^{2+}$. ACTH (at 10^{-9} M and 10^{-12} M) stimulated $^{45}Ca^{2+}$ efflux from $^{45}Ca^{2+}$ preloaded adrenal fasciculata cells, in a superfusion system. These results indicated that concentrations of ACTH that affect phosphoinositide turnover at 10^{-12} M and steroidogenesis at 10^{-9} M also affect the intracellular translocation of Ca^{2+}. Overall, these data are consistent with a role for phospholipase A$_2$/A$_1$ in an effect of ACTH on adrenal fasciculata cells.

In conclusion there is good evidence for an involvement of phospholipase C in the action of angiotensin II on glomerulosa cells; the action of ACTH on fasciculata–reticularis cells is much less clear-cut but it may involve phospholipase A$_2$/A$_1$ (although not necessarily in the steroidogenic effect of ACTH).

References

Balla, T., Baukal, A.J., Guillemette, G., Morgan, R.O. & Catt, K.J. (1986) Angiotensin-stimulated production of inositol trisphosphate isomers and rapid metabolism through inositol-4-monophosphate in adrenal glomerulosa cells. *Proc. natn. Acad. Sci. U.S.A.* **83**, 9323–9327.

Bangham, D.R., Mussett, M.W. & Stacke Dunne, M.P. (1962) The third international standard for corticotropin. *Bull. Wld Hlth Org.* **27**, 395–408.

Berridge, M. & Irvine, R.F. (1984) A novel second messenger in cellular signal transduction. *Nature, Lond.* **312**, 315–321.

Bird, I.M., Smith, A.D. & Schulster, D. (1987) HPLC analysis of inositol monophosphate isomers formed on angiotensin II stimulation of rat adrenal glomerulosa cells. *Biochem J.* **248**, 203–208.

Cheitlin, R., Buckley, D.I. & Ramachandran, J. (1985) The role of extracellular calcium in corticotropin-stimulated steroidogenesis. *J. biol. Chem.* **260**, 5323–5327.

Connolly, T.M., Wilson, D.B., Bross, T.E. & Majerus, P.W. (1986) Isolation and characterisation of the inositol cyclic phosphate products of phosphoinositide cleavage by phospholipase C. *J. biol. Chem.* **261**, 122–126.

Dixon, J.F. & Hokin, L.E. (1985) The formation of inositol 1,2-cyclic phosphate on agonist stimulation of phosphoinositide breakdown in mouse pancreatic minilobules. *J. biol. Chem.* **260**, 16068–16071.

Enyedi, P., Buki, B., Mucsi, I. & Spat, A. (1985) Polyphosphoinositide metabolism in adrenal glomerulosa cells. *Molec cell. Endocrinol.* **41**, 105–112.

Farese, R.V., Sabir, M.A., Larson, R.E. & Trudeau, W. (1983) Further observations on the increases in inositide phospholipids after stimulation by ACTH, cAMP and insulin and on discrepancies in phosphatidylinositol mass and $^{32}PO_4$-labelling during inhibition of hormonal effects by cycloheximide. *Cell. Calcium* **4**, 195–218.

Farese, R.V., Larson, R.E. & Davis, J.S. (1984) Rapid effects of angiotensin II on polyphosphoinositide metabolism in the rat adrenal glomerulosa. *Endocrinology* **114**, 302–304.

Farese, R.V., Rosi, C.N., Babischkin, J., Farese, M.G., Fosters, R. & Davis, J.S. (1986) Dual activation of the inositol trisphosphate calcium and cyclic nucleotide intracellular signalling systems by adrenocorticotropin in adrenal rat cells. *Biochem. Biophys. Res. Commun.* **135**, 742–748.

Hanning, R., Tait, S.A.S. & Tait, J.F. (1970) *In vitro* effects of ACTH, angiotensins, serotonin and potassium on steroid output and conversion of corticosterone to aldosterone by isolated adrenal cells. *Endocrinology* **87**, 1147–1167.

Irvine, R.F., Anggard, E.E., Letcher, A.J. & Downes, C.P. (1985) Metabolism of inositol 1,4,5-trisphosphate and inositol 1,3,4-trisphosphate in rat parotid glands. *Biochem. J.* **229**, 505–511.

Moyle, W.R., Kong, Y.C. & Ramachandran, J. (1973) Steroidogenesis and cyclic adenosine 3'5'-monophosphate accumulation in rat adrenal cells. Divergent effects of ACTH and its o-nitrophenyl sulfenyl derivative. *J. biol. Chem.* **248**, 2409–2417.

Rafferty, B., Zanelli, J.M., Rosenblatt, M. & Schulster, D. (1983) Corticosteroidogenesis and adenosine-3'5'-monophosphate production by the amino-terminal (1–34) fragment of human parathyroid hormone in rat adrenocortical cells. *Endocrinology* **113**, 1036–1042.

Ramachandran, J., Lee, C.Y., Keri, G. & Kenez-Keri, M. (1980) Studies of Adrenocorticotropin receptors. In *Polypeptide Hormones*, pp. 295–308. Eds R. F. Beers, Jr & E. G. Bassett. Raven Press, New York.

Richardson, M.C. & Schulster, D. (1972) Corticosteroidogenesis in isolated adrenal cells: effect of ACTH, adenosine 3'5'-monophosphate and β^{1-24}ACTH, diazotized to polyacrylamide. *J. Endocr.* **55**, 127–139.

Schimmer, B.P. (1980) Cyclic nucleotides in hormonal regulation of adrenocortical function. In *Advances in Cyclic Nucleotide Research*, Vol. 13, pp. 181–214. Eds P. Greengard & G.A. Robinson. Raven Press, New York.

Schulster, D. & Salmon, D.M. (1984) A dual pathway for ACTH steroidogenic action in purified adrenocortical cells. *J. Receptor Res.* **4**, 301–313.

Schulster, D., Rafferty, B. & Williams, B.C. (1984) Corticotropin-induced desensitization: steroidogenic and cyclic AMP responses in superfused adrenocortical cells. *Molec. cell. Endocrinol.* **36**, 43–51.

Seelig, S. & Sayers, G. (1973) Isolated adrenal cortex cells: ACTH agonists, antagonists; cyclic AMP and corticosterone production. *Archs Biochim. Biophys.* **154**, 230–239.

Storring, P.L., Witthaus, G., Gaines Das, R.E. & Stamm, W. (1984). The International Reference Preparation of tetracosactide for bioassay: characterization and estimation of its (1–24)corticotrophin-tetracosa-peptide content by physicochemical and biological methods. *J. Endocr.* **100**, 51–60.

Whitley, St. J.G., Bell, J.B.G., Chu, F.W., Tait, J.F. & Tait, S.A.S (1984) The effects of ACTH, serotonin, K^+ and angiotensin analogues on ^{32}P incorporation into phospholipids of the rat adrenal cortex: basis for an assay method using z.glomerulosa cells. *Proc. R. Soc. Lond.* B **222**, 273–294.

Williams, B.C., McDougall, J.G., Tait, J.F. & Tait, S.A.S. (1981) Calcium efflux and steroid output from superfused rat adrenal cells: effects of potassium, ACTH, 5-hydroxytryptamine, cyclic AMP and angiotensins II and III. *Clin. Sci.* **61**, 541–551.

J. Reprod. Fert., Suppl. **37** (1989), 311–317

Printed in Great Britain
© 1989 Journals of Reproduction & Fertility Ltd

Protein phosphorylation in the corpus luteum*

E. T. Maizels, R. C. Ekstrom, J. B. Miller† and M. Hunzicker-Dunn

Department of Molecular Biology, Northwestern University Medical School, Chicago, IL 60611, U.S.A. and †Department of Obstetrics and Gynecology, University of Illinois College of Medicine at Chicago, Chicago, IL 60612, U.S.A.

Summary. Soluble luteal extracts were incubated with putative second messengers or regulators of protein kinases in the presence of [γ-^{32}P]ATP, and proteins were separated by SDS–PAGE. There was a novel phosphorylation of a protein of M_r 80 000 which was stimulated by phospholipid and 1,2-diacylglycerol but, unlike classical C-kinase phosphorylating activity, was increased by EGTA and reduced by Ca^{2+}. This phospholipid/diolein-stimulated phosphorylation of a M_r 80 000 protein was detectable in rat and pig luteal extracts and was enhanced 2-fold in rabbit CL by administration of oestradiol-17β *in vivo*. These results suggest that the luteotrophic functions of oestradiol in rabbit CL are mediated in part by regulating either the kinase and/or the M_r 80 000 substrate.

Keywords: corpus luteum; phosphorylation; C-kinase; oestradiol-17β

Introduction

One of the key regulatory mechanisms that has been implicated in protein hormone action is protein phosphorylation. Indeed, most signal transduction pathways involve one or more protein phosphorylation events. The kinases catalysing these phosphorylation events may be regulated via the traditional cAMP pathway via activation of cAMP-dependent protein kinases (cAMP-kinase) or via other second messenger pathways via activation of the phospholipid, Ca^{2+}-dependent C-kinases, the Ca^{2+}–calmodulin protein kinases, the growth factor-regulated tyrosine kinases, as well as a variety of other kinases (Edelman *et al.*, 1987).

In the corpus luteum (CL) of most species, luteal functions are regulated predominantly by the gonadotrophin LH. The effects of LH would be expected to be mediated via cAMP (Hunzicker-Dunn & Birnbaumer, 1976) and the cAMP-kinases (Hunzicker-Dunn, 1981) or modulated via the C-kinase pathway (Davis & Clark, 1983; Noland & Dimino, 1986; Wheeler & Veldhuis, 1987). In addition, oestrogens have long been recognized as important luteotrophic factors in rabbits (Keyes & Nalbandov, 1967; Bill & Keyes, 1983) and rats (Takayama & Greenwald, 1973; Gibori *et al.*, 1977). The importance of oestrogen as a luteotrophin is best exemplified by the rabbit, in which progesterone production and luteal maintenance proceeds in the total absence of LH when oestrogen is present (Bill & Keyes, 1983). Although a classical second messenger/protein kinase pathway is not predicted to mediate the effects of oestrogen, recent studies suggest that oestradiol enhances the Ca^{2+}–calmodulin-dependent phosphorylation of an M_r 100 000 protein in soluble luteal extracts of rats (Rao *et al.*, 1987).

Based on the prominent regulatory role of phosphorylation in hormone actions, studies were undertaken to elucidate in-vitro regulators of phosphorylating activities in soluble extracts of luteal tissues.

---

*Reprint requests to Dr M. Hunzicker-Dunn.

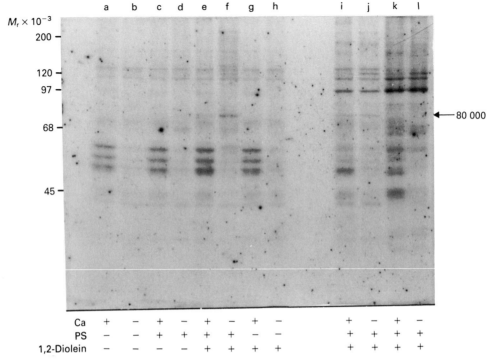

Fig. 1. Autoradiogram showing in-vitro phosphorylation of soluble luteal proteins of pregnant rat (lanes a–h), rat adrenal proteins (lanes i, j) and rat testis proteins (lanes k, l). Phosphorylation reactions were conducted according to Protocol B as described in 'Materials and Methods'. Additions to the incubations are indicated at the concentrations described in 'Materials and Methods': Ca, calcium. Lanes marked '+' contain 0·5 mM-CaCl$_2$, 0·05 mM-EGTA; lanes marked '–' contain 0·55 mM-EGTA and no added CaCl$_2$; PS, phosphatidylserine.

Materials and Methods

Materials. Biochemical reagents were purchased from Sigma Chemical Co. (St Louis, MO), unless otherwise indicated. [γ-^{32}P]ATP, ammonium salt (sp. act. 1000–4000 Ci/mmol) was purchased from ICN Chemical and Radioisotope Division (Irvine, CA). Sodium dodecyl sulphate–polyacrylamide gel electrophoresis (SDS–PAGE) protein standards were from Boehringer Mannheim Biochemicals (Indianapolis, IN) and electrophoresis reagents were purchased from Bio-Rad (Richmond, CA).

Tissue preparation. Ovaries from non-pregnant pigs were obtained from a local slaughter house, transported to the laboratory on ice, and vascular CL were dissected. For rat luteal tissue, outbred Sprague–Dawley rats weighing ~200 g were obtained from Charles River Breeding Laboratories, Inc. and placed in cages with breeding males. About 20 days later, the female rats were killed by cervical dislocation and the CL were dissected out. Adrenal glands and testes were removed from mature male rats. New Zealand White rabbits (7 kg) were obtained from Langshaw Farms (Augusta, MI). Pseudopregnancy was induced on Day 0 with an i.v. injection of 100 i.u. hCG (Ayerst Laboratories, Inc., NY) dissolved in 0·9% (w/v) NaCl. Rabbits were implanted s.c. in the neck on Day 0, 7 or 9 with a Silastic capsule, prepared as described by Holt *et al.* (1975), and containing 1·0 cm crystalline oestradiol-17β. On Day 10, rabbits were killed by cervical dislocation, ovaries were removed, and CL were dissected out. All tissues were maintained on ice before homogenization. Dissected tissues were homogenized in 36 volumes of a buffer containing 10 mM-Tris–HCl, pH 7·5, 4 mM-MgCl$_2$, 0·1 mM-ethyleneglycol-bis-(β-amino ethyl ester)-N,N,N',N'-tetraacetic acid (EGTA), 0·32 M-sucrose with a ground-glass homogenizer. A supernatant fraction (soluble extract) was obtained by centrifuging the homogenate at 105 000 g for 60 min at 4°C. Protein concentrations in the soluble extract were measured by the method of Lowry *et al.* (1951), using crystalline BSA as a standard.

In-vitro phosphorylation studies. Phosphorylation of tissue-extract proteins was carried out using Protocol A or B. In Protocol A, phosphorylation was conducted in an incubation volume of 100 μl containing 75 μg of the soluble extract (±9%) in a reaction buffer consisting of 50 mM-Tris–HCl, pH 7·0, 10 μM-ATP, 10 mM-MgCl$_2$, and 15 μCi [γ-^{32}P]ATP. Incubations were initiated with the addition of [γ-^{32}P]ATP and were for 10 min at 37°C. Incubations

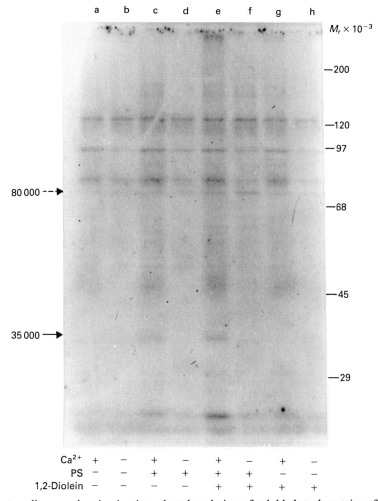

Fig. 2. Autoradiogram showing in-vitro phosphorylation of soluble luteal proteins of pigs. See legend to Fig. 1 for rest of details.

were terminated by the addition of a 3-fold concentrated SDS stop solution containing 6% SDS, 150 mM-Tris–HCl, pH 8·75, 30% glycerol, 15% β-mercaptoethanol, 6 mM-ethylenediamine tetraacetic acid (EDTA), and 0·04% bromphenol blue, heating at 100°C for 5 min. ^{32}P-labelled cellular proteins were separated by SDS–PAGE, using a 5% acrylamide stacking gel and a 10·5% acrylamide separating gel as described by Rudolph & Krueger (1979). After electrophoresis, gels were stained, destained, dried, and placed with Kodak X-Omat XRP-5 X-ray film. Molecular weights were estimated on each gel from migration rates of protein standards (chymotrypsinogen, BSA, ovalbumin, glutamate dehydrogenase, fumarase, lactate dehydrogenase) relative to the dye front.

In Protocol B, phosphorylation of tissue extract proteins was carried out in an incubation volume of 200 µl containing 100 µl of the extract and 100 µl of reaction buffer containing 100 mM-α-glycerol phosphate buffer, pH 7·0, 2 mM-dithiothreitol, 20 mM-MgCl$_2$ and 10 µM-ATP. Preincubation was performed for 3 min at 37°C and then experimental incubation was initiated by the addition of [γ-^{32}P]ATP (5·0 µCi per 0·2 ml sample) in the presence or absence of various test additions. Additions included phospholipid (phosphatidylserine, 50 µg/ml), diacylglycerol (1,2-diolein, 1·25 µg/ml), and CaCl$_2$ (0·5 mM), EGTA (0·55 mM final) or Ca–EGTA buffer (2·5 mM total EGTA, various free Ca^{2+} concentrations). Incubation was performed for 1 min at 37°C, then terminated by addition of 100 µl SDS stop solution (3% SDS, 150 mM-Tris–HCl, pH 6·8, 2·4 mM-EDTA, 3% β-mercaptoethanol, 30% glycerol and 0·5% bromphenol blue) and heat denaturation (100°C, 5 min). ^{32}P-labelled cellular proteins were separated by SDS–PAGE as described above, only using a 4% acrylamide stacking gel and an 8·5% acrylamide separating gel. Molecular weight standards for SDS–PAGE included myosin heavy chain, β-galactosidase, phosphorylase b, BSA, ovalbumin, carbonic anhydrase and soybean trypsin inhibitor. Quantitation of phosphate incorporation on autoradiographs was by densitometric scanning using a Zeineh laser densitometer with a Hewlett-Packard 3390 A integrator.

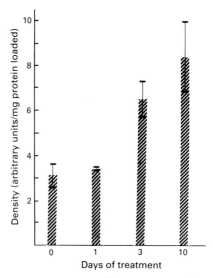

Fig. 3. Effect of in-vivo oestradiol-17β on the ^{32}P content of the M_r 80 000 protein in soluble luteal extracts of rabbits. Phosphorylation reactions were conducted according to Protocol B. The ^{32}P content of the M_r 80 000 protein phosphorylated in the presence of phosphatidylserine, diolein and EGTA was estimated by laser densitometry, as described in 'Materials and Methods'. Values are mean ± range of individual animals (N = 2).

Results

Studies were undertaken to elucidate phosphorylating activities in soluble luteal extracts attributable to various second messengers. Phosphorylation reactions conducted with rat soluble luteal extracts in the absence or presence of Ca^{2+} demonstrated Ca^{2+}-dependent phosphorylation, presumably mediated by Ca^{2+}–calmodulin-dependent protein kinases, of 3 prominent proteins with M_r 60 000, 56 000, and 54 000, as well as of the previously described M_r 100 000 substrate (Maizels & Jungmann, 1983; Rao *et al.*, 1987; Nairn & Palfrey, 1987) migrating just above the M_r 97 000 marker (Fig. 1, lanes a, c, e, g).

Phosphorylations were also performed in the presence of various lipid effectors in order to demonstrate C-kinase-mediated protein phosphorylations. Although a classical C-kinase substrate with requirements for Ca^{2+}, phospholipid and unsaturated diacylglycerol was not evident in the rat luteal extract (Fig. 1, lane e), a novel phosphorylation activity was seen at M_r 80 000 (Fig. 1, lane f) in the presence of EGTA which exhibited phospholipid and diacylglycerol dependence. Three or more higher molecular weight proteins (M_r 120 000–200 000) also showed enhanced phosphorylation in the presence of phospholipid, diacylglycerol and EGTA. This phospholipid-dependent phosphorylating activity observed in the presence of EGTA was also present in soluble ovarian extracts from immature rats (Maizels & Hunzicker-Dunn, 1986). Inclusion of 10^{-7} M or greater free Ca^{2+} reduced the ^{32}P content of the M_r 80 000 substrate (Maizels & Hunzicker-Dunn, 1986).

Evidence that this variant C-kinase pattern of responsiveness to Ca^{2+} seen in ovarian cells was not the result of procedural artefacts was seen by the observation that the classical C-kinase response pattern, in which phosphorylations were stimulated by Ca^{2+} and phosphatidylserine alone or Ca^{2+}, 1,2-diacylglycerol and phosphatidylserine, was observed in soluble rat brain extracts (not shown) and in soluble pig CL extracts at M_r 35 000 (Fig. 2, lanes c, e). The variant C-kinase response, in which phosphorylation activity required diacylglycerol and phosphatidylserine but was inhibited by Ca^{2+}, was also observed in soluble extracts of pig CL at M_r 80 000 (Fig. 2, lane f)

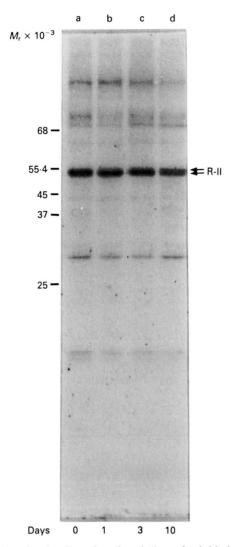

Fig. 4. Autoradiogram showing in-vitro phosphorylation of soluble luteal protein in rabbits. Phosphorylation was conducted according to Protocol A. Ten-day pseudopregnant rabbits were treated for 0 (lane a), 1 (lane b), 3 (lane c) or 10 (lane d) days with oestradiol-17β and 15 μg (±9%) protein were loaded into each lane. The same soluble extracts were used to generate the results shown in Fig. 3.

but was absent in other steroidogenic tissues like rat adrenal (Fig. 1, lanes i, j) and rat testis (Fig. 1, lanes k, l).

Soluble luteal extracts of rabbits also exhibited prominent phosphorylation of the M_r 80 000 substrate stimulated by diacylglycerol and phosphatidylserine and inhibited by Ca^{2+} at 10^{-7} M or greater (not shown). Treatment of pseudopregnant rabbits with oestradiol-17β caused a marked, time-dependent increase in the ^{32}P content of the M_r 80 000 substrate, most pronounced after 10 days of oestradiol treatment (Fig. 3). The increase in ^{32}P content of the M_r 80 000 protein caused by oestradiol-17β was not a generalized effect of this steroid, because it had no effect on the ^{32}P content of various protein substrates, including the prominent type II regulatory subunit (R-II) of cAMP-kinase seen at M_r 51 000 and 52 000 (Fig. 4) and the M_r 100 000 Ca^{2+}–calmodulin kinase substrate (not shown).

Conclusions

CL contain phosphorylating activities attributable to various second messenger-regulated protein kinase-mediated mechanisms. In this report we have described a novel phosphorylating activity demonstrated by a prominent substrate at M_r 80 000 which exhibited some characteristics in common with the recognized Ca^{2+}-dependent phospholipid-dependent class of C-kinases, namely requirements for phospholipid and unsaturated diacylglycerol, but was reduced by the presence of Ca^{2+} at concentrations greater than 10^{-7} M. This phospholipid-dependent, Ca^{2+}–inhibited phosphorylation of the M_r 80 000 substrate was observed in soluble luteal extract of rats, pigs and rabbits. Most notably, exposure of pseudopregnant rabbits to oestradiol-17β *in vivo* increased the observed phospholipid/diolein-stimulated increase in ^{32}P content of the luteal M_r 80 000 substrate (2-fold). Oestradiol did not consistently alter in-vitro phosphorylation activities in rabbit CL regulated by other effector kinase pathways (cAMP-kinase; Ca^{2+}–calmodulin-kinase). The novel phospholipid/diolein-stimulated Ca^{2+}-reduced phosphorylating activity we observed in luteal tissues may be consistent with the type II isoenzyme of C-kinase present in rat ovarian cells (Huang *et al.*, 1987) which shows less Ca^{2+} sensitivity (Huang *et al.*, 1986). Although neither the identity nor the functional role of the M_r 80 000 protein are known, its presence in luteal tissues and regulation by oestradiol-17β in rabbits suggest that it may be important to luteal functions. In rabbit CL, although the absolute requirement for oestrogen has long been recognized, this is the first instance in which exogenous oestradiol treatment of intact rabbits (in which CL already are exposed to endogenous follicular oestradiol) produced a demonstrable effect, i.e. increased ^{32}P content of the M_r 80 000 protein.

Supported by NIH grants HD-11356 to M.H.D. and HD-00447 to J.B.M.

References

Bill, C.H. & Keyes, P.L. (1983) 17β-Estradiol maintains normal luteal function of corpora lutea throughout pseudopregnancy in hypophysectomized rabbits. *Biol. Reprod.* **28**, 608–617.

Davis, J.S. & Clark, M.R. (1983) Activation of protein kinase in the bovine corpus luteum by phospholipid and Ca^{2+}. *Biochem. J.* **214**, 569–574.

Edelman, A.M., Blumenthal, D.K. & Krebs, E.G. (1987) Protein serine/threonine kinases. *Ann. Rev. Biochem.* **56**, 567–613.

Gibori, G., Antczak, E. & Rothchild, I. (1977) The role of estrogen in the regulation of luteal progesterone secretion in the rat after day 12 of pregnancy. *Endocrinology* **100**, 1483–1495.

Holt, J.A., Keyes, P.L., Brown, J.M. & Miller, J.B. (1975) Premature regression of corpora lutea in pseudopregnant rabbits following removal of polydimethyl-siloxane capsules containing 17β-estradiol. *Endocrinology* **97**, 76–82.

Huang, K.P., Nakabayashi, H. & Huang, F.L. (1986) Isozymic forms of rat brain Ca^{2+}-activated and phospholipid-dependent protein kinase. *Proc. natn. Acad. Sci. U.S.A.* **83**, 8535–8539.

Huang, F.L., Yoshida, Y., Nakabayashi, H., Knopf, J.L., Young, W.S., III & Huang, K-P. (1987) Immuno-

chemical identification of protein Kinase C isozymes as products of discrete genes. *Biochem. Biophys. Res. Commun.* **149**, 946–952.

Hunzicker-Dunn, M. (1981) Selective activation of rabbit ovarian protein kinase isozymes in rabbit ovarian follicles and corpora lutea. *J. biol. Chem.* **256**, 12185–12193.

Hunzicker-Dunn, M. & Birnbaumer, L. (1976) Adenylyl cyclase activities in ovarian tissues II. Regulation of responsiveness to LH, FSH, and PGE_1 in the rabbit. *Endocrinology* **99**, 185–197.

Keyes, P.L. & Nalbandov, A.V. (1967) Maintenance and function of corpora lutea in rabbits depend on estrogen. *Endocrinology* **80**, 938–946.

Lowry, O.H., Rosebrough, N.J., Farr, A.L. & Randall, R.J. (1951) Protein measurement with the Folin phenol reagent. *J. biol. Chem.* **193**, 265–275.

Maizels, E.T. & Hunzicker-Dunn, M. (1986) Calcium-independent phospholipid-stimulated protein phosphorylation activity in immature rat ovarian extract. *Endocrinology* **118**, (Suppl.), 103, Abstr. 290.

Maizels, E.T. & Jungmann, R.A. (1983) Ca^{2+}-calmodulin-dependent phosphorylation of soluble and nuclear proteins in the rat ovary. *Endocrinology* **112**, 1895–1902.

Nairn, A.C. & Palfrey, H.C. (1987) Identification of the major M_r 100 000 substrate for calmodulin-dependent protein kinase III in mammalian cells as elongation factor-2. *J. biol. Chem.* **262,** 17299–17303.

Noland, T.A., Jr & Dimino, M.J. (1986) Characterization and distribution of protein kinase C in ovarian tissue. *Biol. Reprod.* **35,** 863–872.

Rao, M.C., Palfrey, H.C., Nash, N.T., Greisman, A., Jayatilak, P.C. & Gibori, G. (1987) Effects of estradiol on calcium-specific protein phosphorylation in the rat corpus luteum. *Endocrinology* **120,** 1010–1018.

Rudolph, S.A. & Krueger, B.K. (1979) Endogenous protein phosphorylation and dephosphorylation. *Adv. cyclic Nucleotide Res.* **10,** 107–133.

Takayama, M. & Greenwald, G.S. (1973) Direct luteotropic action of estrogen in the hypophysectomized-hysterectomized rat. *Endocrinology* **92,** 1405–1413.

Wheeler, M.B. & Veldhuis, J.D. (1987) Catalytic and receptor-binding properties of the calcium-sensitive phospholipid-dependent protein kinase (protein kinase C) in swine luteal cytosol. *Molec. cell. Endocr.* **50,** 123–129.

J. Reprod. Fert., Suppl. **37** (1989), 319–327

Printed in Great Britain
© 1989 Journals of Reproduction & Fertility Ltd

Mechanism of action of GnRH-induced oocyte maturation

N. Dekel, E. Aberdam, S. Goren*, B. Feldman and R. Shalgi†

*Department of Hormone Research, The Weizmann Institute of Science, Rehovot, Israel; and Departments of *Physiology and Pharmacology and †Embryology and Teratology, Sackler School of Medicine, Tel Aviv University, Tel Aviv, Israel*

Keywords: GnRH; oocyte maturation; protein kinase C; cell-to-cell communication

Introduction

Meiosis of the mammalian oocyte is initiated during fetal life. It proceeds up to the diplotene stage of the first prophase and is arrested at birth. The chromosomes in meiotically arrested oocytes decondense and a nuclear structure known as the germinal vesicle (GV) is formed. Meiotic arrest persists until sexual maturity, when at each cycle in one or more oocytes, dependent on the species, the reduction division starts again. The GV in these oocytes disappears, the chromatin is recondensed, the pairs of homologous chromosomes are separated and one half of the chromosomes is eliminated by the formation of the first polar body. The whole series of events, initiated by GV breakdown (GVB) and completed with polar body formation, leads to the production of a mature fertilizable oocyte. This process is therefore defined as oocyte maturation. Maturation of the oocyte is an essential prelude to fertilization since the oocyte cannot be fertilized before completion of meiosis.

The physiological stimulus for resumption of meiosis is provided by luteinizing hormone (LH; Lindner *et al.*, 1974). LH-induced oocyte maturation is preceded by a decrease in intraoocyte concentrations of cAMP (Schultz *et al.*, 1983; Dekel, 1987). On the other hand, experimental conditions that inhibit the decrease or elevate the levels of cAMP within the oocyte prevent the resumption of meiosis (Cho *et al.*, 1974; Dekel & Beers, 1978, 1980; Dekel *et al.*, 1981; Schultz *et al.*, 1983; Aberdam *et al.*, 1987). Taken together, these observations suggest that intracellular levels of cAMP regulate the meiotic status of the oocyte. Furthermore, since microinjection of a cAMP-dependent protein-kinase inhibitor can induce maturation in oocytes, by-passing the drop in intracellular levels of cAMP, it seems that maintenance of meiotic arrest probably involves activation of a cAMP-dependent protein kinase (Bornslaeger *et al.*, 1986).

It was reported several years ago, that gonadotrophin-releasing hormone (GnRH) can successfully promote oocyte maturation. The observation that GnRH could mimic LH action, inducing meiosis resumption, was initially reported by Hillensjö & LeMaire (1980). These investigators found that exposure of isolated ovarian follicles to GnRH or its agonist analogues *in vitro* results in maturation of the oocytes within these follicles. The direct stimulatory action of GnRH on the ovary has also been demonstrated *in vivo*. Both oocyte maturation and ovulation were induced in hypophysectomized rats following administration of GnRH agonists (Corbin & Bex, 1981; Ekholm *et al.*, 1981; Erickson *et al.*, 1983). The action of GnRH on rat oocytes has been extensively studied by us in hypophysectomized rats treated with a GnRH agonist analogue (GnRHa) and in follicle-enclosed oocytes exposed to GnRHa *in vitro*. The results of these studies, as well as relevant findings of other investigators, are summarized in this paper.

Characterization of GnRH action

As reported by others (Hillensjö & LeMaire, 1980; Ekholm *et al.*, 1981; Corbin & Bex, 1981) we have also demonstrated that GnRH agonist analogues are potent inducers of resumption of meiosis in follicle-enclosed oocytes *in vitro*, as well as stimulators of oocyte maturation and ovulation *in vivo*, in hypophysectomized rats (Dekel *et al.*, 1983, 1985).

GnRHa induced resumption of meiosis in follicle-enclosed oocytes in a dose-dependent manner with an ED_{50} at a concentration of 2×10^{-9} M. The stimulation of GVB by a maximal effective dose of GnRHa (10^{-7} M) was complete by 8 h of incubation. Induction of GVB by LH was relatively faster with 95% of the oocytes resuming meiosis after 5 h of incubation (Dekel *et al.*, 1983).

The effect of GnRHa on the oocytes *in vivo* has been studied with immature, hypophysectomized, PMSG-primed rats. Mature oocytes were initially detected in the ovaries of the GnRHa-treated rats (2 µg/rat) at 2 h after administration of the hormone whereas the response to hCG (4 i.u./rat) was observed after 4 h. However, full response to both hormones was obtained at 10 h. Even though the kinetics of response to these hormones were very similar, a clear difference in efficiency of GnRHa and hCG was observed. The maximal number of ovulated oocytes after hCG treatment was 50 ± 7 (mean $\pm$ s.e.m.; N = 8) per rat, with only 29 ± 4 (N = 13) oocytes released in response to GnRHa treatment ($P < 0.05$) (Dekel *et al.*, 1985).

Mechanism of GnRH action

Since GnRH and its analogues seem to mimic the effect of LH on the ovary in terms of oocyte maturation and ovulation, we investigated whether LH and GnRH agonists share any common steps in their mechanism of action. Our initial experiments were directed towards analysis of the receptor specificity for these two hormones. We found that the concomitant addition of a potent GnRH antagonist, [D-pGlu^1,DpClPhe^2,D-Trp^{3,6}]GnRH (from Dr D. Coy, Tulane University, LA, U.S.A.), at a concentration of 10^{-5} M, totally blocked the stimulatory effect of GnRHa (Table 1). However, this antagonist failed to inhibit GVB when added to follicle-enclosed oocytes together with LH (Dekel *et al.*, 1983). Since a potent GnRH antagonist blocked GnRH but not LH actions on the ovary, it seems that GnRH does not share its receptors with LH. These findings are compatible with the demonstrations of stereospecific, tissue-specific high-affinity gonadal sites for GnRH (Clayton & Catt, 1981).

Incubation of ovarian follicles with LH results in an immediate rise in cAMP concentration (Dekel *et al.*, 1985). In a previous study we have demonstrated that follicular cAMP plays a mediatory role in the induction of oocyte maturation by LH (Dekel & Sherizly, 1983). Unlike LH, GnRH action did not involve elevation of cAMP concentrations in the ovarian follicle (Fig. 1). These findings suggest that GnRHa and LH use different mediatory systems for the transduction of similar signals (Dekel *et al.*, 1985).

Since cAMP does not rise after exposure of the ovarian follicle to GnRH it seems that cAMP-dependent protein kinase A is not involved in the mechanism of GnRH action in this system. Protein kinase C, on the other hand is independent of cAMP. This enzyme has been reported to mediate GnRH action in the pituitary (Hirota *et al.*, 1985; Harris *et al.*, 1985; Naor *et al.*, 1985). The possible involvement of protein kinase C in the regulation of oocyte maturation has been tested (Aberdam & Dekel, 1985).

Activation of protein kinase C is dependent on the inositol phospholipid turnover. This reaction is initiated by the cleavage of a phosphodiester linkage and production of diacylglycerol, which is the biological activator of protein kinase C. This reaction is catalysed by phospholipase C. We found that in follicles incubated in the presence of 0·5 U of phospholipase C/ml, 100% of the

Table 1. Effect of GnRH antagonist on LH- or GnRHa-induced GVB in follicle-enclosed rat oocytes

Additions to medium			GVB	
oLH (0·1 µg/ml)	GnRHa (10^{-7} M)	GnRH antagonist (10^{-5} M)	% of oocytes	Total no. of oocytes
—	—	—	2	65
+	—	—	93	96
—	+	—	97	149
—	—	+	3	33
—	+	+	11	56
+	—	+	99	79

Isolated follicles were incubated in the presence of the indicated concentrations of ovine LH (oLH) or GnRHa with or without GnRH antagonist. After 20 h the oocytes were recovered and examined for the presence or absence of GVs.

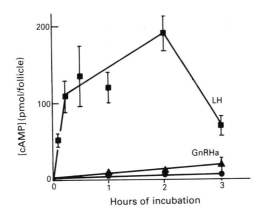

Fig. 1. Cyclic AMP accumulation by rat ovarian follicles in response to GnRHa or LH. Follicles were isolated from intact PMSG-primed immature rats and incubated in the presence or absence of GnRHa (10^{-7} M) or ovine LH (5 µg/ml). Cyclic AMP was determined in samples of 2 follicles and the results are presented as means ± s.e.m. of 5 replicates of 3 different experiments. (From Dekel *et al.*, 1985.)

oocytes were stimulated to resume meiotic maturation (Fig. 2). We further demonstrated that the membrane permeable derivative of diacylglycerol, 1-oleoyl 2-acetyl glycerol, as well as a tumour-promoting phorbol ester (TPA), which is known to activate protein kinase C by substituting for its physiological substrate, also induced the resumption of meiosis in follicle-enclosed oocytes (ED_{50} of 120 and 1·2 µg/ml, respectively). All these activators of protein kinase C not only induced initiation of the meiotic process, which is indicated by the disappearance of the GV, but also stimulated the oocytes to proceed to the second metaphase forming the first polar body (Aberdam & Dekel, 1985). Since the two most potent activators of protein kinase C as well as phospholipase C mimicked GnRHa stimulation, we suggest that GnRH-induced oocyte maturation is probably mediated by protein kinase C. This idea gains further support from our current experiments conducted using the newly synthesized inhibitors of protein kinases, the isoquinolinesulphonamide derivatives, H-7, H-8 and HA 1004 (Hidaka *et al.*, 1984). Our preliminary experiments demonstrate that these agents effectively inhibit GnRHa-induced oocyte maturation. Furthermore, the relative inhibitory effect of these agents on GnRHa action directly corresponds to their binding affinities towards protein kinase C (N. Dekel, unpublished).

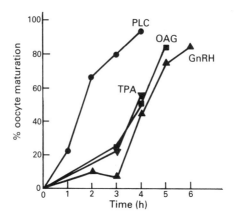

Fig. 2. Induction of rat oocyte maturation by GnRHa and activators of protein kinase C. Follicles were incubated with GnRHa (10^{-7} M), phospholipase C, PLC (15 mU), 1-oleoyl 2-acetyl glycerol, OAG (180 µg/ml) or tumour-promoting phorbolester, TPA (2 µg/ml). After the indicated periods the oocytes were recovered and examined for maturation (GVB). Each experimental point represents the pooled results of 3 individual experiments in which at least 90 oocytes were examined.

Protein kinase C activation is thought to be biochemically dependent on calcium. The involvement of calcium in oocyte maturation has been studied in several mammalian species (Tsafriri & Bar-Ami, 1978; Leibfried & First, 1979; Paleos & Powers, 1981; Jagiello *et al.*, 1982; Powers & Paleos, 1982; Maruska *et al.*, 1984; Bae & Channing, 1985; Racowsky, 1986). The results of these studies are confusing since they demonstrate both inhibition and induction, as well as no effect of calcium on meiosis resumption. In an attempt to elucidate this issue we have tested the effect of calcium on GnRHa-induced oocyte maturation. Our results demonstrate that the presence of extracellular calcium is essential for GnRHa-induced oocyte maturation which is further potentiated by increasing concentrations of this ion in the medium (Fig. 3). Furthermore, they also indicate that in the presence of divalent ionophores, A 23187 or ionomycin, calcium can mimic GnRHa action and induce, on its own, maturation of follicle-enclosed oocytes (Fig. 3). Taken together, the data presented in this and our previous studies are compatible with the following sequence of events. The binding of GnRHa to its receptors activates receptor-gated channels leading to an increase in intracellular calcium. This, in turn, leads to the activation of protein kinase C that by, an as yet unknown mechanism, initiates oocyte maturation.

Within the ovarian follicle the oocyte is surrounded by the cumulus and granulosa cells. It has been suggested that cAMP is transferred from the granulosa/cumulus compartment to the oocyte to maintain it in meiotic arrest. It has been further proposed that LH action, which involves the elevation of cAMP in the surrounding follicular cells, leads to the disruption of cell-to-cell communication that is followed by a decrease in oocyte cAMP. This decrease in cAMP removes the putative tonic inhibition of oocyte maturation and is considered as a sufficient signal for the resumption of meiosis (reviewed by Dekel, 1986, 1987). In all the studies described in this paper, both *in vivo* and *in vitro*, the oocytes were enclosed by the ovarian follicles. Since the follicle is a

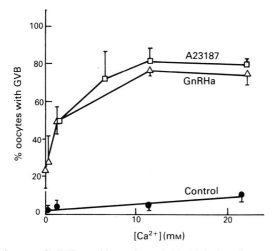

Fig. 3. Effect of calcium on GnRHa and ionophore A 23187-induced oocyte maturation of rats. Follicles were incubated in the presence of GnRHa (10^{-7} M) or ionophore A 23187 (10^{-6} M) with the indicated calcium concentrations. After 24 h the oocytes were recovered and examined for maturation (GVB). Each experimental point represents the pooled results of 3 individual experiments with at least 90 oocytes.

complex structure composed of heterologous cell populations it makes it difficult to determine the cellular target for GnRHa. It is likely that the hormone acts on the granulosa/cumulus compartment, since specific receptors for GnRHa on rat granulosa cells have been demonstrated (Clayton *et al.*, 1979; Jones *et al.*, 1980) and biological response of granulosa and cumulus cells to the hormone has been reported (Clark *et al.*, 1980; Hsueh & Jones, 1981; Dekel *et al.*, 1985).

By which mechanism could the cumulus–granulosa cells mediate GnRHa-action to induce oocyte maturation? Like LH, GnRHa could interfere with cell-to-cell communication and reduce the supply of the inhibitory cAMP from the somatic follicular compartment to the oocyte. We have found that GnRHa uncouples the oocyte from the cumulus cells soon after exposure of the follicle to this hormone *in vitro* (50% of decrease in the level of communication after 3 h). The dose–response curve of GnRHa-induced breakdown of communication is in the same range of concentrations that were found to trigger oocyte maturation ($ED_{50} = 5 \times 10^{-10}$ M and 2×10^{-9} M, respectively). These results (B. Feldman & N. Dekel, unpublished) suggest that GnRHa-induced oocyte maturation could be mediated by interaction of the hormone with the granulosa–cumulus compartment in the ovarian follicle. We cannot, however, exclude direct action of GnRHa on the oocyte.

Fertilizability of oocytes undergoing maturation in response to GnRHa

The studies discussed above demonstrated that GnRH, like LH, can stimulate the oocyte to mature, and can trigger the follicle to release the mature oocyte. LH action results in the release of a functional fertilizable oocyte; after sperm penetration this ovum will develop into a normal embryo. The diagnosis of GnRH-induced oocyte maturation in all the studies mentioned so far is based only on morphological markers such as GVB or polar body formation (Hillensjö & LeMaire, 1980; Ekholm *et al.*, 1981; Dekel *et al.*, 1983). One of our more recent studies was designed to assess the ability of oocytes undergoing maturation in response to GnRH to be fertilized (Dekel & Shalgi, 1987).

Fertilization rate of the control groups of oocytes isolated from intact or hypophysectomized PMSG-primed, hCG-induced ovulators was 88·3 ± 3·3 and 90·0 ± 2·8 respectively. The success rate of fertilization of oocytes undergoing maturation and ovulation *in vivo* in response to GnRHa was not significantly different (Fig. 4a). Fertilization rate of oocytes exposed to GnRHa *in vitro* was lower than that of control oocytes isolated from the oviducts of intact PMSG/hCG-treated rats (Fig. 4b), but did not differ significantly from that of oocytes exposed *in vitro* to LH ($P > 0·1$) (Dekel & Shalgi, 1987). Our study demonstrates that the potential of oocytes, undergoing maturation in response to GnRHa stimulation, to be fertilized is similar to that of oocytes stimulated by LH/hCG. Moreover, we further demonstrated that their ability to develop into a 2-cell embryo is also similar (Dekel & Shalgi, 1987). We have found that 2-cell embryos obtained from oocytes undergoing maturation in response to GnRHa and LH are equally potent to implant in uteri of foster mothers (25·5% and 22·3%, respectively) and subsequently develop into live embryos (16·8% and 14·9%, respectively) (R. Shalgi & N. Dekel, unpublished). Our findings cannot point towards any impaired fertilizability of oocytes exposed to GnRH. They do indicate that oocytes undergoing maturation in response to GnRH have the potential to develop into normal embryos as do LH-stimulated oocytes.

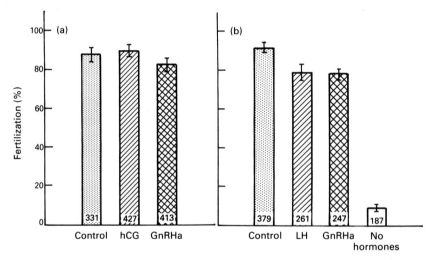

Fig. 4. Fertilization rates of oocytes undergoing maturation (a) *in vivo* and (b) *in vitro*. In (a) ovulated oocytes were recovered from oviducts of hypophysectomized PMSG-primed rats treated with GnRHa or hCG. The oocytes were exposed *in vitro* to spermatozoa recovered from the uteri of mature cyclic rats soon after mating. In (b) mature oocytes were recovered from follicles following their incubation *in vitro* in the absence or presence of GnRHa or LH. The oocytes were exposed *in vitro* to spermatozoa recovered from the uteri of mature cyclic rats soon after mating. Ova were examined for fertilization 24 h later. Ovulated oocytes recovered from intact PMSG/hCG-treated rats were used as controls. The total number of ova examined for each group is indicated at the bottom of the bars. The pooled results of (a) 9 and (b) 14 different experiments are presented as the mean ± s.e. of the fraction of fertilized ova. At least 20 (a) and 21 (b) individual cultures were examined for each treatment group.

Concluding remarks

While the role of LH in regulation of oocyte maturation is very well documented, the physiological relevance of GnRH action in this system is not yet clear. The studies on GnRH, discussed above, have all been performed in the rat, and an important question is whether such findings can be extended to other species. Attempts to answer this question by investigating whether ovarian GnRH receptors are present has yielded negative results for women (Clayton & Huhtaniemi, 1982), sheep, cattle and pigs (Brown & Reeves, 1983). However, direct ovarian effects of GnRH agonists have been shown in the pig (Massicotte *et al.*, 1980), cow (Milvae & Hansel, 1980) and man (Tureck *et al.*, 1982) and specific but 'low affinity' GnRH-agonist receptors have been demonstrated in human corpus luteum (Popkin *et al.*, 1983). It is possible that inability to demonstrate receptors for GnRH in ovaries of some species results from technical problems associated with such studies because, even in rat ovaries, GnRH receptors are few in number.

Even if the presence of ovarian GnRH receptors is demonstrated, any attempt to suggest a direct role for this hormone in regulation of ovarian functions should take into consideration that hypothalamic GnRH reaches the ovary in concentrations that are too low to elicit any biological response. Are the ovarian cells a possible alternative source for GnRH? The presence of a GnRH-like protein in ovaries of domestic species and the rat has been reported (Aten *et al.*, 1986, 1987). These findings raise the possibility that this substance may play a paracrine regulatory role in the ovary of animals of several species.

The meiotic status of the oocyte is regulated by concentrations of cAMP within the oocyte. The mechanisms by which cAMP exerts its action have not been studied and the cascade of events initiated following the maturation-associated decrease in intra-oocyte cAMP is obscure. The attempts to resolve this issue should be based on the following set of assumptions. The inhibitory action of cAMP is probably exerted via protein kinase A. This kinase in turn could phosphorylate specific protein(s) which maintain meiotic arrest. To allow resumption of meiosis this protein(s) should be dephosphorylated. Dephosphorylation of such protein(s) may result simply from the decreased levels of cAMP, leading to inactivation of the protein kinase A. Alternatively, there could be a positive stimulus which would antagonize the inhibitory action of protein kinase A. A combination of both these mechanisms is also possible.

Nishizuka (1986) has reported that in various cell types protein kinase C-induced responses are profoundly blocked by signals that produce cAMP. Conversely, in other types of cells protein kinase C itself inhibits the adenylate cyclase system. Our findings suggest that protein kinase C may be involved in the mechanism of induction of oocyte maturation. In that case it is possible that the oocyte represents another cell type in which protein kinase A and protein kinase C counteract each other. The reciprocal relationships between these two enzymes is an intriguing possibility that we are now investigating.

These studies were supported by grants from the Israel Academy of Science and Humanities, United-States Binational Science Foundation and the Minerva Foundation Munich, West Germany.

References

Aberdam, E. & Dekel, N. (1985) Activators of protein kinase C stimulate meiotic maturation of rat oocytes. *Biochem. Biophys. Res. Commun.* **132**, 570–574.

Aberdam, E., Hanski, E. & Dekel, N. (1987) Maintenance of meiotic arrest in isolated rat oocytes by the invasive adenylate cyclase of Bordetella pertussis. *Biol. Reprod.* **36**, 530–535.

Aten, R.F., Williams, A.T. & Behrman, H.R. (1986) Ovarian gonadotropin-releasing hormone-like protein(s): demonstration and characterization. *Endocrinology* **118**, 961–966.

Aten, R.F., Ireland, J.J., Weems, C.W. & Behrman, H.R. (1987) Presence of gonadotropin releasing hormone-like protein in bovine and ovine ovaries. *Endocrinology* **120**, 1727–1733.

Bae, I. & Channing, C.P. (1985) Effect of calcium ion on maturation of cumulus-enclosed pig follicular oocytes isolated from medium-sized Graafian follicles. *Biol. Reprod.* **33**, 79–87.

Bornslaeger, E.A., Mattei, P. & Schultz, R.M. (1986) Involvement of cAMP-dependent protein kinase and protein phosphorylation in regulation of mouse oocyte maturation. *Devl Biol.* **114**, 453–462.

Brown, J.L. & Reeves, J.J. (1983) Absence of specific LHRH receptors in ovine, bovine and porcine ovaries. *Biol. Reprod.* **29**, 1179–1182.

Cho, W.K., Stern, S. & Biggers, J.D. (1974) Inhibitory effect of dibutyryl cAMP on mouse oocyte maturation *in vitro. J. exp. Zool.* **187**, 383–386.

Clark, M.R., Thibier, C., Marsh, J.M. & LeMaire, W.J. (1980) Stimulation of prostaglandin accumulation by luteinizing hormone-releasing hormone (LHRH) and LHRH analogs in rat granulosa cells in vitro. *Endocrinology* **107**, 17–23.

Clayton, R.N. & Catt, K.J. (1981) Gonadotropin-releasing hormone receptors: characterization, physiological regulation and relationship to reproductive function. *Endocrine Rev.* **2**, 186–209.

Clayton, R.N. & Huhtaniemi, I.T. (1982) Absence of gonadotropin-releasing hormone receptors in human gonadal tissue. *Nature, Lond.* **299**, 56–59.

Clayton, R.N., Harwood, J.P. & Catt, K.J. (1979) Gonadotropin-releasing hormone analogue binds to luteal cells and inhibits progesterone production. *Nature, Lond.* **282**, 90–92.

Corbin, A. & Bex, F.J. (1981) Luteinizing hormone releasing hormone agonists induce ovulation in hypophysectomized proestrous rats: direct ovarian effect. *Life Sci.* **29**, 185–192.

Dekel, N. (1986) Hormonal control of ovulation. In *Biochemical Action of Hormones*, vol. 13, pp. 57–90. Ed. G. Litwack. Academic Press, New York.

Dekel, N. (1987) Interaction between the oocyte and the granulosa cells in the preovulatory follicle. In *Endocrinology and Physiology of Reproduction*, pp. 197–209. Eds D. T. Armstrong, H. G. Freisen, P. K. C. Leung, W. Moger & K. B. Ruf. Plenum Press, New York.

Dekel, N. & Beers, W.H. (1978) Rat oocyte maturation in vitro: relief of cyclic AMP inhibition by gonadotropins. *Proc. natn Acad. Sci. U.S.A.* **75**, 4369–4373.

Dekel, N. & Beers, W.H. (1980) Development of the rat oocyte *in vitro*: inhibition and induction of maturation in the presence or absence of the cumulus oophorus. *Devl Biol.* **75**, 247–254.

Dekel, N. & Shalgi, R. (1987) Fertilization *in vitro* of oocytes undergoing maturation in response to a GnRH analogue. *J. Reprod. Fert.* **80**, 531–535.

Dekel, N. & Sherizly, I. (1983) Induction of maturation in rat follicle-enclosed oocyte by forskolin. *FEBS Lett.* **151**, 153–155.

Dekel, N., Lawrence, T.S., Gilula, N.B. & Beers, W.H. (1981) Modulation of cell-to-cell communication in the cumulus-oocyte complex and the regulation of oocyte maturation by LH. *Devl Biol.* **86**, 356–362.

Dekel, N., Sherizly, I., Tsafriri, A. & Naor, Z. (1983) A comparative study of the mechanism of action of luteinizing hormone and gonadotropin releasing hormone analog on the ovary. *Biol. Reprod.* **28**, 161–166.

Dekel, N., Sherizly, I., Phillips, D.M., Nimrod, A., Zilberstein, M. & Naor, Z. (1985) Characterization of the maturational changes induced by a GnRH analogue in the rat ovarian follicle. *J. Reprod. Fert.* **75**, 461–466.

Ekholm, C., Hillensjö, T. & Isaksson, O. (1981) Gonadotropin-releasing hormone agonists stimulate oocyte meiosis and ovulation in hypophysectomized rats. *Endocrinology* **108**, 2022–2024.

Erickson, G.F., Hofeditz, C. & Hsueh, A.J.W. (1983) GnRH stimulates meiotic maturation in preantral follicles of hypophysectomized rats. In *Factors Regulating Ovarian Function*, pp. 257–261. Eds G. S. Greenwald & P. F. Terranova. Raven Press, New York.

Harris, C.E., Staley, D. & Conn, P.M. (1985) Diacyl-glycerol and protein kinase C: potential amplifying mechanism for Ca^{2+}-mediated GnRH stimulated LH release. *Molec. Pharmacol.* **27**, 532–536.

Hidaka, H., Inagaki, M., Kawamoto, S. & Sasaki, Y. (1984) Isoquinolinesulfonamides, novel and potent inhibitors of cyclic nucleotide dependent protein kinase and protein kinase C. *Biochemistry, N.Y.* **23**, 5036–5041.

Hillensjö, T. & LeMaire, W.J. (1980) Gonadotropin releasing hormone agonists stimulate meiotic maturation of follicle-enclosed rat oocytes *in vitro. Nature, Lond.* **287**, 145–146.

Hirota, K., Hirota, T., Aguilera, G. & Catt, K.J. (1985) Hormone induced redistribution of calcium activated phospholipid-dependent protein kinase in pituitary gonadotrophs. *J. biol. Chem.* **260**, 3243–3246.

Hsueh, A.J.W. & Jones, P.B.C. (1981) Extrapituitary action of gonadotropin-releasing-hormone. *Endocrine Rev.* **2**, 437–461.

Jagiello, G., Ducayan, M.B., Downey, R. & Jonassen, A. (1982) Alternation of mammalian oocyte meiosis I with divalent cations and calmodulin. *Cell Calcium* **3**, 153–162.

Jones, P.B.C., Conn, P.M., Marian, J. & Hsueh, A.J.W. (1980) Binding of gonadotrophin-releasing hormone agonist to rat ovarian granulosa cells. *Life Sci.* **27**, 2125–2132.

Leibfried, L. & First, N.L. (1979) Effect of divalent cations on *in vitro* maturation of bovine oocytes. *J. exp. Zool.* **210**, 575–580.

Lindner, H.R., Tsafriri, A., Lieberman, M.E., Zor, U., Koch, Y., Bauminger, S. & Barnea, A. (1974) Gonadotrophin action on cultured Graafian follicles: induction of maturation division of the mammalian oocyte and differentiation of the luteal cell. *Recent Prog. Horm. Res.* **30**, 79–138.

Maruska, D.V., Leibfried, M.L. & First, N.L. (1984) Role of calcium and the calcium-calmodulin complex in resumption of meiosis, cumulus expansion, viability and hyaluronidase sensitivity of bovine cumulus oocyte complexes. *Biol. Reprod.* **31**, 1–6.

Massicotte, J., Veilleux, R., Lavoie, M. & Labrie, F. (1980) An LHRH agonist inhibits FSH-induced cyclic AMP accumulation and steroidogenesis in porcine granulosa cells in culture. *Biochem. Biophys. Res. Commun.* **94**, 1362–1366.

Milvae, R. & Hansel, W. (1980) A luteolytic effect of GnRH on bovine luteal cells in vitro. *J. Anim. Sci.* **51**, (Suppl. 1), 306 Abstr. 484.

Naor, Z., Zer, J., Zakut, H. & Hermon, J. (1985) Characterization of pituitary calcium activated, phospholipid-dependent protein kinase: redistribution by gonadotropin-releasing hormone. *Proc. natn. Acad. Sci. U.S.A.* **82**, 8203–8208.

Nishizuka, Y. (1986) Studies and perspectives of protein kinase C. *Science, N.Y.* **233**, 305–312.

Paleos, G.A. & Powers, R.D. (1981) The effect of calcium on the first meiotic division of the mammalian oocyte. *J. exp. Zool.* **217**, 409–416.

Popkin, R.M., Bramley, T.A., Currie, A.J., Shaw, R.W.,

Baird, D.T. & Fraser, H.M. (1983) Specific binding of luteinizing hormone-releasing hormone to human luteal tissue. *Biochem. Biophys. Res. Commun.* **114,** 750–756.

Powers, R.D. & Paleos, G.A. (1982) Combined effect of calcium and dibutyryl cyclic AMP on germinal vesicle breakdown in the mouse oocyte. *J. Reprod. Fert.* **66,** 1–8.

Racowsky, C. (1986) The releasing action of calcium upon cyclic-AMP-dependent meiotic arrest in hamster oocyte. *J. exp. Zool.* **239,** 263–275.

Schultz, R.M., Montgomery, R.R. & Belanoff, J.R. (1983) Regulation of mouse oocyte meiotic maturation: implication of a decrease in oocyte cAMP and protein dephosphorylation in commitment to resume meiosis. *Devl Biol.* **97,** 264–273.

Tsafriri, A. & Bar-Ami, S. (1978) Role of divalent cations in the resumption of meiosis of rat oocytes. *J. exp. Zool.* **205,** 293–300.

Tureck, R.W., Mastroianni, L., Blasco, L., Jr & Strauss, J.F., III (1982) Inhibition of human granulosa cells progesterone secretion by a gonadotropin releasing hormone agonist. *J. clin. Endocr. Metab.* **54,** 1078–1080.

J. Reprod. Fert., Suppl. **37** (1989), 329–333

Summary

W. Hansel

Department of Physiology, New York State College of Veterinary Medicine, Cornell University, Ithaca, NY 14853-6401, U.S.A.

Introduction

Conference summaries are often disappointing to those who prepare them, as well as to captive audiences who must listen to them. Necessarily, one can discuss only a small portion of the data presented at a conference such as this and each participant has his own perceptions of which findings are the most important. Often, the really important contributions do not become evident for several years. Perhaps the greatest value of workshops such as this is the emergence of one or two facts that serve to alter the courses of individual research programmes. The chances that a summary will focus on these facts are small indeed!

Placental luteotrophins

The workshop began, appropriately enough, with a discussion of the genetic control of chorionic gonadotrophin (hCG) and placental lactogen (hPL) production in the human placenta (Boime)*. The remarkable relationship between the production and regulation of these hormones and placental differentiation was a major feature of these results. Cytotrophoblasts first produced the α-subunit of hCG; later, as the cells changed from mononucleate to binucleate forms, β-subunit synthesis occurred. hPL synthesis occurred later and did not reach maximal levels until term. Genetic control of β-subunit synthesis is remarkably complex, involving as many as 6 genes.

The remaining 5 presentations in the sessions on placental luteotrophins all reported identification of factors from embryos or placentae of cattle, mice, rabbits and women that stimulate maternal progesterone production. Hansel pointed out that peripheral progesterone concentrations are higher in the blood of pregnant than non-pregnant cattle as early as Day 10 of pregnancy and well before the presumed day (Day 16) of pregnancy recognition. This finding was to be a recurring theme in the workshop and appears to occur in rabbits, monkeys and women. Apparently, these species are not aware that they need only block the luteolytic mechanisms of the normal cycle to 'rescue' the corpus luteum and ensure a normal pregnancy!

Hansel and O'Neill each discussed in some detail the potential role of platelet-activating factor (PAF), as perhaps the earliest pregnancy recognition signal in mice, cattle and women. PAF itself proved not to be directly luteotrophic when added to dispersed bovine luteal cells. However, several products of platelet activation, including serotonin and platelet-derived growth factor, were luteotrophic and could play roles *in vivo* in stimulating progesterone production. A thrombocytopenia during early pregnancy was demonstrated for cattle as had previously been shown for mice and PAF was shown to be a potent autacoid for the preimplantation mouse embryo.

Hickey, Izhar and Gadsby each identified potentially important luteotrophins from allantoic fluid and fetal placental tissues. The substance isolated from bovine allantoic fluid is a glycoprotein having an M_r of 68 000 and is present in very low concentrations. A substance of similar molecular weight, as well as a low molecular weight luteotrophic substance, were identified in

---

*Presentations are referred to by the name of the first author so that thay can be traced in the Contents list at the front of the volume.

granule-enriched preparations of bovine fetal cotyledons. The rabbit placental luteotrophin, found in fetal placenta-conditioned media, proved to be a heat-stable, trypsin-sensitive peptide with an M_r of 6000–8000; this factor, along with ovarian oestradiol, is required to maintain normal levels of luteal progesterone synthesis during the second half of pregnancy in the rabbit.

In a closely related paper presented in a later session, Saxena also described a luteotrophin produced by rabbit blastocysts from Day 4 of pregnancy. The purified blastocyst protein caused luteinization of, and progesterone production by, monkey granulosa cells. The material was hCG, or perhaps more appropriately, LH-like in character. This luteotrophin was also secreted by human blastocysts cultured for more than 7 days following fertilization.

Immunology of pregnancy

This session, which included presentations on maternal immunological recognition of pregnancy in sheep, horses, rodents and women, produced some of the most animated discussion of the entire workshop. Hansen presented data to show that, in sheep, a major reason for maternal tolerance of the conceptus is the production of immunosuppressive substances, including low and high molecular weight classes of agents, at the maternal–conceptus interface.

However, Antczak felt that there was little evidence for the maternal immunological recognition of pregnancy in most species, except during early pregnancy among and between species of the genus *Equus*. In the mare, strong antibody responses, directed against the major histocompatibility complex antigens produced by the invasive chorionic girdle cells, are seen. However, these maternal anti-fetal antibody responses do not appear to affect fetal development adversely, nor are they required for successful pregnancy. In the ensuing discussion it was stated that no antigenic response against a trophoblast antigen has ever been demonstrated—perhaps because the placenta produces no 'new' molecules.

Toder presented evidence that non-specific stimulation of the maternal immune system by complete Freund's adjuvant improved reproductive success in allogeneic mice having increased pregnancy losses and suggested that fertility in habitually aborting women might be improved in this way. Tachi proposed that, in the rat, macrophages are involved in the immunological recognition of the conceptus. When blastocysts and macrophages were co-cultured, two macrophage populations emerged; rounded macrophages that did not produce leucotriene C_4 and elongated ones that did.

Placental and luteal cells

In these sessions, Bazer, Thatcher and Sharp each presented excellent reviews of current knowledge of the events that inhibit luteolysis during early pregnancy in sheep, pigs, cattle and horses. A major feature of discussions was the ability of proteins, particularly the ovine and bovine conceptus secretory proteins (oTP-1 and bTP-1), to inhibit uterine prostaglandin (PG) F-2α production in the ewe and the cow. The conceptus secretory proteins had no influence on interoestrous intervals in the pig, and a mechanism controlling the direction (exocrine or endocrine) of uterine PGF-2α secretion was suggested as a control mechanism for this species. In the mare, conceptus membranes were shown to produce a low molecular weight ($M_r > 1000$ and < 6000) inhibitor of PGF synthesis.

These presentations and the paper by Stewart, who showed that there is a high degree of homology between oTP-1 and bovine interferon α-2, and that intrauterine infusion of interferon inhibited uterine PGF-2α production and corpus luteum regression in the ewe, were among the highlights of the workshop.

Sasser presented interesting new data on pregnancy-specific protein B, which appears to be produced by the binucleate trophoblast cells and thus may enter the maternal circulation when these cells invade the endometrium. Protein B has an M_r of 78 000, has 7 isoelectric variants and contains 3·7% hexose and 3·1% sialic acid. RIAs for this protein provide an accurate pregnancy test after Day 25, but persistent titres during the post-partum period may present a practical problem.

Kraicer studied progesterone uptake after decidual induction in rats. This uptake proved to be due to a widespread change in vascular permeability. The anti-oestrogen clomiphene blocked the decidual cell response. Following uptake, progesterone was receptor bound and concentrated in the nucleus within 1 h.

Steroidogenesis

Sessions 6 and 7 concerned the control of steroidogenesis in rat Leydig cells, human cytotropho-blasts and granulosa cells, rat ovarian cells and bovine mono- and binuclear placental cells. Poorly understood interactions between the LH–cAMP and the polyphosphoinositol–Ca^{2+}–protein kinase C second messenger systems appear to be involved in control of steroidogenesis in all of these tissues except the bovine placenta. Shemesh and Ullman each presented evidence that progesterone production in bovine monoculate and binucleate trophoblastic cells is controlled primarily by Ca^{2+} and protein kinase C. In contrast, Nulsen emphasized that common cyclic AMP-mediated mechanisms regulate the expression of genes involved in steroid hormone synthesis in the human placenta.

Cooke showed that LH stimulates both the lipoxygenase and cyclooxygenase pathways in Leydig cells and that inhibitors of the lipoxygenase pathway of arachidonic acid metabolism inhibit testosterone and cyclic AMP production. Orly used an antibody to mitochondrial cholesterol side-chain cleavage cytochrome P-450 to study this enzyme during follicular development; it was found that gonadotrophin treatment does not necessarily lead to induction of P-450, even when functional receptors are available.

Finally, Farin presented a clear analysis of the dynamic changes that occur in steroidogenic and non-steroidogenic cells in the ovine ovary during the oestrous cycle and pregnancy. Small luteal cells increase in numbers and large luteal cells increase in size during the cycle. Evidence to support the concept that the small theca-derived luteal cells are converted into large luteal cells under the influence of LH was presented. It appears that the cells of the sheep corpus luteum become larger, less numerous and less responsive to LH as pregnancy advances, as seems to be the case in corpora lutea of cows.

Peptides and prostaglandins

In these sessions, some particularly interesting new developments were reported, including the discovery and characterization of an antigonadotrophic, GnRH-like molecule by Behrman. This protein completely inhibits GnRH binding to rat ovarian membranes and also inhibits progester-one synthesis *in vitro* in dispersed bovine luteal cells. Bramley studied GnRH agonist binding sites in human luteal tissue during the menstrual cycle and early pregnancy. There appear to be major differences in receptor and/or ligand structure between pituitary and extra-pituitary receptors.

Flint ably summarized the evidence for a luteolytic role for ovarian oxytocin in the ewe and showed that continuous intravenous infusions of oxytocin caused down regulation of uterine oxytocin receptors and prolonged the oestrous cycle. However, Schams was unable to extend the life-span of the bovine corpus luteum by infusion of oxytocin. As a result of these and other exper-iments, he concluded that oxytocin does not appear to play an essential role in corpus luteum regression in cattle. These findings were supplemented by the report of Fields who traced the changes in populations of oxytocin-containing secretory vesicles in the large luteal cells of cows during the oestrous cycle and pregnancy. The population of these vesicles rises sharply between Days 7 and 11 of the oestrous cycle and declines on Days 17 and 19. Oxytocin–neurophysin-containing vesicles are low in early pregnancy, but similar granules containing an unknown substance occur with increasing frequency after this time. During the oestrous cycle, PGF-2α has been shown to cause exocytosis of the secretory granules.

In a final paper Lahav reported that PGF-2α suppresses LH-induced cyclic AMP accumulation in corpora lutea of gonadotrophin-treated immature rats. The inhibitory effect was not abolished by phospholipase C activation or by alteration of intra- or extracellular calcium. The exact mechanism involved therefore remains unexplained.

Environment and the early embryo

Heap presented the results of some most interesting recent studies using passive immunization of mice with monoclonal antibodies to progesterone. In these studies he was able to block pregnancy very soon after fertilization and to overcome this effect by administered progesterone. The monoclonal antibody acts primarily by disruption of the cell division programme in the uterine epithelium. Spitz reported that the antiprogestagen drug RU 486 (mifepristone) acts at multiple sites; it blocks progesterone receptors in the endometrium, inhibits the pituitary–hypothalamic axis and directly affects steroidogenesis. At high doses RU 486 is an antiglucocorticoid.

Lamming reported the results of a statistical study of milk progesterone values. These studies again emphasized the high early embryo mortality rate seen in dairy cattle. It was also shown that progesterone concentrations were higher in pregnant than non-pregnant cows from Day 8. A small decline in milk progesterone seen in a number of studies in pregnant animals at Day 12 was identified as characterizing a significant (unknown) physiological event.

Two interesting papers by Lewis and Kindahl concerning prostanoid synthesis by the bovine blastocyst during early pregnancy in the cow provided new evidence for the existence of an endometrial inhibitor of the synthesis of the cyclooxygenase products. This inhibitory activity was greater in endometria from pregnant than non-pregnant cows.

Schallenberger summarized extensive data concerning concentrations of LH, FSH, progesterone, oestradiol, oxytocin, PGF-2α, PGE-2 and PGI-2 in frequently collected vena cava and aorta blood samples from cyclic cattle. The data again pointed to maternal recognition of pregnancy in cattle within a few days of conception. An unidentified conference participant was heard to remark that if the conference had lasted 1 more day, someone would surely have reported the occurrence of pregnancy recognition before fertilization! Concentrations of oestradiol-17β and oxytocin were lower in pregnant than in cycling animals by Days 4–7. It was disappointing that none of these workers measured any representatives of the cyclooxygenase pathway of arachidonic acid metabolism, since several papers presented in this conference and a number of previous studies implicate these compounds in the control of ovarian and testicular steroidogenesis.

Intracellular signalling

In the final session on intracellular signalling, four participants presented new data emphasizing the importance of the Ca^{2+}–polyphosphoinositol–protein kinase C second messenger system in the rat ovary, adrenal and pituitary. The studies of Schulster on signal transduction in isolated rat adrenal glomerulosa and fasciculata-reticularis cells were of special interest, since they paralleled, in some respects, the studies being carried out on separated ovine and bovine small and large luteal cells. The rat glomerulosa cells responded to the Ca^{2+}-mobilizing hormone, angiotensin II, with increased phosphoinositol metabolism. Fasciculata-reticularis cells responded to ACTH agonists with an increased phosphoinositol–glycerophosphoinositol pool. The effects were seen over a dose range of ACTH that gave no increased cAMP output. The Ca^{2+}-dependent phospholipase A_2 is active in fasciculata-reticularis cells, but not in glomerulosa cells. It was suggested that the phosphoinositols may play a major physiological role in steroidogenesis in these cells.

Similar data were presented for phosphoinositol turnover in pituitary cells in response to GnRH by Naor and to GnRH or PGF-2α in rat luteal cells by Leung. Leung showed that the inhibitory actions of GnRH and PGF-2α on gonadotrophin-induced progesterone production in the rat ovary may be mediated by Ca^{2+} and protein kinase C. Gonadotrophin secretion by cultured rat pituitary cells in response to GnRH occurs in two phases and Naor showed that the first phase is mediated by inositol triphosphate (IP_3) and intracellular Ca^{2+} mobilization. The second sustained phase of exocytosis is mediated by Ca^{2+} influx controlled by voltage-sensitive and insensitive channels. Maizels discussed all of the second messengers, including protein kinase C and oestrogen in the corpus luteum and concluded that the corpus luteum contains protein kinases responsive to a variety of second messengers, as well as oestrogen. Dekel showed that GnRH directly induces development of mature fertilizable oocytes by a receptor mechanism involving Ca^{2+} activation of protein kinase C.

Future developments

This has clearly been a most productive workshop; significant advances in our knowledge of the factors involved in early pregnancy recognition and corpus luteum maintenance have been reported and at least 5 major unsolved problems have emerged. These may be summarized as follows:

(1) The role of platelet-activating factor (PAF) as an early pregnancy recognition signal and as an autacoid for the preimplantation embryo, in species other than the mouse, needs to be clarified.

(2) The roles (if any) of the luteotrophic principles produced by early cow, rabbit, and human conceptuses need to be established.

(3) The exact relationships of the conceptus secretory proteins to the interferons need to be established and better ways of producing biologically useful amounts of these proteins must be developed.

(4) The complex interrelationships between the cyclic AMP and the protein kinase C second messenger systems in luteal and placental cells must be more clearly defined and tested *in vivo*.

(5) The role of luteal oxytocin in corpus luteum function and the factors that control its secretion in a variety of species need to be more firmly established.

Final solutions to these difficult problems will require new experimental approaches and, in particular, the use of new techniques. New animal models, such as the 'donkey-in-mare' embryo described in this workshop need to be developed. New cell lines, such as bovine binucleate tropho-blastic cells that have unique mechanisms for regulating steroidogenesis, need to be developed. Maximum use must be made of new instrumentation, including cell sorters, and fluorometers with imaging capabilities that enable precise and rapid monitoring of intracellular Ca^{2+} concentrations in individual cells. Finally, new genetic engineering approaches, such as the production and use of 'anti-sense' genes for key compounds, such as oxytocin in luteal cells, need to be developed and utilized.

INDEXES

AUTHORS

Entries in **bold** type indicate citations in the reference sections.

SUBJECTS

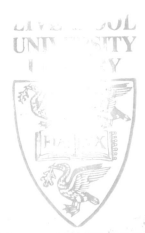